Immunotherapies for Allergic Disease

Immunotherapies for Allergic Disease

Edited by

Linda S. Cox, MD

Allergy and Asthma Center
Ft. Lauderdale
FL, United States

Assistant Clinical Professor of Medicine
University of Miami School of Medicine and
Nova South eastern University School of Osteopathic Medicine
Miami, FL, United States

ELSEVIER

Elsevier
Radarweg 29, PO Box 211, 1000 AE Amsterdam, Netherlands
The Boulevard, Langford Lane, Kidlington, Oxford OX5 1GB, United Kingdom
50 Hampshire Street, 5th Floor, Cambridge, MA 02139, United States

Immunotherapies for Allergic Disease
Copyright © 2020 Elsevier Inc. All rights reserved.

Notices

ISBN: 978-0-323-54427-6

Publisher: Mica Haley
Acquisition Editor: Robin Carter
Editorial Project Manager: Megan Ashdown
Production Project Manager: Kiruthika Govindaraju
Cover Designer: Alan Studholme

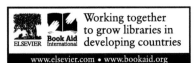

Working together
to grow libraries in
developing countries

www.elsevier.com • www.bookaid.org

Contents

SECTION 2   Allergic diseases

Marcella Aquino, MD, Stephanie Lynn Mawhirt, DO and
Luz Fonacier, MD

Contributors

Marcella Aquino, MD
Hasbro Children's Hospital, Department of Pediatrics, Division of Allergy & Immunology, Associate Professor of Pediatrics, Warren Alpert Medical School of Brown University, 593 Eddy Street, Providence, Rhode Island, United States

Cecilia Berin, PhD
Division of Pediatric Allergy and Immunology, Icahn School of Medicine at Mount Sinai, New York, NY, United States; Pediatrics, Mount Sinai School of Medicine, New York, NY, United States

Luisa Brussino, MD
Università degli Studi di Torino, Dipartimento di Scienze Mediche, AO Ordine Mauriziano Umberto I, Torino, Italy

Giorgio Walter Canonica, MD
Department of Biomedical Sciences, Humanitas Univeristy, Pieve Emanuele (MI), Italy; Personalized Medicine, Asthma and Allergy, Humanitas Research Hospital IRCCS, Rozzano (MI), Italy

Christopher A. Coop, MD
Department of Allergy and Immunology, Allergist, Allergy and Immunology Clinic, Wilford Hall Ambulatory Surgical Center, San Antonio, TX, United States

Stephen R. Durham, FRCP
Allergy and Clinical Immunology, Royal Brompton Hospital, London, United Kingdom; Allergy and Clinical Immunology, National Heart and Lung Institute, Imperial College London, United Kingdom

Anne K. Ellis, MD, MSc, FRCPC
Departments of Medicine and Biomedical & Molecular Sciences, Queen's University, Kingston, ON, Canada; Allergy Research Unit, Kingston General Health Research Institute, Kingston, ON, Canada

Robert E. Esch, PhD
Faculty, Biology, School of Natural Sciences, Lenoir-Rhyne University, Hickory, NC, United States

Elizabeth Feuille, MD
Assistant Professor, Division of Pediatric Pulmonology, Department of Pediatrics, Weill Cornell Medicine, New York, NY, USA

Ira Finegold, MD
Professor of Medicine, Icahn School of Medicine at Mount Sinai Hospital, New York, NY, United States; Chief Division of Allergy, Department of Medicine, Mount Sinai West, New York, NY, United States

Luz Fonacier, MD
Professor of Medicine, NYU Long Island School of Medicine, Mineola, NY, United States; Head of Allergy, Internal Medicine, NYU Langone Health, NYU Winthrop Hospital, Mineola, NY, United States; Training Program Director, Allergy and Immunology, NYU Winthrop Hospital, Mineola, NY, United States

Theodore M. Freeman, MD
San Antonio Asthma and Allergy Clinic, Owner, Allergy Immunology, San Antonio, TX, United States

David B.K. Golden, MD
Associate Professor of Medicine, Johns Hopkins University, Baltimore, MD, United States

Natasha C. Gunawardana, MRCP
Allergy and Clinical Immunology, Royal Brompton Hospital, London, United Kingdom; Allergy and Clinical Immunology, National Heart and Lung Institute, Imperial College London, United Kingdom

Robert G. Hamilton, PhD, DABMLI, FAAAAI
Professor, Division of Allergy and Clinical Immunology, Departments of Medicine and Pathology, Johns Hopkins University School of Medicine, Baltimore, MD, United States

Enrico Heffler, MD, PhD
Department of Biomedical Sciences, Humanitas Univeristy, Pieve Emanuele (MI), Italy; Personalized Medicine, Asthma and Allergy, Humanitas Research Hospital IRCCS, Rozzano (MI), Italy

Hsi-en Ho, MD
Division of Pediatric Allergy and Immunology, Icahn School of Medicine at Mount Sinai, New York, NY, United States

Pål Johansen, PhD
Department of Dermatology, University Hospital Zurich & University of Zurich, Zurich, Switzerland

Jasper H. Kappen, MD, PhD, MSc
Allergy and Clinical Immunology, Immunomodulation and Tolerance Group, Imperial College London, London, United Kingdom; MRC & Asthma UK Centre in Allergic Mechanisms of Asthma, London, United Kingdom; Allergy and Clinical Immunology, National Heart and Lung Institute, Imperial College London, London, United Kingdom; Department of Pulmonology, STZ Centre of Excellence for Asthma & COPD, Sint Franciscus Gasthuis and Vlietland Group, Rotterdam, The Netherlands

Thomas M. Kündig, MD
Department of Dermatology, University Hospital Zurich & University of Zurich, Zurich, Switzerland

Wenyin Loh, MBBS, MRCPCH
Allergy and Immune Disorders, Murdoch Children's Research Institute, Melbourne, VIC, Australia; Allergy Service, Department of Paediatrics, KK Women's and Children's Hospital, Singapore, Singapore

Stephanie Lynn Mawhirt, DO
Professor of Clinical Medicine, NYU Langone Long Island School of Medicine, NYU Winthrop Rheumatology, Allergy & Immunology, Mineola, NY, United States

Drew Murphy, MD
Chief Medical Officer, Allergy, Asthma Allergy and Sinus Center, West Chester, PA, United States

Harold S. Nelson, MD
Professor of Medicine, National Jewish Health and University of Colorado Denver School of Medicine, Denver, CO, United States

Stefania Nicola, MD
Università degli Studi di Torino, Dipartimento di Scienze Mediche, AO Ordine Mauriziano Umberto I, Torino, Italy

Anna Nowak-Wegrzyn, MD, PhD
Professor of Pediatrics, Division of Pediatric Allergy and Immunology, Department of Pediatrics, NYU Langone School of Medicine, New York, NY, United States

Reynold A. Panettieri, Jr., MD
Rutgers Institute for Translational Medicine and Science, Rutgers University, New Brunswick, NJ, United States

Neha Patel, MD
Allergy/Immunology, Dept of Medicine, UMKC School of Medicine, KC, MO, United States

Marta Paulucci, MSc
Department of Dermatology, University Hospital Zurich & University of Zurich, Zurich, Switzerland

Brooke I. Polk, MD
Assistant Professor, Pediatrics, Washington University, St Louis, MO, United States

Francesca Puggioni, MD
Department of Biomedical Sciences, Humanitas Univeristy, Pieve Emanuele (MI), Italy; Personalized Medicine, Asthma and Allergy, Humanitas Research Hospital IRCCS, Rozzano (MI), Italy

Giovanni Rolla, MD
Università degli Studi di Torino, Dipartimento di Scienze Mediche, AO Ordine Mauriziano Umberto I, Torino, Italy

Lanny J. Rosenwasser, MD
Allergy/Immunology, Dept of Medicine, UMKC School of Medicine, KC, MO, United States

Umit Murat Sahiner, MD, Prof of Pediatrics, Pediatric Allergist
Allergy and Clinical Immunology, Immunomodulation and Tolerance Group, Imperial College London, London, United Kingdom; Hacettepe University School of Medicine, Pediatric Allergy Department, Ankara, Turkey

Gabriela Senti, MD
Direction Research and Education University, University Hospital Zurich, Zurich, Switzerland

Mohamed H. Shamji, PhD, FAAAAI
Allergy and Clinical Immunology, Immunomodulation and Tolerance Group, Imperial College London, London, United Kingdom; MRC & Asthma UK Centre in Allergic Mechanisms of Asthma, London, United Kingdom; Allergy and Clinical Immunology, National Heart and Lung Institute, Imperial College London, London, United Kingdom

Jeffrey R. Stokes, MD
Professor, Pediatrics, Washington University in St. Louis School of Medicine, St. Louis, MO, United States

Mimi L.K. Tang, MBBS, PhD, FRACP, FRCPA, FAAAAI
Allergy and Immune Disorders, Murdoch Children's Research Institute, Melbourne, VIC, Australia; Department of Allergy and Immunology, The Royal Children's Hospital, Melbourne, VIC, Australia; Department of Paediatrics, University of Melbourne, Melbourne, VIC, Australia

Mark W. Tenn, BHSc
Departments of Medicine and Biomedical & Molecular Sciences, Queen's University, Kingston, ON, Canada; Allergy Research Unit, Kingston General Health Research Institute, Kingston, ON, Canada

Omursen Yildirim, MD, Specialist ENT
Allergy and Clinical Immunology, Immunomodulation and Tolerance Group, Imperial College London, London, United Kingdom; Istanbul Bilim University, ENT department, Istanbul, Turkey

Background

Allergen immunotherapy: a historical progression

Ira Finegold, MD [1,2]

[1]*Professor of Medicine, Icahn School of Medicine at Mount Sinai Hospital, New York, NY, United States;* [2]*Chief Division of Allergy, Department of Medicine, Mount Sinai West, New York, NY, United States*

The history of immunotherapy over the past century is a fascinating story of a treatment that begins with mostly empirical and anecdotal observations for the first 50 years. In the following half century, scientifically controlled high-grade studies supported the observations of the first 50 years. It is also a saga of many brilliant and dedicated investigators. This chapter begins with the historical development and then examines specific goals and how they were achieved.

Historical development

The 19th century was the beginning of the explosion of the vast knowledge of the immune system. Nineteenth century scientists discovered that the immune system could be used to protect people from disease by vaccination, inoculation, or injections of different substances. It followed that these early observations could be applied to combat allergic disease. Antihistamines and corticosteroids were more than 100 years away.

Seasonal allergy was first described by a French-Italian physician, Leonardo Botallo, in 1565.[1] It was not until 1819, that Bostock,[2] in London, described a classic case of hay fever based on his own symptoms. An American physician, Morrill Wyman,[3] identified ragweed as a cause of what was called autumnal catarrh by sniffing ragweed pollen and published this information in 1872. One year later, Blackely[4] published his observations that hay fever was caused by grass pollen. He even performed crude pollen counts. As Jenner[5] had shown in the previous century that treatment by inoculation (vaccination) with cow pox protected the patient from small pox. This breakthrough led to inoculation of other substances to prevent or treat illness. By 1900, Curtis[6] was using watery extracts of pollens to immunize patients with rhinitis and/or asthma. Dunbar[7] had shown that not only were mucous membranes such as the conjunctivae sensitive but the skin of hay fever patients was sensitive as well. He also demonstrated that the injection of pollen toxin gave rise, in animals, to the production of what was termed antitoxin. He recognized that after treating patients with the pollen extracts, soluble precipitates could be found in the serum.

Immunotherapies for Allergic Disease. https://doi.org/10.1016/B978-0-323-54427-6.00001-8

In 1910, Noon[8] began experiments with subcutaneous injections of pollen extracts. He referred to his pollen preparations as a toxin. Noon's hypothesis was that by injecting small amounts of this pollen toxin, he could induce a state of immunity and the patient would get better. The plan of his experiment "was to obtain numerical measure of the sensitiveness of the patients to the pollen toxin and to observe whether this was increased or decreased by subcutaneous inoculations of various quantities of pollen toxin." The pollen extract was prepared by extraction with distilled water aided by freezing and thawing several times. Then the extracts were boiled for 10 minutes in sealed glass tubes using the method of Dunbar. Noon found that boiling did not decrease activity of his pollen preparations. He used several different species of grass and found all of them "capable of exciting an energetic reaction when instilled into the conjunctival sac of hay fever patients." Timothy grass, *Phleum pratense*, was found to yield the most active extract and that is what he used in his experiments. He began with 1 g of pollen in 50 mL of water. One drop of that mixture, diluted five thousandfold, was found to be sufficient to excite a distinct reaction in the more sensitive patients.

He defined a unit of pollen toxin as that amount of "pollen toxin which could be extracted from the thousandth part of a milligram of *Phleum* pollen." Using these defined units, he found that the most sensitive patients reacted to four units, the least sensitive to 70 units. Normal individuals failed to respond to the strongest extract, of 20,000 Noon units.

This two-page article with a crude hand drawn graph (Fig. 1.1) was the first paper to show evidence that this therapy could be successful for the treatment of "hay fever" in Great Britain. Noon's article "Prophylactic Inoculation Against Hay Fever" defined hay fever "as a form of recurrent catarrh affecting certain individuals during the months of May, June, and July." He ascribed it to what he termed a "soluble toxin found in the pollen of grasses." He thought his patients had an "idiosyncrasy of being sensitive to this toxin which is innocuous to normal individuals." Further, he reproduced this "idiosyncrasy" by dropping a small amount of an extract of grass pollen into the suspected individual's eye. He used this conjunctival challenge test for diagnosis and response to therapy. This test was not new, having originally been described by Blakely[9] as a way of proving that pollen caused hay fever.

He began his subcutaneous injection with small doses every 3–4 days and increased the dose as well as the time interval between doses. Fig. 1.1 shows his initial chart for treatment in 1910 and 1911. He found out in the early stages of immunization, an overdose could induce a severe attack of hay fever lasting nearly 24 hours which was not observed in the later stages. He was able to show that after the inoculations there was an increase in tolerance. Before he could continue this pioneering work, he succumbed to tuberculosis in 1913.

John Freeman continued Noon's work.[10] He wrote a personal note about Noon and included interesting facts such as his sister collected the grass pollen for Noon's studies.[11]

Noon made the first attempt at standardizing doses by establishing the Noon unit based on weight per volume. One year later, across the Atlantic Ocean, in New York,

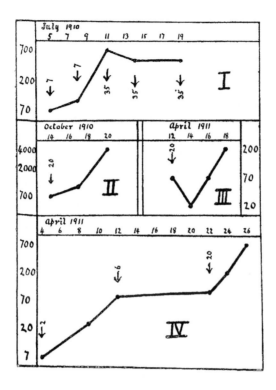

FIGURE 1.1

The numbers at the sides denote the resistance of the patient, given in terms of the strength of pollen extract, one drop of which was sufficient to excite a conjunctival reaction. The arrows indicate subcutaneous inoculations of pollen extract, quantities given in the units described in the text. I and II refer to one patient at different periods of treatment; III shows the response obtained after about a month's treatment in another case; and IV, the early stages of treatment.

Cooke[12] presented his results on grass pollen immunotherapy. Robert A. Cooke was the chief American proponent of allergy as early as 1910. His 1916 landmark paper[13] dealt with human allergies, summarizing 5 years of work with 621 cases of "human protein sensitization." He looked at inheritance patterns and concluded that "Sensitized individuals transmit to their offspring not their own specific sensitization but an unusual capacity for developing bioplastic reactivities to any foreign proteins." When Cooke was honored at a dinner on February 27, 1958,[14] on the 40th Anniversary of the founding of the first allergy clinic in New York, he spoke about the factors that led him to medicine and allergy. The first factor was his great grandfather, the first Dr Cooke who was a physician in the Revolutionary War. He was the last Dr Cooke in a continuing lineage of eldest son physicians. The second factor he cited was that he had asthma since the age of 8 years. He found out when he was sent to boarding school in 1890 that his asthma disappeared and could be traced to animals at his home, particularly horses. The third factor that committed him to his future allergy career was an exposure to diphtheria in 1908 that required him to have an injection of horse antitoxin. This injection resulted in severe anaphylaxis. Epinephrine injections and artificial respiration saved his life.

In 1910, Cooke, an asthmatic, and Vander Veer, a hay fever sufferer, began studies of "hypersensitivities in humans." Cooke related that in 1911 he began the experiments that culminated in his article with Albert Vander Veer, in 1915, on "Human Sensitization."[12] In 1911, he had "extracted a pollen protein that caused skin reactions in his patients.[15] Among the contributions Cooke and Vander Veer made were inheritance of sensitization; development of the intradermal skin test; methods of collecting pollen and making extracts for testing and treatment, antibodies in hay fever, constitutional reactions, drug idiosyncrasy, elucidation of house dust as an important allergen; and classifications of hypersensitiveness. He was able to show that pillows containing animal hair could result in asthma. He also established common house dust as a cause of asthma. He preferred his own method of standardization by nitrogen content as determined by the Kjeldahl method. This eventually became the protein nitrogen unit still in use today. Cooke was a master investigator who developed the basic methods of subcutaneous immunotherapy as it is practiced today. His contributions to the field of allergy are without parallel.

During this period, other important events occurred. In 1921, Prausnitz and Kustner[16] discovered a factor that was present in serum of allergic individuals that could be transferred. In 1923, Cooke along with Longcope, Schloss, Vander Veer, Coca, Spain, and Alexander met in his office and organized the Society for the Study of Asthma and Allied Conditions. This Society along with the Western allergists eventually formed the American Academy of Allergy.[17]

Early materials and methods

Over the next few decades, following Noon's and Cooke's reports, the materials and methods for allergen immunotherapy were defined and refined. In 1912, Om Schloss[18] applied the skin test to food allergy. Wodehouse[19] developed extract preparation methods. Chandler Walker[20] extended desensitization to substances other than pollen. In 1922, *Journal of Immunology*, founded by Arthur Coca, published, for the first time, an entire issue dedicated to allergy. This landmark issue contained a number of articles of major significance. Among them was Cooke's paper on constitutional (systemic) reactions.[21] This paper described causes and treatment of systemic reactions. For treatment of constitutional reactions, Cooke advocated adrenalin 1:1000, 1 cc injected in adults and 0.4−0.6 cc in children. He wrote: "The writer has never seen any ill effects from these large doses of Adrenalin and is confident that if it is used early enough and in large enough doses, the serious results of a reaction can be avoided."

Another paper in that issue by Coca[22] reported on improved methods of allergen extraction, and to this day Coca's solution or modifications of it are still in use.

Table 1.1 Landmark achievements and individuals in the history of allergen immunotherapy.

Jenner	First demonstration of vaccine principles	1788
Blackley	First attempt at SIT by pollen application to abraded skin	1880
Richet and Portier	Experimental description of anaphylaxis	1902
Noon and Freeman	First successful pollen SIT trial	1911
Hollister,G and Stier, R	Prepare their first lot of allergenic extract	
Cooke	Discovery of house dust as ubiquitous allergen, blocking antibodies, and more	1922, 1935
Loveless	First demonstration that venom was superior to whole body for treatment of hymenoptera anaphylaxis	1956
Lowell and Frankin	First double-blind controlled SIT trial with purified extracts	1965
Ishazaka and Ishizaka, Johannsson et al.	Discovery of IgE	1967
Hopkins Group	Ragweed and venom immunotherapy	1974
Lockey, R	IT safety	1989
Cohen S.	Immunotherapy and allergy historian	1991
Nelson H.	Optimum dosing and extract stability	1996
Finegold	IT clinical advocacy and marketing	1996
Passalaqua et al.	Double-blind controlled SLIT trial for dust mite	1998
Durham et al.	Sustained efficacy of both SCIT and SLIT using grass pollen	1999,2010
Cox	Parameters of IT, value, transition to SLIT	2003

Note the acronym IT has been replaced with AIT per an AAAAI/EAACI document on AIT nomenclature.[1] Adapted from Fitzhugh DJ, Lockey RF. History of immunotherapy: the first 100 years. Immunol Allergy Clin N Am. 2011;31:149.

Allergens were prepared by some institutions for their own use, and allergen extract manufacturers appeared as early as 1921 (Table 1.1).[23]

Even though Cooke had mentioned the possibility of reactions with intradermal testing, in that same 1922 issue, Brown discussed whether puncture or intradermal tests were better.[24] In the last paper of that journal, Cooke described the desensitizing effects of allergen injections. He wrote[25]: "The writer has had numerous opportunities to make such a study following subcutaneous injections in hay fever and asthma for therapeutic purpose. The effect of those injections has usually been a specific lessening of the general cutaneous reactivity, which, however, never approached extinction."

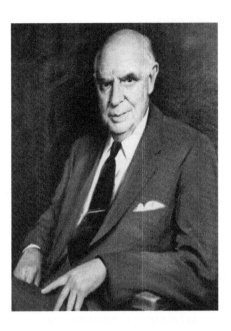

"Robert A. Cooke, MD, Mount Sinai West"

Specific treatment: allergic rhinitis

By 1927, Vander Veer, Cooke, and Spain[27] had published a summary article on the diagnosis and treatment of seasonal hay fever. This article summarized pollen seasons, sensitivity of patients according to five classes or categories. They analyzed the results of 1070 cases. They described local reactions and 96 constitutional reactions in the 1070 cases (9% of patients or 1% of all injections). Treatment recommended for severe reactions was 0.5 cc of epinephrine subcutaneously, and in extreme cases intravenously. Improvement occurred in 85% of the patients treated (in a preantihistamine era) and 15% were unsuccessful. In their series, 30% of allergic rhinitis patients had allergic asthma, 75% of this subgroup were improved. This was preseasonal therapy of at least 3 months duration. These investigators also described encouraging results using continuing (perennial) therapy instead of only preseasonal. Some patients did not respond to treatment, so there was a constant debate in the 1960s about whether allergen immunotherapy was effective. Lowell and Franklin's report on the benefits of ragweed immunotherapy for allergic rhinitis was in the affirmative.[28] Fontana et al. reported soon after Lowell and Franklins study that immunotherapy was not effective.[29] The Hopkins group,[30] in 1968, reported a study demonstrating efficacy to be dose related utilizing defined extracts. In this study, they also demonstrated that low dose was the same as placebo. A metaanalysis confirmed efficacy of IT for allergic rhinitis.[31]

Allergic asthma

Cooke[32] felt bacterial infection played a role in asthma exacerbations. He was a proponent of culturing respiratory bacteria from patients and injecting killed extracts of these bacteria in the patient. This treatment persisted until studies in the mid-1950s with asthmatic patients failed to show a difference when bacterial vaccines were administered.[33–36] Autogenous bacterial vaccines were supplanted by commercially prepared bacterial respiratory vaccines. In the late 1990s, production of these products ceased in the United States.

Johnstone and Dutton[85] showed that 14 years after immunotherapy was stopped there was less asthma in the immunotherapy-treated group. The specific immunotherapy group had more patients without asthma than the control group. The number of patients who continued to have asthma was higher in the control group than in the immunotherapy-treated groups. Warner in 1978,[36] and Rak[37] in 1991, observed decreases in allergen-induced late asthmatic responses and associated bronchial inflammation, respectively, in children and adults. Additional studies were published indicating efficacy not only for rhinitis but for asthma. The PAT study exemplifies these data.[38] Two separate metaanalyses confirmed these observations.[39,40].

Other studies show the value of immunotherapy, that is, cost efficacy. It became clear that patients with asthma treated with immunotherapy had fewer hospitalizations and unscheduled visits.[41]

Insect venom immunotherapy

Venom desensitization may be considered one of the most effective forms of subcutaneous immunotherapy. This was not always the case. For a number of years, injections of whole body mixes of hymenoptera were used for the treatment of patients who had sustained severe stinging insect reactions. But in 1974, Lichenstein, Valentine et al.[42] showed that venom was significantly more effective than treatment with whole body extracts. With the publication of this paper, venom therapy became the only acceptable treatment for hymenoptera venom hypersensitivity. Fire ant extract is still made from whole body preparation and has been showed to be effective.[43]

However, the true heroine of venom treatment is Mary Hewitt Loveless. In 1935, following a vacation in Europe, she met Dr Cooke in New York on her way back to California. She did not originally plan this stopover. But she stayed on with Dr Cooke for the next 3 years, completing a fellowship with him. Over the next 20 years or so she investigated such areas as blocking antibodies, serum responses to pollen injections, reaginic antibodies, and repository immunotherapy.[44] In the mid-1950s, after a colleague's mother had two near fatal reactions to insect stings, she became interested in using hymenoptera venom for treatment. Since venom was not commercially available, she personally caught hymenoptera and dissected out their venom sacs. Having been trained by Cooke and his colleagues, and later on by Heidelberger at Columbia University, she was quite able to make venom containing extract and administer desensitizing doses. Her successful results were published in 1956.[45] Whether it was lack of commercial venoms, or being a female physician, allergist, and immunologist in a male-dominated specialty, her results were never actively pursued or accepted, leaving no effective treatment for the next 22 years. Since the Hopkins Group's paper,[46] hymenoptera sensitivity has been successfully treated with immunotherapy saving countless lives. Ross et al. confirmed efficacy in a metaanalysis[47] of venom immunotherapy data.

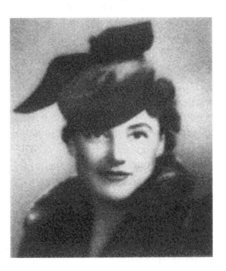

"Mary Loveless, MD reference 44"

Food allergy immunotherapy

As early as 1908, Schofield[48] reported the use of minute amounts of egg to treat egg allergy. By 1930, Freeman[49] reported that with the use of subcutaneous immunotherapy (SCIT) a state of tolerance was induced in a fish-allergic patient. The use of SCIT to peanut, although effective, resulted in an unacceptable side effect profile.[50] Recent reports have highlighted efficacy of oral immunotherapy and sublingual immunotherapy (SLIT) for various food allergies, including egg, milk, hazelnut, and peanut. Regimens have varied from rush protocols, generally being performed in a hospitalized setting, to slow updosing, which in some cases is performed with dosing at home.[51]

Decreasing side effects of immunotherapy

Beginning in the 1930s there were experiments with adjuvants and attempts to modify the allergens. These were attempts to increase immunogenicity and decrease allergenicity. There were data, early in the development of this new therapy, that injecting allergens into allergic patients was not innocuous. Cooke described constitutional reactions in his text book and stated that they were rarely fatal.[52] Modifying allergy injectable materials was an effort to decrease risk of reactions by prolonged absorption of the allergen. Methods such as injecting extracts in mineral oil were efforts to slow absorption and retain the allergen locally in the tissues. When this practice was shown to lead to plasmacytomas in mice, it was abandoned.[53] Aluminum hydroxide was added to allergens.[54] The resulting precipitate was less allergenic and allowed for slow absorption. However, immunogenicity probably suffered as well. Standardization was not available. Some patients also developed lumps under their skin at injection sites. These extracts are slowly disappearing in the United States. Later on, formalin mixed with extracts led to polymerized allergens that preserved immunogenicity. These were termed allergoids. Patterson[55] showed efficacy but the allergoid vaccines were not approved by the FDA. However, allergoid-based immunotherapy is currently used in Europe. Other methods utilized recombinant DNA technology to produce recombinant allergens[56] and breaking down the allergen to peptides.[57] In 2006, a combined approach of using an allergoid of ragweed attached to L tyrosine depot and adjuvanated with monophosphoryl lipid A was developed.[58] The advantages are a short effective course and low allergenicity. It appears to be quite safe.[59] This vaccine is used in Europe. Additional studies in the United States are planned.[60] Repository immunotherapy was pioneered by Mary Loveless in the 1940s, and subsequently by many others. Currently, there is resurgence in using modified allergens with adjuvants in an attempt to improve safety and decrease the number of injections per year.

Potency/standardization

The need for quantifying the strength of extracts with regard to biologic potency was a perplexing problem beginning in 1911. Noon, as described above, based the Noon unit on weight per volume, which is still in effect for many extracts. Cooke defined the protein nitrogen unit. While this unit measured protein content, it did not give an accurate measurement of the biologic potency. In order to evaluate potency, one needed to skin test with the extracts in known allergic patients. Cooke's protein nitrogen unit system is still used by some allergists but weight per volume strength is more common. The goal has been to standardize extracts by potency with known standards. Reagents for in vitro testing had to be developed. Once IgE was identified,[61,62] standardization based on IgE inhibition in vitro could be established. Currently, there are 19 standardized extracts commercially available. During the decades of empirical immunotherapy, various dosing schedules and durations, as well as dubious indications for immunotherapy existed. An early attempt in 1931 by the Joint Committee of Survey and Standardizations (the Western Association for the Study of Allergy and the Eastern Society for the Study of Asthma and Allied Conditions) failed to come up with any standards based on the available technology at that time.[63] The two major allergy societies, AAAAI and ACAAAI, established the Joint Council of Allergy and Immunology, which in turn led to the formation of the Joint Committee on Practice Parameters. With the publication of the first Practice Parameters for Immunotherapy in 2003[64] an accepted codified up-to-date approach now existed. There have been subsequent updates.[65] As reagents improved, with appropriate dosing schedules, and physician awareness increased, the rare fatality from subcutaneous immunotherapy decreased. For the last 10 years per AAAAI/ACAAI AIT fatality survey Epstein et al. JACI 2019 there have been at least 7 fatalities since 2008.

Mechanisms of allergy

The state of the field of allergy was summarized in 1955 by Sherman when he addressed the attendees at the 11th annual meeting of the American Academy of Allergy on the subject of Reaginic and Blocking Antibodies.[66] Reagin was thought to be the substance that conferred allergy and blocking antibodies, the response to allergy treatment. At that time Sherman stated, "I think it is safe to say that there has been no significant correlation between blocking antibody titers and clinical results." Reagin was identified by Ishizakas[61] and Johansen[62] as IgE in 1967. How allergy shots worked was still unknown. Earlier, Cooke had described blocking antibody that arose as a response to immunotherapy. But it too was undefined and not always detectable in patients who improved with immunotherapy. The induction of blocking antibodies was one of the first explanations for clinical improvement with allergen immunotherapy.[67] Eventually, IgG4 was identified as immunoglobulin class containing blocking antibody. It was thought that blocking antibody competed for the determinants on the allergen and the more blocking antibody present, from repeated injections, the better the clinical result. Studies also showed that as repeated injections were given, specific IgE increased and then subsequently decreased. But this was not known until the 1960s−1980s when great strides were made in defining the immune changes that occurred with immunotherapy (Table 1.2).

Other changes include specific IgG increases; early, predominantly IgG1; late, predominantly IgG4; nonspecific loss of immunologic responsiveness in basophils. Lymphocytes and peripheral blood mononuclear cells experience (1) decreased lymphocyte proliferation; (2) generation of allergen-specific CD8 T cells; (3) an increase in cutaneous cells expressing human leukocyte antigen-DR and CD25 (interleukin-2 receptor); (4) a decrease in stimulated release of macrophage inhibitory factor, histamine releasing factors, IL-4, platelet activating factor, and tumor necrosis factor, and eosinophilic chemotactic activity; and (5) an increase in stimulated mRNA levels, interleukin-2, interferon groups about the importance of this field and providing the best treatment information.[51]

Table 1.2 A summary of mechanisms from the immunotherapy practice parameters third update.[68]

Summary Statement 1	The immunologic response to subcutaneous immunotherapy is characterized by decreases in the sensitivity of end organs and changes in the humoral and cellular responses to the administered allergens.
Summary Statement 2	Reduction in end-organ response with immunotherapy includes decreased early and late responses of the skin, conjunctiva, nasal mucosa, and bronchi to allergen challenge; decreased allergen-induced eosinophil, basophil, and mast cell infiltration; blunting of mucosal priming; and reduction of nonspecific bronchial sensitivity to histamine.
Summary Statement 3	Shortly after initiation of immunotherapy, there is an increase in CD41CD251 regulatory T lymphocytes secreting IL-10 and TGF-b associated with immunologic tolerance, which is defined as a long-lived decrease in allergen-specific T cell responsiveness. With continued immunotherapy, there is some waning of this response, and immune deviation from TH2 to TH1 cytokine response to the administered allergen predominates.
Summary Statement 4	Specific IgE levels initially increase and then gradually decrease. Levels of specific IgG1, IgG4, and IgA increase. None of these changes in antibody levels have been shown to consistently correlate strongly with clinical improvement.
Summary Statement 5	Increases in allergen-specific IgG levels are not predictive of the degree or duration of efficacy of immunotherapy. However, functional alterations in allergen-specific IgG levels, such as changes in avidity, affinity, or both for allergen, might play a role in determining clinical efficacy.

Length of treatment

Then there were questions as to duration of treatments and persistence of immunotherapy effects. It was the early work of Johnstone[69] that showed effects of immunotherapy could persist for 14 years. But this was not the same for all patients. In fact there were patients who did not improve with immunotherapy. This difference in response was not understood. Finally in 1999, Durham elegantly showed that improved symptoms, with immunotherapy with grass pollen in adults, persisted at least 3 years after three or more years of immunotherapy[70] (Fig. 1.2).

Durham et al. subsequently studied the optimal duration of SLIT and found 3 years more effective than 2 years of treatment.[2,3]

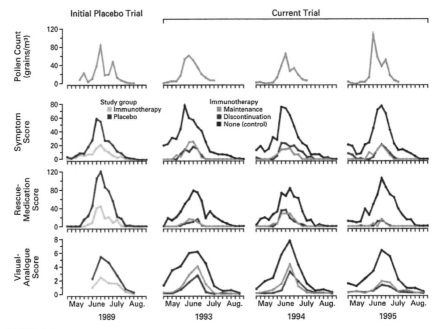

FIGURE 1.2

Median Weekly Pollen counts and Symptom, Rescue-medication, and visual Analogue scores for the Initial Placebo Trial (1989) and for the current trial (1993–1995). Analysis of the area under the curve with the Mann-Whitney U test revealed no significant differences between the maintenance group and the discontinuation group (see Table 1.2); the median scores in both of these group were markedly lower than those in the control group. For comparison, results are also shown for the initial placebo-controlled trial of immunotherapy (1989). Tick marks on the X-axes indicate one-week intervals. Data for 1989 are from Varney et al.[4]

Routes of immunotherapy

Alternate routes of immunotherapy have been tried over the years. Oral immunotherapy was first attempted more than 100 years ago by Schoffield who treated an egg-allergic patient with very low doses of egg.[48] However, it was not until the late 1980s that well-controlled studies began to emerge from European allergists. They were clearly able to show efficacy of this method. There appears to be a chasm between the United States and much of Europe, where sublingual immunotherapy is now used more frequently than subcutaneous immunotherapy. There are numerous well-controlled studies. A World Allergy Organization position paper[71] speaks to the strength of this form of immunotherapy. Certainly, from the perspective of the patient, the home dosing (beyond initial dose) protocol of sublingual immunotherapy is attractive; however, questions still remain with regard to sublingual immunotherapy. These questions include efficacy compared with subcutaneous immunotherapy schedules, mixes, and duration of treatment.

At present (January 2018) in the United States, there are four preparations for sublingual immunotherapy approved by the Food and Drug Administration of the United States. Countless other patients have been treated by sublingual immunotherapy using conventional extracts off-label. In addition to the sublingual method, other routes have been studied such as intranasal, epicutaneous and intralymphatic. None of these has been approved for use in United States (except for intranasal flu).

Concluding thoughts

At the end of their two-part review of asthma, allergy, and immunotherapy[72] Cohen and Evans make two noteworthy points namely that although immunotherapy began with decades of loosely controlled trial and error studies which evolved into better conducted ones, there were still needs to be met. These were "(1) epidemiological studies of the scope and design required for an in-depth understanding of the natural history of asthma and allergic disease and (2) large-scale clinical trials from which to construct critical criteria for exact indications, materials, and methods in the conduct of immunotherapeutic regimens." The second point was the "enormous impact and influence that allergen immunotherapy had on the launching, development, and continuation of allergy as a medical specialty."

Nelson[73] in one of his many presentations and papers on immunotherapy summarized the achievements with these comments. "Over the last century immunotherapy has evolved to a present state where:

- It has been proven to be effective in allergic rhinitis, allergic asthma, hymenoptera sensitivity, and some atopic dermatitis
- Effective doses have been defined
- It has been shown to modify the underlying immune defect both in preventing progression and inducing persisting benefit
- The immunologic basis is increasingly understood, allowing for tailoring approaches to immunotherapy"

This chapter has sought to present some insights into the work of some of the key individuals who have contributed to the success of the specialty of allergy, asthma, and immunology. A key difference between the Board-Certified Allergist and other physicians who may treat allergies is that the Board-Certified Allergist-Immunologist has been trained and continues to be trained in the theory, science, and art of immunotherapy. Immunotherapy remains to this day, the most unique and powerful tool in the armamentarium of the practicing allergist even though there have been great improvements in additional immune modulators.

References

1. Botallo Simons FE. *Ancestors of Allergy*. New York: Global Medical Communications; 1994.
2. Bostock J. Case of periodical affection of the eyes and chest. *Med Chir Trans*. 1819;10: 161.
3. Wyman M. *Autumnal Catarrh*. Cambridge, MA: Hurd and Houghton; 1872.
4. Blackley CH. *Experimental Researches on the Causes and Nature of Catarrhus Aestivus*. London: Bailliere, Tindall and Cox; 1873.
5. Jenner E. *An Inquiry into the Causes and Effects of the Variolae… Sampson Low*. London: Soho; 1798.
6. Curtis HH. The immunizing cure of hay fever. *Med News*. 1900;77:16.
7. Dunbar WP. The present state of our knowledge of hay-fever. *J Hyg*. 1902;13:105.
8. Noon L. Prophylactic inoculation against hay fever. *Lancet*. 1911;1:1572.
9. Blakely CH. *Hay Fever; its Causes, Treatment and Effective Prevention*. London: Balliere; 1880.
10. Freeman J. Vaccination against hay fever; report of results during the last three years. *Lancet*. 1914;1:1178.
11. Leonard Noon FJ. *Int Arch Allergy*. 1953;4:282–284.
12. Cooke RA, Vander Veer A. Human sensitization. *J Immunol*. 1916;1:201–305.
13. Cooke RA. He treatment of hay fever by active immunization. *Laryngoscope*. 1915; 25(108).
14. Siegel S. Dinner in honor of Robert A. Cooke, M.D. *Proc NY Allergy Soc NY state J Med*. 1959;59:289–302.
15. Rackemann FM. Robert Anderson Cooke. 1880–1960. *Trans Assoc Am Physicians*. 1961;74:11–13.
16. PrausnitzC KH. Studien uber Uberempfindlichkeit. *Centralb Bacteriol 1 Abt Orig*. 1921; 86:160.
17. Siegel. *Personal Communication*.
18. Schloss OM. A case of allergy to common foods. *Am J Dis Child*. 1912;111:341.
19. Wodehouse RP. Immunochemical study and immunochemistry of protein series. *J Immunol*. 1917;11VI. Cat hair, 227;VII. Horse dander, 237;VIII dog hair,243.
20. Walker IC. Studies on the sensitization of patients with bronchial asthma (Study series III-XXXVI). *J Med Res*. 1917;35–37.
21. Cooke RA. Studies in specific hypersensitiveness. III. On constitutional reactions:the dangers of the diagnostic cutaneous test and therapeutic injection of allergens. *J Immunol*. 1922;7:119–146.
22. Coca AF. Studies in specific hypersensitiveness. V. The preparation of fluid extracts and solutions for use in the diagnosis and treatment of the allergies with notes on the collection of pollens. *J Immunol*. 1922;7:163–178.
23. Moffitt DD. *History and Growth. The Fill*. Jubilant Hollister-Stier; Winter 2014.
24. Brown A. 1. The diagnostic cutaneous reaction in allergy. Comparison of the intradermal method (Cooke) and the scratch method (Schloss). *J Immunol*. 1922;7:97–111.
25. Cooke RA. Studies in specific hypersensitiveness. IX. On ther phenomenon of hyposensitization (The clinically lessened sensitiveness of allergy). *J Immunol*. 1922;7:219–242.
26. Fitzhugh DJ, Lockey RF. History of immunotherapy: the first 100 years. *Immunol Allergy Clin N Am*. 2011;31:149.

27. Vander Veer A, Cooke RA, Spain WC. Diagnosis and treatment of seasonal hay fever. *Am J Med Sci.* 1927;174:101.
28. Lowell FC, Franklin W. A double blind study of the effectiveness and specificity of injection therapy in ragweed hay fever. *N Engl J Med.* 1965;273:675.
29. Fontana VC, Holt Jr LE, Mainland D. Effectiveness of hyposensitization therapy in ragweed hay-fever in children. *JAMA.* 1967;195:109.
30. Norman PS, Winkenwerder WL, Lichtenstein LM. Immunotherapy of hay fever with ragweed antigen E: comparisons with whole pollen extracts and placebos. *J Allergy.* 1968;42:93.
31. RN Ross RN, Nelson HS, Finegold I. Effectiveness of specific immunotherapy in the treatment of allergic rhinitis: an analysis of randomized, prospective, single-or double-blind, placebo-controlled studies. *Clin Ther.* 2000;22:342.
32. Cooke RA. *Infective Asthma with Pharmacopeia* (Chapter 7). In: *Allergy in Theory and Practice.* Cooke RA: WB Saunders Co; 1947:151.
33. Frankland AW, Hughes WH, Garrill RH. Autogenous bacterial vaccines in the treatment of asthma. *Br Med J.* 1955;2:941.
34. Helander E. Bacterial vaccines in the treatment of bronchial asthma. *Acta Allergol.* 1959; 3:47.
35. Johnstone DE. Study of the value of bacterial vaccines in the treatment of bronchial asthma associated with respiratory infections. *AMA J Dis Child.* 1957;94:1.
36. Price JF, Warner JO, Hey EN, Turner MW, Soothill JF. A controlled trial of hyposensitization with adsorbed tyrosine Dermatophagoides pteronyssinus antigen in childhood asthma: in vivo aspects. *Clin Allergy.* 1984;14:209−219.
37. Rak S, Lowhagen O, Venge P. The effect of immunotherapy on bronchial hyperresponsiveness and eosinophil cationic protein in pollen-allergic patients. *J Allergy Clin Immunol.* 1988;82:470−480.
38. Jacobsen L, Niggemann B, Dreborg S, et al. Specific immunotherapy has long-term preventive effect of seasonal and perennial asthma: 10-year follow-up on the PAT study. *Allergy.* 2007;62:943−948.
39. Abramson MJ, Puy RM, Weiner JM. Is allergen immunotherapy effective in asthma? A meta-analysis of randomized controlled trials. *Am J Respir Crit Care Med.* 1995;151(4): 969−974.
40. Ross RN, Nelson HS, Finegold I. Effectiveness of specific immunotherapy in the treatment of asthma: a meta-analysis of prospective, randomized, double-blind, placebo-controlled studies. *Clin Ther.* 2000;22:329.
41. Hankin CS, Cox L, Lang D, et al. et al., Allergy immunotherapy among Medicaid-enrolled children with allergic rhinitis: patterns of care, resource use, and costs. *J Allergy Clin Immunol.* 2008;121:227.
42. Lichenstein LM, Valentine MD, Sobotka AK. A case for venom treatment in anaphylactic sensitivity to Hymenoptera sting. *N Engl J Med.* 1974;290:1223−1227.
43. Freeman TM, Hylander R, Ortiz A, Martin ME. Imported fire ant immunotherapy: effectiveness of whole body extracts. *J Allergy Clin Immunol.* 1992;90:210−215.
44. Cohen S. Loveless on wasp venom allergy and immunity. Part 1. The allergy Archives. *J Allergy Clin Immunol.* 2003;112:1252.
45. Loveless MH, Feckler WR. Wasp venom allergy and immunity. *Ann Alllergy.* 1956;14: 347−366.
46. Hunt KJ, Valentine MD, Sobotka AK, et al. A controlled trial of insect hypersensitivity. *N Engl J Med.* 1978;299:157.

47. Ross RN, Nelson HS, Finegold I. Effectiveness of specific immunotherapy in the treatment of hymenoptera venom hypersensitivity: a meta-analysis. *Clin Ther.* 2000;22:351.
48. Schofield AT. A case of egg poisoning. *Lancet.* 1908;1:716.
49. Freeman J. "Rush" inoculation. *Lancet.* 1930;1:744.
50. Pajno GB, Caminiti L, Ruggeri P, et al. Oral immunotherapy for cow's milk allergy with a weekly up-dosing regimen: a randomized single blind controlled study. *Ann Allergy Asthma Immunol.* 2010;105:376.
51. Finegold I, Dockhorn RJ, Ein D, et al. Immunotherapy throughout the decades: from Noon to now. *Ann Allergy Asthma Immunol.* 2010;105:328.
52. Cooke RA. *Allergy in Theory and Practice.* Philadelphia and London: WB Saunders Company; 1947:203.
53. Potter M, Boyce CR. Induction of plasma cell neoplasms in strains BALB/c mice with mineral oil and mineral oil adjuvants. *Nature.* 1962;193:1086.
54. Nelson HS. Long-term immunotherapy with aqueous and alum precipitated grass extracts. *Ann Allergy.* 1980;45:333.
55. Patterson R, Suszko IM, Pruzansky JJ, et al. Polymerized ragweed antigen E. II in vivo elimination studies and reactivity with IgE antibody systems. *J Immunol.* 1973;110:1413.
56. Valenta R, Duchene M. BirknerVS, et al. Look up. *J Clin Investig.* 1997 99: 1673. Look for a better date.
57. Norman PS, Togias A. Potential new forms of immunotherapy. In: Lockey RF, Bukantz S, eds. . *Allergens and Allergen Immunotherapy.* 2nd ed. New York: Marcel Dekker, Inc.; 1999. Revised and Expanded.
58. Patel P, Salapatek AM. Pollinex Quatro: a novel and well tolerated , ultra short course of allergy vaccine. *Expert Rev Vaccines.* 2006;5:617.
59. Baldrick P, Richardson D, Woroniecki SR, Pollinex Quatro Ragweed. Safety evaluation of a new allergy vaccine adjuvanated with monophosphoryl lipid A (MPL) for the treatment of ragweed pollen allergy. *J Appl Toxicol.* 2007;27:399.
60. *Allergy Therapeutics Sept 2016 Report on Website.*
61. Ishizaka K, Ishizaka T. Identification of Υ E-antibodies as a carrier of reaginic activity. *J Immunol.* 1967;99:1187−1198.
62. Johannson SG. Raised levels of a new immunoglobulin class (IgND) in asthma. *Lancet.* 1967;ii:951−953.
63. Report of the Joint Committee on Standards. *J Allergy.* 1935;6:408.
64. Joint Task Force on Practice Parameters. Allergen immunotherapy: a practice parameter. *Ann Allergy Asthma Immunol.* 2003;90:S1−S40.
65. Cox L, Li JT, Nelson H, Lockey R. Allergen immunotherapy: a practice parameter second update. *J Allergy Clin Immunol.* 2007;120:S25−S85.
66. Sherman WB. Reaginic and blocking antibodies. *J Allergy.* 1957;28:62.
67. Cook RA, Barnard JH, Stull HS. Seerological evidence of immunity with coexisting sensation in a type of human allergy. (Hay fever). *J Exp Med.* 1935;62:733.
68. Cox L, Nelson H, Lockey R. Allergen immunotherapy: a practice parameter third update. *Allergy Clin Immunol.* 2011;127(Supplement):S1−S55.
69. Johnstone DE, Dutton A. The value of hyposensitization therapy for bronchial asthma in children − a 14-year study. *Pediatrics.* 1968;42:793−802.
70. Durham SR, Walker SM, Varga EM, et al. Long-term clinical efficacy of grass-pollen immunotherapy. *N Engl J Med.* 1999;341:468−475. https://doi.org/10.1056/NEJM199908123410702.

71. Canonica GW, Bousquet J, Casale T, et al. Sub-lingual immunotherapy: world allergy position paper 2009. *Wold Allergy Org J*. 2009;2(233).
72. Cohen SG, Evans RA. Allergy and immunotherapy; a historical review: Part I. *Allergy Proc*. 1991;12(6):407−415.
73. Nelson HS. *ACAAI Presentation 2011 Annual Meeting*.

References: In addition the references listed below excellent sources of material about the history of immunotherapy can be found in:

1. Cohen SG, Evans RE. Allergen immunotherapy in historical prospective. In: Lockey, Bukantz, eds. *Allergens and Immunotherapy*. NY: Marcel Decker, Inc.; 1999:1−37.
2. Cohen SG, Samter M. *Excerpts from Classics in Allergy*. 2nd ed. Carlsbad, CA: Symposia Foundation; 1992.
3. Lockey RF, Bukantz S. *Allergens and Allergen Immunotherapy*. Revised and Expanded. 2nd ed. New York: Marcel Dekker, Inc.; 1999.
4. Calderon MA, Casale T, Cox L, et al. Allergen immunotherapy: a new semantic framework from the European academy of allergy and clinical immunology/American academy of allergy, asthma and immunology/PRACTALL consensus report. *Allergy*. 2013;68: 825−828.
5. Scadding GW, Calderon MA, Shamji MH, et al. Effect of 2 Years of treatment with sublingual grass pollen immunotherapy on nasal response to allergen challenge at 3 Years among patients with moderate to severe seasonal allergic rhinitis: the GRASS randomized clinical trial. *JAMA*. 2017;317:615−625.
6. Cox LS. Sublingual immunotherapy for allergic rhinitis: is 2-year treatment sufficient for long-term benefit? *JAMA*. 2017;317:591−593.

Definition of an allergen

2

Robert G. Hamilton, PhD, DABMLI, FAAAAI

*Professor, Division of Allergy and Clinical Immunology, Departments of Medicine and Pathology,
Johns Hopkins University School of Medicine, Baltimore, MD, United States*

In its simplest form, an allergen may be defined as any substance (most commonly a protein, glycoprotein, lipoprotein) that is capable of inducing the production of IgE antibody in a genetically predisposed individual and evoking an allergic immune response.[1] By its nature, an allergen is an antigenic molecule that is viewed as foreign to the immune system and the IgE antibody it produces binds onto high affinity cellular Fc receptors on mast cells and basophils. The production of IgE antibodies and arming of mast cells and basophils defines an individual as sensitized. Reexposure to the same allergenic substance may or may not elicit an allergic reaction depending on the number of IgE antibodies cross-linked. This elicitation of an allergic reaction depends principally on the IgE antibody concentration that determines the density of IgE antibodies on the mast cell and basophil (effector cell) surface. Three other associated factors involve the affinity or strength of binding, the precise epitope specificity on the allergen, and the percentage of the total IgE that is specific for the target allergenic molecule. Sufficient cross-links of IgE antibody on the cell surface result in cell activation and release of mediators that in turn can produce a spectrum of allergic symptoms depending upon the release of the vasoactive mediators.[2]

Classification of allergens

Allergenic materials that are used as in vivo diagnosis (skin testing), immunotherapy, and in vitro serological reagents are principally complex physiological extracts of biological source materials that contain a mixture of proteins, carbohydrates, lipids, glycoproteins, and other substances, some of which may not be allergenic. They are often described according to their routes of exposure as aeroallergens, injected allergens, and ingested allergens. Alternatively, they can be broadly classified according to their source material that encompasses epidermal and animal proteins, drugs, foods [fruits, vegetables, seeds, legumes, nuts, spices, fish, shellfish, mollusks, egg and fowl, meat, milk, and additives], insect and parasite excretions, venoms, plant [grass, weed, and tree] pollens, microorganisms [molds], mites, and occupational products [natural rubber latex]. Each group has its unique challenges in reproducibly collecting the source material and optimizing extraction protocols. As a biological substance, there is

Immunotherapies for Allergic Disease. https://doi.org/10.1016/B978-0-323-54427-6.00002-X

inherently variability in the allergenic content of the source material that is changing with environmental climate alterations as well as natural biological variation. This leads to allergen extracts with variable composition (identity and purity) and potency (strength and content) (see Chapter 3).

In the United States, of the nearly 500 allergen extract specificities used in in vivo diagnosis and treatment, 19 have been standardized, which allows for a more consistent measure of potency and composition across manufacturers.[3] Nonstandardized extracts in the United States are labeled by a variable weight (mass) to volume ratio or quantity of protein per volume (e.g., protein nitrogen unit per mL). As no United States Food and Drug Administration validated methods or requirements exist for determining the potency of a nonstandardized extract, there is variability among different allergen manufacturers. This variability poses a problem when patients transfer from one allergist/immunologist practice to another (i.e., due to insurance change, move, etc.). The European Union (European Medicinal Agency, EMA manufacturing guideline is accommodating special allergenic products, such as recombinant allergens, synthetic peptides, allergoids, and conjugates.[4]

Naming allergenic products

The convention for naming of allergens was originally proposed by Marsh et al. in 1986[5] and has received international agreement.[6] Using "rAra h 8.0101," the cross-reactive Bet v 1 family protein in peanut (*Arachis hypogaea*) as an example, "r" refers to recombinant protein produced in microorganisms such as bacteria as opposed to extraction from an actual natural peanut source. "Ara" are the first three letters of the Latin scientific genus for peanut (*Arachis*). "h" is the first letter of the species name (hypogaea). "8" is the allergen number that indicates the order in which the allergen was first reported. "0.01" is the isoallergen number that indicates that the allergen has >67% amino acid sequence identity with another reported Ara h 8 molecule. The "01" is a variant in which the different sequences of the allergens have >90% sequence identity. The World Health Organization and International Union of Immunological Societies (WHO/IUIS) allergen nomenclature database includes a peer-reviewed listing of the available allergens at "www.allergen.org." It provides a link to nucleotide and protein databases from the National Center for Biotechnology Information, UniProt database, and Protein Databank of macromolecular structures.[7]

There are a number of other databases that classify allergens according to protein families that share a similar amino acid, secondary and tertiary structure. The family of molecules may also share related biological functions.[8] The structural database for allergenic proteins (SDAP, https://fermi.utmb.edu/) provides a listing of allergen sequences, IgE antibody binding sites or epitopes, and models of molecular structures. Of the known protein families ($n = 16,395$) (http://pfam.xfam.org/) based on their amino acid sequences, known allergens have been identified in only 130 families. Among these, the clinically most important allergens can be found in an even smaller number of 30—40 protein families The AllFam database ([9]; http://

www.meduniwien.ac.t/allergens/allfam/) provides a listing of the allergen families. The clinically important allergen families include the profilins, PR10-like allergens, nonspecific lipid transfer proteins, serum albumins, tropomyosins, polcalcins, lipocalins, and parvalbumins. Each allergen family is described in detail elsewhere in separate chapters in the EAACI Molecular Allergology User's Guide.[10] A comprehensive database of allergenic molecule-related information is found in the Allergome website (http://www.allergome.org/). It is nonpeer-reviewed and has accumulated allergen-related facts since the early 1960s. It provides free searches of all allergens that have been reported to date and provides details on the allergenic molecules' variants, structures, allergen sources, and epidemiologic statistics.

Properties of allergens

What properties of a molecule predisposes it to elicit IgE antibody and become an allergen? Is there an inherent primary amino acid sequence, secondary folding of the polypeptide chain, tertiary three-dimensional structure, or quaternary complex consisting of several polypeptide chains that causes it to be recognized as foreign and elicit IgE antibodies? Is there a functional property that is unique to allergens? These fundamental questions are at the basis of continuing research. Several attributes of an allergen have become evident. Allergenic molecules tend to be abundant in nature. They occur sufficiently often in the environment to provide opportunity for exposure through injection or contact with the skin or GI tract. They are generally soluble in water and thus extractable; however, some are lipid soluble. The more structurally stable the molecule, the greater its potential to become a potent allergen that can elicit a severe allergic reaction. Allergens often possess enzymatic activity (e.g., proteases, venoms, and glycosidases), which promotes their ability to penetrate epithelium. They are often lipid binding (lipocalins, lipid transfer proteins), defense-related (PR-10 family, lipid transfer proteins, glycolases), motility/signaling (profilin, tropomyosin), and calcium-regulating proteins (polcalcin, parvalbumin). Although any molecule has the potential to become an allergen, the degree of relatedness to comparable molecules in the human body as determined by their primary amino acid and overall secondary and tertiary structure is possibly the most important property that causes the molecule to elicit an IgE antibody immune response.[11–13]

Rationale for the use of single allergens and allergenic extracts

Although allergenic extracts are assumed to be comprehensive with regard to containing all the relevant allergenic molecules in particular natural source material, there are applications where the use of native and recombinant allergenic molecules can be useful. These are depicted in Fig. 2.1 and examples are provided in Table 2.1. In cases, where particular allergenic molecules are in low abundance following an aqueous

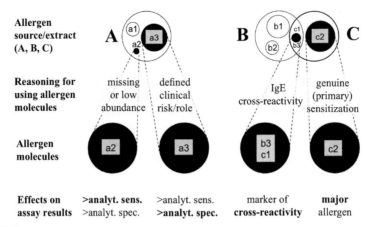

FIGURE 2.1

Rationale for the use of single allergens in contrast with allergen extracts. Specific examples for each application are provided in Table 2.1.

Reproduced with permission from Hamilton RG, Matsson PNJ, Adkinson Jr NF, et al. Analytical Performance Characteristics, Quality Assurance, and Clinical Utility of Immunological Assays for Human Immunoglobulin E Antibodies of Defined Allergen Specificities. ILA20, 3rd ed. Wayne, PA: Clinical and Laboratory Standards Institute; 2017.

extraction or they exhibit weak stability (e.g., Cor a 1—hazelnut extract, Glym4—soy extract; omega-5 gliadin—wheat extract), recombinant or natural allergen has been added to the complex extract mixture to enhance its performance as a diagnostic and therapeutic reagent. The presence of an IgE antibody response to particular allergenic molecules provides information about the potential for a severe allergic reaction following additional allergen exposure (e.g., storage proteins Ara h 1, 2, 3, 6, vs. whole peanut extract; Cor a 9 and 14 vs. hazelnut extract). IgE antibody responses to certain allergens can help clarify a patient's sensitization pattern and provide clear evidence for cross-reactivity to aid in the interpretation of an IgE antibody response (e.g., Bet v 1 homologues in birch pollen allergic individuals with positive peanut (Ara h 8) and or peach (Pru p 1) responses). IgE antibody responses to certain allergenic molecules can identify a genuine (species specific) sensitization (e.g., Cor a 9 and 14 vs. hazelnut extract). These are special in vitro applications of allergenic molecules that are increasingly used clinically to aid in clarifying sensitization patterns obtained with the use of allergen extracts. No single or mixture of allergenic components is currently being used in North America as immunotherapy drugs.

Concluding thoughts

The allergen is the principal biological material that provides specificity both in the diagnosis and immunotherapy treatment of select human allergic diseases. Allergen extracts derived from natural sources that can be used for allergy diagnostic testing

Table 2.1 Utility of allergen molecules as reagents from various allergen sources/extracts (left column), reasons, and improved assay performance (upper row) will vary due to the individual diagnostic question and the specific allergen applied.

Examples (allergen source, allergen carrier)	Increased analytic sensitivity	Increased analytical specificity/ selectivity	Cross-reactive allergens	Species/ family-specific major allergens
Cat		**Fel d 2**	**Fel d 2**	**Fel d 1**
Hazelnut	**Cor a 1** (Bet v 1-homolog)	**Cor a 14** (2S albumine), **Cor a 9** (11S globulin) **Cor a 8** (LTP, mediterranean)		
Kiwi	**Act d 8** (Bet v 1-homolog)		**Act d 8** (Bet v 1-homolog)	
Peach	**Pru p 1** (Bet v 1-homolog)	**Pru p 3** (LTP, marker, mediterranean)	**Pru p 1** (Bet v 1-homolog), **Pru p 4** (profilin)	
Peanut	Ara h 10, Ara h 11 (oleosins)	**Ara h 1** (7S globulin) **Ara h 2** (2S albumin) **Ara h 3** (11S globulin) Ara h 6/7 (2S albumin) **Ara h 9** (LTP, mediterranean)	Ara h 8 (Bet v 1-homolog), Ara h 5[a]	
Soy	**Gly m 4** (Bet v 1-homolog)	**Glym 5** **Gly m 6**		
Wheat	**Tri a 19** (omega-5-gliadin)			
Meat	**Alpha-GAL**	**Alpha-GAL**		
Bee venom	Api m 3, Api m 4, Api m 10	**Api m 1**, Api m 3, Api m 4, Api m 10		**Api m 1**, Api m 3, Api m 4, Api m 10
Wasp venom	**Ves v 5**	**Ves v 1, Ves v 5**		**Ves v 1, Ves v 5**
Birch (hazel, alder, birch pollen) and		**Bet v 1**	**Bet v 2**[a], **Bet v 4**[b]	**Bet v 1**

Continued

Table 2.1 Utility of allergen molecules as reagents from various allergen sources/extracts (left column), reasons, and improved assay performance (upper row) will vary due to the individual diagnostic question and the specific allergen applied.—*cont'd*

Examples (allergen source, allergen carrier)	Increased analytic sensitivity	Increased analytical specificity/ selectivity	Cross-reactive allergens	Species/ family-specific major allergens
beech trees (beech, oak pollen)				
Oleaceae (ash, olive pollen)		**Ole e 1**	Ole e 2[a], Ole e 3[b]	**Ole e 1**
Poaceae (pollen from moderate climate grasses)		**Phl p 1, Phl p 5**	**Phl p 12**[a], **Phl p 7**[b]	**Phl p 1, Phl p 5**
Mugwort pollen		**Art v 1**	Art v 4[a], Art v 5[b]	**Art v 1**
Ragweed pollen		**Amb a 1**	Amb a 8[a], Amb a 10[b]	**Amb a 1**

Bolded letters indicate availability as reagents mainly non-USA, (e.g., Europe, Japan); regular letters: not (yet) available as reagents.
[a] *Profilin (pan-allergen in pollen and plant foods).*
[b] *Procalcin (pan-allergen in pollen, see Table 7 for definitions).*
Reproduced with permission from Hamilton RG, Matsson PNJ, Adkinson NF Jr, et al. Analytical Performance Characteristics, Quality Assurance, and Clinical Utility of Immunological Assays for Human Immunoglobulin E Antibodies of Defined Allergen Specificities. ILA20, 3rd ed. Wayne, PA: Clinical and Laboratory Standards Institute; 2017.

(both in vitro and in vivo, which will help guide allergist/immunologist determine the best treatment approach for optimal patient care. Single (e.g., rBet v 1 for immunotherapy of birch pollen allergic individuals) or cocktails of recombinant allergen vaccines or engineered hypoallergenic molecules are a future application of technology but their use is dependent on licensing and the required clinical validation studies. Thus, they remain a distant goal for use in immunotherapy. It still needs to be demonstrated that single allergenic molecules or cocktails of recombinant allergens can effectively modulate the symptoms in cases where complex allergen extracts have been successfully used. Judicious application of allergenic molecules will continue in the diagnostic work-up of allergic patients, especially for food allergies (e.g., peanut and hazelnut). They provide information related to potential cross-reactions, risk of severe reactions, potential reduction or elimination of food challenges, and the presence of a genuine sensitization. Above all, the clinical relevance of allergic sensitization as determined by the presence of allergen-specific IgE, independent of method (skin test/serology) or diagnostic allergen source (extracts or molecules), can only be determined by the physician based on the individual's clinical history and not by the test alone.[14] IgE antibody is necessary but not sufficient for accurate diagnosis of allergic disease without a clear positive clinical history of symptoms following an allergen exposure.

References

1. https://en.wikipedia.og/wiki/allergen.
2. MacGlashan D. IgE receptor and signal transduction in mast cells and basophils. *Curr Opin Immunol*. 2008;20:717−723.
3. Bonertz A, Roberts G, Slater JE, Bridgewater J, Rabin RL, et al. Allergen manufacturing and quality aspects for allergen immunotherapy in Europe and the United States: an analysis from the EAACI AIT Guidelines Project. *Allergy*. 2018;73:816−826.
4. European Medicines Agency Evaluation of Medicines Guideline on The Clinical Development Of Products For Specific Immunotherapy For The Treatment Of Allergic Diseases. http://www.ema.europa.eu/docs/en_GB/document_library/Scientific_guideline/2009/09/WC500003605.pdf. In: 20 November 2008 ed. London2008. Accessed 06/03/2009.
5. Marsh DG, Goodfriend L, King TP, Lowenstein H, Platts-mills TA. Allergen nomenclature. *Bull World Health Org*. 1986;64:767−774.
6. Radauer C, Nandy A, Ferreria F, Goodman RE, Larsen JN, Lidholm J, et al. Update of the WHO/IUIS Allergen Nomenclature Database based on analysis of allergen sequences. *Allergy*. 2014;69:413−419.
7. Radauer C, Bublin M, Wagner S, Mari A, Breiteneder H. Allergens are distributed into few protein families and possess a restricted number of biochemical functions. *J Allergy Clin Immunol*. 2008;121:847−852.
8. Breitneder H. Allergen families and databases. In: *EAACI Molecular Allergology User's Guide*Pediatric Allergy Immunol. Vol. 27. 2016:39−44.
9. Kleine-Tebbe J, Ollert M, Radauer C, Jakob T. Introduction to Molecular Allergology: protein families, databases and potential benefits. In: Kleine-Tebbe J, Jakob T, eds. *Molecular Allergy Diagnostics*. Cham Switzerland: Springer; 2015 (Chapter 1).
10. Matricardi PM, Kleine-Tebbe J, Hoffmann HJ, Valenta R, Hilger C, et al. EAACI molecular allergology user's guide. *Pediatric Allergy Immunol*. 2016;27:1−250.
11. Bonertz A, Roberts G, Slater JE, Bridgewater J, Rabin RL, Hoefnagel M. Allergen manufacturing and quality aspects for allergen immunotherapy in Europe and the United States: an analysis from the EAACI AIT Guidelines Project. *Allergy*. April 2018;73(4):816−826.
12. Jenkins JA, Breiteneder H, Mills EN. Evolutionary distance from human homologues reflects allergenicity of animal food proteins. *J Allergy Clin Immunol*. 2007;120:1399−1405.
13. Aalberse RC. Structural features of allergenic molecules. *Chem Immunol Allergy*. 2006;91:134−146.
14. Cox L, Williams B, Sicherer S, et al. Pearls and pitfalls of allergy diagnostic testing: report from the American College of Allergy, Asthma and Immunology/American Academy of Allergy, Asthma and Immunology specific IgE test task force. *Ann Allergy Asthma Immunol*. 2008;101(6):580−592.
15. Hamilton RG, Matsson PNJ, Adkinson Jr NF, et al. *Analytical Performance Characteristics, Quality Assurance, and Clinical Utility of Immunological Assays for Human Immunoglobulin E Antibodies of Defined Allergen Specificities*. ILA20. 3rd ed. Wayne, PA: Clinical and Laboratory Standards Institute; 2017.

Allergen standardization and manufacturing

3

Robert E. Esch, PhD

Faculty, Biology, School of Natural Sciences, Lenoir-Rhyne University, Hickory, NC, United States

Introduction

There are currently four licensed companies that manufacture and market allergen extracts in the United States for diagnostic and therapeutic use (see Table 3.1). Together, they manufacture hundreds of substances derived from a variety of allergen sources including pollens, fungi, epithelia, insects, and foods. Before the 1970s, allergenic products were the only FDA-regulated products that were not required to be standardized. This was partly because it was a practice for allergists to manufacture their own diagnostic and therapeutic extracts utilizing source materials provided by regional suppliers. In addition, there were provisions in the Federal regulations (21 CFR 680.3.e.) allowing use of nonstandardized extracts with potency designations such as weight per volume (w/v) and protein nitrogen units (PNU) that did not convey information about the extract's potency or composition. However, if a specific potency test for the product was available, the regulatory authorities required the extract manufacturers to utilize it.[1,2]

During the past 30 years, through the collaboration of licensed manufacturers, CBER, and academicians, 19 allergenic extracts have been standardized (see Table 3.2).

Classification and manufacture of allergen extracts in the United States

Allergen source materials

The hundreds of different allergen source materials from which extracts are made can be grouped into a limited number of product classes: pollens, fungi, mites and insects (including hymenopteran venoms), animal epithelia, and foods.[3,4] The physical and biological characteristics of the source material allow manufacturers to employ related processing equipment and controls in the extract manufacturing process.

Table 3.1 U.S. Licensed allergenic products manufacturers.

Manufacturer	City, State
ALK/Center Laboratories	Round Rock, TX
Allermed	San Diego, CA
Stallergenes-Greer	Lenoir, NC
Hollister-Stier	Spokane, WA

Table 3.2 Standardized allergenic products licensed in the United States.

Standardized allergenic extracts	Potency units	Analyte(s)/Test method
Hymenoptera venoms		
Honey bee (*Apis mellifera*) Yellow hornet (*Dolichovespula arenaria* White-faced hornet (*Dolichovespula maculata*) Paper wasp (*Polistes* spp.) Yellow jacket (*Vespula* spp.) Mixed vespid (*Vespula* + *Dolichovespula*)	μg protein/mL	Total protein/Lowry method Hyaluronidase/enzyme assay Phospholipase A,B/enzyme assay
House-dust mites		
Dermatophagoides farina *Dermatophagoides pteronyssinus*	AU/mL = BAU/mL	Multiple allergens/IgE-ELISA inhibition
Cat extracts		
Cat hair (*Felis catus (domesticus)*) Cat pelt (*Felis catus (domesticus)*)	BAU/mL	Fel d 1/Radial immunodiffusion
Short ragweed pollen		
Short ragweed (*Ambrosia artemisiifolia*)	W/V AU/mL	Amb a 1/Radial immunodiffusion Multiple allergens/IgE-ELISA inhibition
Grass pollens		
Bermuda grass (*Cynodon dactylon*) Redtop grass (*Agrostis gigantea (alba)*) June (Kentucky blue) grass (*Poa pratensis*) Orchard grass (*Dactylis glomerata*) Perennial ryegrass (*Lolium perenne*) Timothy grass (*Phleum pretense*) Meadow fescue (*Festuca pratensis (elatior)*) Sweet vernal grass (*Anthoxanthum odoratum*)	BAU/mL	Multiple allergens/IgE-ELISA inhibition

Pollens

Pollens are the most common allergenic extract used for allergy diagnostic testing and immunotherapy.[3] Pollen extracts derived from more than 300 plant species are manufactured in the United States. Some common pollens from grasses, trees, and "weeds" that cause allergy in humans are listed in Table 3.3. Pollen source materials are collected in the field by vacuum collection, in a greenhouse by water setting, or the flower heads may be cut, dried, ground, and sieved in the laboratory.[4,5] Vacuum collection is performed in fields with pure stands during pollination. Water setting involves transporting plant stems and flowers to a greenhouse shortly before pollination, setting them in water and allowing the plants to pollinate over days onto paper surrounding the plants. After the pollen has been shed, they are collected by vacuum. In cut-dried-ground-and-sieved pollen, mature flowering heads of the plant are collected just before pollination, and dried and ground to release the pollen. The pollen is separated from other plant parts by passing them through sieves of varying mesh sizes. The procedure used depends on the factors such as accessibility to the plants, presence of other pollinating plants, and weather. Contamination by plant parts is usually limited to <1% except for pollen collected using the cut-dried-ground-and-sieve method can contain 5%−10% plant parts.

Fungi

More than 200 fungal allergen extracts are produced by US-licensed manufacturers and each manufacturer employs different techniques for cultivating, harvesting, and processing fungi.[4,6] Common allergenic fungi are listed in Table 3.4. Fungal source materials must be derived from well-defined, pure seed cultures. The seed cultures derived from a specific strain are grown on defined growth medium and used to inoculate larger batch cultures. Strains that produce mycotoxins need to be avoided unless their removal can be validated through processing. Media free of animal-derived material or allergen-free components are preferable. If animal-derived material is used, documentation that they were from herds free of transmissible spongiform encephalopathies is needed. It is common for manufacturers to use culture media and conditions for growth (temperature, pH, cultivation time, photoperiod, and aeration) to maximize the production of spores and vegetative growth at harvest time. The fungus is inactivated, usually with phenol, before harvesting to ensure the safety of manufacturing personnel and to prevent contamination of the manufacturing environment. Fungal cells, mycelia, and spores are separated from the culture using sieving, filtration, centrifugation, or a combination of these methods. The spent medium containing secreted allergens can also be harvested and processed. The recovered cellular and/or extracellular fractions are further processed to produce a final, dried product that is suitable for subsequent extraction. A variety of techniques can be used including homogenization, ultrafiltration, dialysis, acetone treatment, freeze-drying, and milling.

Table 3.3 Examples of common allergenic pollens: representative genera are members of the same botanical family or subfamily from which pollen are used to prepare licensed allergen extracts for diagnosis and immunotherapy. Manufacturers may offer extracts derived from one or more species of each listed genus.

	Taxonomic group	Representative genera
Grass pollens	*Pooideae*	*Poa* (bluegrass), *Bromus* (brome), *Dactylis* (orchard), *Festuca* (fescue), *Lolium* (perennial rye), *Agrostis* (redtop), *Anthoxanthum* (vernal), *Avena* (cultivated oat), *Holcus* (velvet), *Phalaris* (canary), *Phleum* (timothy), *Agropyron* (quack), *Elymus* (wild rye), *Secale* (cultivated rye), *Triticum* (cultivated wheat).
	Chloridoideae	*Cynodon* (Bermuda), *Bouteloua* (grama), *Distichlis* (salt).
	Panicoideae	*Paspalum* (Bahia), *Sorghum* (Johnson), *Panicum* (Para), *Zea* (corn),
Tree pollens	Aceraceae	*Acer* (maples and box elder)
	Betulaceae	*Alnus* (alder), *Betula* (birches), *Corylus* (hazelnut)
	Cupressaceae	*Cupressus* (cypress), *Juniperus* (junipers and cedars), *Taxodium* (bald cypress)
	Fabaceae	*Acacia* (mimosa), *Robinia* (locust) *Prosopis* (mesquite)
	Fagaceae	*Quercus* (oaks), *Fagus* (beech)
	Hamamelidaceae	*Liquidambar* (sweet gum)
	Juglandaceae	*Carya* (hickory and pecan), *Juglans* (walnut)
	Moraceae	*Morus* (mulberry), *Broussonetia* (paper mulberry)
	Myricaceae	*Myrica* (bayberry)
	Oleaceae	*Olea* (olive), *Fraxinus* (ash), *Ligustrum* (privet)
	Pinaceae	*Pinus* (pines)
	Platanaceae	*Platanus* (sycamore)
	Salicaceae	*Populus* (cottonwood and poplars), *Salix* (willows)
	Ulmaceae	*Ulmus* (elms) *Celtis* (hackberry)
"Weed" pollens	Chenopodiaceae	*Atriplex* (scales and saltbush), *Chenopodium* (lamb's quarter), *Salsola* (Russian thistle), *Kochia* (firebush), *Allenrolfea* (iodine bush).
	Asteraceae: *Artemisia*	*Artemisia* (mugworts, wormwood, and sages)
	Asteraceae: *Ambrosia*	*Ambrosia* (ragweeds), *Xanthium* (cocklebur), *Iva* (poverty weed and marsh elders), *Baccharis* (groundsel tree)
	Amaranthaceae	*Amaranthus* (careless weed and pigweeds)
	Plantaginaceae	*Plantago* (plantain)
	Polygonaceae	*Rumex* (dock and sorrel)
	Urticaceae	*Urtica* (nettle), *Parietaria* (pellitory)

Table 3.4 Examples of common allergenic fungi: representative genera are members of the same botanical class or order from which fungal source materials (cells, mycelium and spores) are used to prepare licensed allergen extracts for diagnosis and immunotherapy. Manufacturers may offer extracts derived from one or more species of each listed genus.

	Taxonomic group	Representative genera
Zygomycetes	Mucorales	Mucor, Rhizopus
Ascomycetes	Saccharomycetes	Candida, Saccharomyces, Geotrichum
	Dothideomycetes	Cladosporium, Alternaria, Curvularia, Dreschslera, Bipolaris, Helminthosporium, Stemphylium, Ulocladium, Epicoccum, Phoma, Aureobasidium
	Eurotiomycetes	Aspergillus, Penicillium, Paecilomyces, Trichophyton, Epidermophyton,
	Sordariomycetes	Fusarium, Trichoderma, Acremonium, Trichothecium, Neurospora, Chaetomium, Nigrospora, Trichoderma, Acremonium
	Leotiomycetes	Botrytis
Basidiomycetes	Microbotryomycetes	Rhodotorula
	Ustilagomycetes	Ustilago
	Malassesziomycetes	Malassezia

Mites and insects

Several mite species are responsible for allergic reactions in sensitized patients (see Table 3.5). The house-dust mites belonging to genus *Dermatophagoides* are the most important worldwide. In tropical and subtropical regions, *Blomia* can reach densities equal to that of *Dermatophagoides*. Storage mites, which belong to a wide range of taxonomic groups, are found in stored grains, barn dust, and hay. Mites source materials used for allergen extracts are derived from pure laboratory cultures using defined growth media preferably free of animal-derived material and allergen-free.[7] In the United States, mite bodies are separated from the culture to >99% purity. This is accomplished in a variety of ways including sieving; air classifiers, which separate materials according to their size and density; or the heat-escape method, which collects living mites escaping from cultures exposed to low heat. Alternatively, whole spent cultures containing mite bodies, eggs, larvae, fecal particles, and residual culture media have been shown to be suitable source materials for mite extracts and are routinely used in some countries (primarily in Europe). This approach requires the use of culture media free of potential contaminating allergens.[7a]

Table 3.5 Examples of common allergenic mites and insects: representative genera are members of the same insect order from which source materials (venom or whole bodies) are used to prepare licensed allergen extracts for diagnosis and immunotherapy. Manufacturers may offer extracts derived from one or more species of each listed genus.

	Taxonomic group	Representative genera
Mites	Pyroglyphidae	Dermatophagoides, Euroglyphus (house-dust mites)
	Glycyphagidae	Lepidoglyphus, Blomia (storage mites)
	Acaridae	Acarus, Tyrophagus (grain mites)
Insects	Hymenoptera	Apis (honeybee), Vespula (yellow jackets), Dolichovespula (hornets), Polistes (paper wasps), Bombus (bumblebees), Solenopsis (fire ants), Pogonomyrmex (harvester ants)
	Diptera	Culex, Aedes, Anopheles (mosquitoes), Chrysops (deer flies), Tabanus (horse flies), Culicoides (biting midges), Musca (house fly), Chironomus (midge)
	Hemiptera	Triatoma ("kissing" bugs)
	Blattodea	Blattella, Blatta, Periplaneta (cockroaches)
	Siphonaptera	Ctenocephaledes (fleas)
	Coleoptera	Harmonia (Asian ladybeetle)
	Ephemeroptera	Ephemerella, Drunella, etc. (mayflies)
	Trichoptera	Phylocentropus, Agapetus, etc. Various (caddisflies)

Insects and their venoms

Several species of stinging hymenopterans and their venom proteins are responsible for causing anaphylaxis in sensitized individuals (see Table 3.5). The venoms derived from the honey bee (*Apis mellifera*), paper wasps (*Polistes* spp.), yellow jackets (*Vespula* spp.), and hornets (*Dolichovespula* spp.) are used to manufacture standardized extracts for diagnosis and treatment. Hymenoptera immunotherapy is the only form or immunotherapy that can be "curative," that is, induce long-lasting, if not, permanent immune tolerance. Fire ants (*Solenopsis* spp.) and other stinging ants, for example, *Pogonomyrmex* can be important in certain geographical regions of the United States. Honey bee venom is collected by electrical stimulation by a method developed for commercial scale by Benton et al.[8] The apparatus with an electrical grid covered by a membrane is placed near a hive and when the bee lands on the grid, they expel their venom on the membrane surface. They also release attack pheromones that attract additional bees. The venom is dried and recovered essentially in pure form. Yellow jacket and wasp venom are derived from venom sacs dissected from female insects.[9] Active nests that have not been treated with pesticides or chemicals are collected in bags and the insects kept alive until frozen.

The insects can be anesthetized by refrigeration or carbon dioxide before freezing. On the day of processing, the insects are thawed, females sorted, and venom sacs dissected. The venom sacs are placed in chilled extraction buffer until a specified number of venom sacs per mL of buffer is reached. The venom is recovered from the sacs by sonication or homogenizing followed by clarification (centrifugation and filtration). Yellow jacket (*Vespula* spp.) and Paper Wasp (*Polistes* spp.) venom products may specify the inclusion of multiple species, that is, *V. squamosa, V. vulgaris, V. germanica, V. maculifrons, V. pensylvanica*, and *V. flavopilosa*; or *P.annularis, P. apaches, P. exclamans, P. fuscatus*, and *P. metricus*, respectively. The source material is lyophilized (freeze-dried) and stored frozen until further processing. Honey bee, wasp, and vespid venom extracts are prepared by reconstituting the dried venom source materials in an aqueous buffer to a specified protein concentration. Each species is reconstituted individually and mixed according to product specifications.[10]

Among the thousands of species of ants recognized worldwide, only members of the genera *Solenopsis* (fire ants) and *Pogomyrmex* (harvester ants) are known to cause anaphylaxis. In contrast to bee, wasp, yellow jacket, and hornet whole body extracts, fire ant and harvester ant whole body extracts contain clinically significant amounts of venom allergens.[11,12] Fire ants can be collected from active nests by transferring ant mound soil into buckets, coated with talcum powder, which prevents ants from escaping.[13] The bucket is sealed, sealed and frozen until the ants can be sorted. Alternatively, water can be dripped into the ant colony that induces the ants to carry brood out of the nest and float *en masse* on the water's surface. The ants are scooped into buckets or bags, sealed, and transferred to the laboratory. Once the insects are separated from the soil and other extraneous matter, they are washed, dried, and frozen until extracted. To obtain venom, live ants must be separated from the colony and induced to expel their venom using electric shock. The venom is collected, dried, and stored frozen until reconstituted and processed further. Fire ant venom has been produced experimentally and is not yet commercially available. Nonstandardized, whole body extracts are used for allergy diagnosis and immunotherapy. The venom content of whole-body extracts is highly variable and is about 10 times less potent than the venom, thus the effective dose for immunotherapy has not been clearly established. Availability of fire ant extracts composed of pure venom would significant improve the safety and efficacy of fire ant immunotherapy for individuals who have experienced fire-ant anaphylaxis.

Insects belonging to orders *Diptera* (the flies, mosquitoes, and midges), *Siphonaptera* (the fleas), *Hemiptera* (the true bugs), and *Trichoptera* (the caddisflies) have been described. For biting insects, the saliva may contain allergenic proteins and methods to harvest saliva and salivary glands have been developed.[14] Dissection of salivary glands requires highly trained technicians because the glands are difficult to locate and once located, they are easily ruptured and lost during the operation. Direct collection of insect saliva requires living insects that have been reared in controlled environments without having a blood meal. Saliva from mosquitoes can be collected by confining living female adults in a plexiglass box by placing petroleum jelly on their wings and legs. The proboscis of each mosquito is inserted into a capillary tube filled with distilled water and salivation is induced by applying malathion-acetone solution to the mosquito's thorax. The saliva from the capillary tubes are pooled, lyophilized, and stored frozen until reconstituted. Insect saliva tends to contain a variety of active enzymes and pharmacologically active substances like prostaglandins that must be removed or inactivated before in vivo use. No commercial insect salivary extracts are currently available, and there is limited data (only case reports) that immunotherapy is effective for these insects.

Insects can also cause inhalational allergies. Cockroach (*Blattella germanica* and *Periplaneta americana*) allergens can be a major cause of asthma symptoms in the inner cities of the United States. Cockroaches are raised in controlled environments under conditions that promote reproduction and growth. The insects are killed by freezing and the bodies, fecal pellets, egg cases, and the exuviae (shed skins) can be separated by sieving from the culture media. Most source materials used for extract manufacture utilize the whole bodies because fecal pellets can contain allergens derived from the culture media used to feed the insects. Unfortunately, the extracts are relatively low in potency and the recommended dose is "highest tolerated."[1] Other allergenic insects such as the Asian lady beetle (*Harmonia axyridis*) can be collected during the fall and winter months, as they are drawn to shelters and abandoned homes to seek warmth or "hibernate." The insects are collected into bags and frozen. The collected insects are stored frozen until processed further. Lady beetles can survive being frozen for at least a year, so processing must be initiated quickly before they completely thaw and escape. A defatted dried powder, suitable for extraction, is produced by processing in acetone and drying. Alternatively, the frozen insects can be directly extracted by homogenization in extraction fluid. Due to the high enzymatic activity of cockroach extracts, extraction must be carried out under refrigeration and with extraction fluids containing 50% glycerin to reduce proteolysis. Only glycerinated extracts should be used due to the instability of aqueous formulations.

Animal epithelia

Animal epithelia (dander, hair, and skin) from common pets, farm animals, and rodents are important sources of allergens found both in homes and the workplace (see Table 3.6). An important aspect of handling source materials derived from these sources is to avoid the presence of infectious agents and other contaminants such as external parasites.[4,15] Epithelial materials must be collected from healthy animals free of infectious agents and ectoparasites (ticks, mites, and fleas). Epithelia collected from cows, sheep, goats, or other ungulates need to be from herds free of transmissible spongiform encephalopathies. Differences in allergenic profiles of extracts prepared from epithelial source materials can depend on which fraction(s) are included.[15,16] In the United States, two types of standardized cat extracts are available: cat pelt and cat hair extract. Cat pelt extracts are produced from the full-thickness skin, whereas cat hair is derived from the hair shaved from the skin. Both extracts are standardized based on the major allergen content, Fel d 1, but

Table 3.6 Examples of common allergenic animal epithelia: representative genera are members of the same arthropod order or family from which source materials (venom or whole bodies) are used to prepare licensed allergen extracts for diagnosis and immunotherapy. Manufacturers may offer extracts derived from one or more species of each listed genus.

	Taxonomic group[1]	Representative genera
Mammals	Equidae	*Equus* (horse)
	Bovidae	*Bos* (cow), *Ovis* (sheep), *Capra* (goat)
	Suidae	*Sus* (hog)
	Carnivora	*Felis* (cat), *Canis* (dog)
	Rodentia	*Mus (*mouse), *Rattus* (rat), *Meriones* (gerbil), *Mesocricetus* (hamster), Cavia (Guinea pig)
	Lagomorpha	*Oryctolagus* (rabbit)
Birds	*Galliformes*	*Gallus* (chicken), *Meleagris (*turkey)
	Psittaciformes	*Melopsittacus* (parakeet)
	Anseriformes	*Anas* (duck)
	Passeriformes	*Serinus* (canary)

they differ significantly in their Fel d 3 (cat albumin) content. Fel d 3 may not be a major allergen but is important in some patients. Thus, compositional and qualitative differences can arise from subtle differences between source materials used for extract manufacture. These differences are exemplified by the terms used in the literature to describe skin-derived source materials: pelt, hair, epithelia, dander, dandruff, skin scrapings, cat washes, wool fur, and hides. Another important consideration is the presence of urine and saliva. Both can be important sources of animal allergens and can be found associated with and in varying amounts on hair. Thus, the importance of well-defined, detailed protocols for collecting and processing animal-derived source materials cannot be overemphasized. Finally, these source materials may require additional processing such as defatting to remove lipids, drying and milling to prepare source materials suitable for extraction. Similar differences have been found with dog extract, with one product have adequate amount of one of the major dog allergens (Can f 1) but no detectable Can f 4, which has been identified as a significant allergen in some dog allergic patients.[1–3]

Foods

Source materials derived from foods are obtained fresh from grocery vendors or directly from farmers.[4,17] This helps to ensure that the source material is unadulterated and allows visual confirmation of identity. This is particularly important with fish, which may be mislabeled by some vendors who frequently only use common names to identify their identity. Produce that have been sprayed with pesticides or other chemicals should be avoided unless processes to remove them are implemented and validated. Canned and processed foods should not be used as source materials for food extracts. As with other allergen source materials that tend to degrade or spoil, food source materials are processed, defatted, dried, and milled to prepare a product suitable for extraction later. The processing steps used will vary depending on the food, for example, dairy products, eggs, seeds, nuts, grains, fruits, crustaceans, or meats. Other decisions that must be made include whether to include the skin or seeds; whether the food is cooked or uncooked; and whether the food is intended or use in oral food challenges. Food extracts are primarily distributed for diagnostic use only and are available almost exclusively in glycerinated form.

Allergen extracts

Allergen extracts are marketed in glycerinated, aqueous, alum-precipitated, or lyophilized formulations to practicing allergists.[3] These products, called as manufacturer's stock concentrates, are either standardized or nonstandardized. Standardized products must be tested for safety, sterility, potency and identity, and stability. Standardized allergens are also subject to CBER lot release. Nonstandardized allergens are primarily tested for safety and sterility. Manufacturer's stock concentrates are mixed by practicing allergists to formulate a "name-patient" products, similar to a compound prescription. The treatment set usually includes four or five dilutions sets at varying dilutions. As the compound formulation of prescription sets is considered pharmacy practice it is regulated by individual State Boards of Pharmacy.

The basic concepts of extracting allergens from allergenic source materials into a liquid medium suitable for parenteral use can be quite simple, provided the source materials have been well characterized. The goal is to use an efficient and reproducible process that maintains the quality and potency of the allergens being extracted from the source material. Extraction procedures using slightly alkaline buffers such as bicarbonate buffer pH 8.4 (Coca's extraction fluid) are generally preferred for increasing protein and allergen yields. Some source materials may require adjustments in pH to maintain the solubility and stability of allergens. Extraction times and temperatures can be optimized to increase recovery without risking allergen degradation or promoting microbial growth. Additives such as 0.4% phenol or 50% glycerin can be added to suppress microbial growth during extraction.

Once extraction is complete, the extract is separated from the insoluble portion by centrifugation and/or filtration through a series of filters that are compatible with the product. Filter substrates that adsorb minimal amounts of allergenic components and shed negligible amounts of residual chemical or extractables need to be selected. Additional processing such as dialysis, concentration, or purification steps may be included to remove nonallergenic or unwanted substances or to increase specific allergen content and potency.

Allergen extracts used parenterally must be sterile, which is accomplished by filtration through a sterilizing filter with a nominal 0.2 μm pore size and validated according to the US Pharmacopeia. To maintain sterility in multiple-dose vials, they must contain a preservative that is bacteriostatic and fungistatic. Most manufacturers of allergen extracts use 0.2%–0.4% phenol with or without 50% glycerin and their effectiveness must be validated according to compendial tests described in the US Pharmacopeia.

In general, allergen extracts are available in four types: aqueous, glycerinated, lyophilized, or alum precipitated. Aqueous extracts are the easiest to manufacture and probably the most commonly prescribed dosage form. Their advantages include ease of processing because they are less viscous than glycerinated extracts, they are suitable for intradermal skin testing, and they do not cause as much discomfort when injected as compared to glycerinated extracts. Disadvantages are mainly associated with their limited stability. Glycerinated extracts are manufactured by either including glycerin in the extraction fluid or by adding glycerin after preparing an aqueous extract. In either case, the final glycerin concentration of 50% is achieved to maximize their shelf life. Manufacturers' stock concentrates containing 50% glycerin have shelf lives of up to 36–48 months while aqueous extracts are limited to 12–18 months or less.[1] The longer expiration dating, and the stabilizing effect of glycerin makes glycerinated extracts probably the most desirable type for the allergist. The disadvantage is the patient discomfort it causes at the injection site. Lyophilized extracts are manufactured by extracting source materials in a suitable aqueous buffer, frozen and removing the water from the extract through sublimation under vacuum. The major advantage of lyophilized extracts is their enhanced shelf life while stored in the freeze-dried state. The stability and expiry date depend on the concentration, diluent and medium used to reconstitute the product. The disadvantages include the manufacturing cost and the added handling required in reconstituting the product before use. Today, only the hymenopteran venom extracts are available as lyophilized extracts. Alum-precipitated extracts are manufactured by adding aluminum-potassium sulfate (Alum) to an aqueous extract. The allergens are adsorbed to the Alum matrix at neutral pH, nonadsorbed substances are removed by centrifugation, and the final precipitate is resuspended in an aqueous buffer. The product is used exclusively for immunotherapy and not for diagnostic use. It is widely available in Europe, but only used sparingly in the United States.

The sterile manufacturer's stock concentrates are tested for sterility, toxicity (safety testing in guinea pigs and mice), pH, preservatives (phenol and/or glycerin), and released according to the manufacturer's licenses. Potency is tested only for US standardized extracts, and nonstandardized extracts are labeled according to the "weight-by-volume" (W/V) ratio used for extraction or the PNU of the final extract.

Standardization of allergen extracts in the United States

It has long been accepted that the safe and effective use of allergen immunotherapy is dependent upon a successful allergen standardization program.[3,18,19] Standardization refers to the criteria and methods used to select a standard or reference allergen product use to establish equivalence with manufactured lots before distribution. The approaches that have been proposed, however, have been varied and at times controversial. For example, in the United States, allergen standardization is based on the establishment of a US standard of potency for each product applicable to products manufactured by all companies. In contrast, European regulators allow for the establishment of in-house references and standards that are specific to each manufacturer. Both approaches are employed to minimize the variation in allergen content and potency between manufactured lots. The US system, it can be claimed, goes one step further to minimize the risk of adverse reactions when switching from one manufacturer's product to another's by using a single, national potency standard and the use of bioequivalent doses of standardized allergen vaccines.[20]

ID$_{50}$EAL method of standardization

The method used for assigning potency units to reference preparations in the United States is named the ID$_{50}$EAL method (Intradermal Dilution for 50 mm sum of Erythema diameters determines bioequivalent ALlergy units). For this method,[18,21] at least 15 highly sensitive adult subjects with a history of allergic disease related to exposure to the allergen of interest are initially selected. Skin testing is performed by technicians with demonstrated proficiency, precision, and accuracy of administering intradermal skin tests. Quantitative intradermal skin tests are performed using 0.05 mL of threefold serial dilutions of the prospective reference extract and the dose and the sum of erythema diameters (longest plus midpoint orthogonal diameters) as the response. The dose-response line is generated using four serial threefold dilutions with graded erythema responses (ΣE) which bracket ΣE = 50 mm and includes the endpoint where ΣE = 0. The best-fit regression lines for each subject is calculated using formula $Y = I + mX$, where Y is the sum of erythema diameters (ΣE) at each dose, I is the y-intercept, m is the slope, and X is the logarithm to the base 3 of dose. If the best-fit line yields a high correlation coefficient ($r > 0.90$) and slope ($m \geq 13$), then the subject sensitivity (D_{50}) is calculated using the formula, $D_{50} = (50\text{-}I)/m$. The mean D_{50} and standard deviation (SD) of the mean is calculated and if the SD is within acceptable limits, then the bioequivalent allergy units (BAU/mL) of the prospective reference is calculated using the formula, BAU/mL $= 3^{-(14 - \text{Mean D})}_{50} \bullet 100,000$ (see Fig. 3.1). When a large number of standardized and nonstandardized allergen concentrates (1:10 and 1:20 w/v prick test products in 50% glycerin) were evaluated using this method, most of them fell between 10,000 and 100,000 BAU/mL. Grass and weed pollen extracts were frequently at the higher potency range as compared to tree pollen, animal, and fungal extracts. Once BAUs are assigned to a prospective reference, the relative potencies and BAUs of other products with respect to the reference can be determined either by a relative potency assay based on parallel-line skin test assay or a validated in vitro potency assay acceptable to CBER.[3,18] Because the performance of bioassays in human subjects for lot-release purposes is cumbersome, expensive and can be highly variable, validated in vitro potency assays have been developed for this purpose. Table 3.3 lists in vitro potency tests used for lot release of standardized products in the United States. For those allergen products for which a major allergenic component has

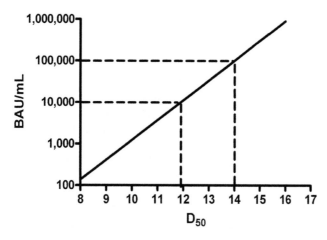

FIGURE 3.1

Relationship between bioequivalent allergy units (BAU) and the mean D_{50} obtained using the $ID_{50}EAL$ method.

been identified and shown to be predictive of relative potency by bioassay, the mass unit content of these major allergens is the basis for standardization. The FDA has accepted the measurement of Amb a 1 and Fel d 1 content for short ragweed pollen and cat extracts, respectively, as potency assays. For products containing multiple major allergens and in cases when a single allergenic component has not been shown to be predictive on in vivo relative potency, the IgE-ELISA inhibition assay using appropriate reference extracts and serum pools has been validated. All manufacturers performing these tests in their laboratories use the same reference reagents standards, and assay methodology because the in vitro assay performance characteristics may vary depending on the reagents used.[16,22] The Laboratory of Immunochemistry at CBER provides such references and standards to the licensed manufacturers and monitors each assay's performance characteristics and manufacturers' results to ensure the consistency and accuracy of the assays.

Standardized hymenoptera venom extracts
Hymenoptera venom extracts, standardized in the 1970s, were the first standardized allergen products licensed in the United States. Two major allergenic proteins identified in the venoms, phospholipase and hyaluronidase, possess enzymatic activity and this became part of the potency testing.[9] The manufacturer's stock lyophilized products are reconstituted to a total protein concentration of 100 µg/mL. For mixed vespid venom containing equal parts of yellow jacket, yellow hornet, and white-faced hornet venoms, the protein concentration is formulated to contain 300 µg/mL total protein. Limits for phospholipase and hyaluronidase enzyme activities are established for lot-release and stability testing. The labeling based on total venom protein content and the availability of lyophilized product has served to ensure a consistent diagnostic and therapeutic product. However, the major vespid

allergen, Ves 5, is not measured, nor are any assays measuring total allergenic activity based on IgE binding is required.

Standardized house-dust mite extracts

The first products to be standardized in the United States using biological potency units were the house-dust mite extract/vaccines (*Dermatophagoides farinae* and *Dermatophagoides pteronyssinus*). The regulatory process was simplified by the fact that there was only a single manufacturer marketing these products for many years. This situation allowed for relatively rapid process for clinical and laboratory evaluation as well as the establishment of a US reference standard. Thus, all subsequent product applications submitted by other manufacturers conformed to the US reference standard and currently marketed house-dust mite products are consistent across the industry. Both the *D. farinae* and *D. pteronyssinus* references are standardized at 10,000 allergy units (AU) per mL and based on lot-release testing using an IgE-ELISA competition assay are marketed at 10,000 AU/mL or 30,000 AU/mL.[23]

Standardized pollen extracts

Short ragweed pollen extracts are labeled based on their Amb a 1 content and the W/V extraction ratio used for their manufacture. Manufacturer's stock concentrates are required to contain at least 130 Units of Amb a 1 per milliliter (1 unit is approximately equal to 1 μg). The radial immunodiffusion (RID) assay currently used for potency testing is based on the diffusion of the antigen from a circular well cut into a gel containing specific antibodies. The precipitin ring of antigen-antibody complexes forms within the gel and grow until equilibrium in reached. The diameters of the rings are a function of antigen concentration. The assay is relatively simple to perform, and consistent results can be obtained between laboratories. The time required to obtain results, especially if repeated tests are needed may take days. The detection limit is about 5 μg/mL which is suitable for measuring specific allergen content in stock concentrates. However, at dilutions greater than about 1: 20 v/v of concentrate or with sample preparations in the nanogram range, more sensitive immunoassays must be used. Efforts are currently being pursued to replace the RID assay with an ELISA to address these limitations.

Before their standardization, grass pollen allergenic extracts in the United States were labeled using the "weight by volume" (W/V) or PNU designation. Table 3.6 gives examples of BAU potencies of previously marketed, nonstandardized grass pollen extracts before they were phased out in 1998.[24] The potencies of the manufacturer's stock concentrates varied from species to species. Bermuda grass was the least potent with potencies in the 4000−14,500/mL range; and meadow fescue grass was the most potent with potencies ranging from 169,000 to 666,000 BAU/mL. Based on the FDA standardization approach, the US Bermuda reference was assigned 10,000 BAU/mL and meadow fescue, Kentucky blue/June, orchard, redtop, perennial rye, sweet vernal, and Timothy references at 100,000 BAU/mL. In addition, the maximum marketable strength of standardized grass pollen extracts was

Table 3.7 BAU/mL of previously marketed, nonstandardized grass pollen extracts.

Pollen	1:10 w/v aqueous	1:20 w/v glycerinated
Bermuda	10,740	4000–14,500
Meadow fescue	287,300–666,000	169,200–378,200
June (Kentucky blue)	56,100–145,400	56,100–91,500
Orchard	134,000–139,200	71,200–110,500
Redtop	141,900–425,000	134,600–219,200
Perennial rye	59,100–302,000	52,900–80,400
Sweet vernal	171,900–234,800	63,900–201,200
Timothy	186,300–291,000	63,000–104,800

limited to 100,000 BAU/mL (10,000 BAU/mL for Bermuda). Thus, standardization of grass pollen extracts established consistency previously not found in grass pollen extracts. At the same time, the potency of standardized extracts became generally lower than previously available nonstandardized extracts (see Table 3.7).

The US system of national potency standards works well with allergenic products that are manufactured using qualitatively similar source materials, for example, pollen extracts and insect venoms. Pollen source materials show qualitative and quantitative variations depending on the collection methods used, collection year, and place.[3] Still, these variations in pollen source material quality can be controlled relatively easily. Furthermore, the extraction procedures for pollen allergenic extracts/vaccines are consistent among US manufacturers. Together, these conditions lead to similar products that allow for a single reference extract that is suitable for the different manufacturers' products. Indeed, it is a common practice for CBER/FDA to use commercially produced allergen products for reference standards. In contrast, allergen products with a wide variation in source material quality and processing methods may not be amenable to this standardization approach.

Standardized cat hair and cat pelt extracts

The standardization of cat epithelia extracts in the United States illustrates how the system can be adjusted to accommodate qualitative differences that may exist between different manufacturers' products. Before biological standardization, products labeled as cat epithelia extracts were derived from hair, dander, pelts, cat washings, or any combination of thereof. Some manufacturers marketed separate cat extracts derived from these different source materials.[15] Cat extracts containing 10 to 19.9 Fel d 1 units/mL were arbitrarily assigned 100,000 AU/mL. Extracts containing 5 to 9.9 Fel d 1 units/mL were arbitrarily assigned 50,000 AU/mL. One important attribute differentiating extracts derived from these various sources is the relative concentrations of the allergens Fel d 1 and cat albumin: products derived from hair, dander, and cat washings possess relatively high Fel d 1: cat albumin ratios while pelt-derived products possess low ratios due to the high concentrations of

Table 3.8 Fel d 1 and cat albumin content of standardized cat extracts.

Manufacturer	Product	Fel d 1	Albumin	Fel d 1: Albumin
A	Cat hair	14.3	11	1.28
B	Cat hair	17.3	84	0.21
C	Cat hair	14.9	122	0.12
D	Cat pelt	15.2	1645	0.009
E	Cat pelt	16.3	5657	0.002

cat albumin (see Table 3.8). To accommodate both types of products, two national reference standards were created based on these compositional differences. All standardized cat extracts are now designated as cat pelt or cat hair extract based on isoelectric focusing (IEF) patterns or specific cat albumin assay showing the presence of non-Fel d 1 components. Subsequently, the $ID_{50}EAL$ method was adopted for the assignment of allergy units to standardized allergenic extracts and vaccines in the United States. Based on this method, it was determined that cat extracts containing 10 to 19.9 Fel d 1 units/mL should be assigned 10,000 AU/mL instead of the current 100,000 AU/mL. To avoid confusion about the change in allergy unit labeling and with the recommendation of APAC, the allergy unit nomenclature was changed to BAU/mL. Thus, in 1992, cat extracts were designated as either cat hair or cat pelt based on the presence of non-Fel d 1 allergens (esp. albumin), and standardized based on their Fel d 1 content, where 10,000 BAU/mL was equivalent to approximately 15 Fel d 1 units/mL.

A standardization algorithm

Clearly, a major objective in allergen product standardization has been to establish US standards of potency using a transparent process where currently marketed nonstandardized allergen products are selected for review and eventual standardization. In 2000, CBER/FDA proposed the allergen standardization algorithm to expedite this process[25] (see Fig. 3.2). In the preliminary phase, an allergen product is selected based on impact criteria that include (a) the availability of stable, preferably lyophilized material for use as long-term reference extract, (b) consistency or inconsistency of currently marketed products, (c) widespread use as a diagnostic and/or therapeutic product in the United States, (d) number of manufacturers marketing the product, (e) potential use in immunotherapy, and (f) public health impact of correct diagnosis and/or adequate treatment. These criteria should not be taken as a means to exclude products from standardization, but rather a way to set priorities and target products for consideration. Once an allergen is identified, and, in the first phase, multiple lots of each manufacturer's product are evaluated for consistency, comparability, and antigenic composition using generally accepted methods. These methods may include testing for IgE binding using well-defined patient sera,

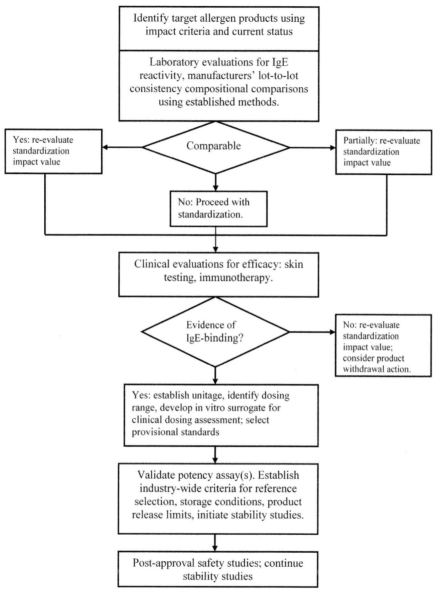

FIGURE 3.2

Standardization algorithm for the standardization of new allergens.

biochemical separation analyses, for example, SDS-PAGE or IEF profiles, and specific allergen measurements using validated assays. After review of the laboratory analyses, a decision is made to proceed to the second or clinical testing phase. Products are tested using the $ID_{50}EAL$ method described previously, and the biological activities of each manufacturer's products are compared. During the first two phases of evaluation, the original impact may be reconsidered or if the marketed products are found to lack allergenic activity, withdrawal of the product from the market may be considered. If a decision is made to proceed with the process, this would be the time to establish potency units and identify an ideal dosing range based on the clinical studies. In vitro tests that correlate with biological activity are identified and provisional standards are selected. In the third (manufacturing) phase, CBER and industry would collaborate to validate the potency tests; establish industry-wide criteria for selecting reference reagents; and define storage conditions and release limits. Stability testing would be initiated to determine shelf life and product expiration dating. Each manufacturer's changes in product specifications, processing methods, labeling, and marketing information would have to be addressed individually using established change control policies. The extent of changes required would depend on the manufacturer's current product quality compared to the newly selected US reference. A reasonable deadline for replacing the obsolete nonstandardized product would be announced to allow for notifying the public and implementing the changes. In the final postapproval phase, stability testing would continue, and safety monitoring will be initiated.

Based on the selection criteria, the first products identified by CBER were cockroach, *Aspergillus fumigatus*, and *Alternaria alternata* allergen extracts/vaccines. Progress has been made with laboratory and clinical testing of cockroach extracts marketed in the United States. CBER found that commercial cockroach extracts were highly variable in total protein, allergen composition, and potency.[26] German cockroach extracts varied in potency from 10 to 783 BAU/mL while American cockroach extracts varied from 10 to 250 BAU/mL. In glycerinated extracts, relative potencies and specific allergen concentrations were significantly correlated. One of the consequences of these findings has been the voluntary removal of aqueous cockroach allergen products from the market based on the low quality of these products. Thus, only the more stable glycerinated cockroach extracts are now available. The availability of standardized cockroach extracts will now depend upon the cooperation of industry to assist CBER in validating and selecting reference standards and reagents. Little to nothing has been accomplished to date with *Aspergillus* and *Alternaria* allergen products. The extreme variability found with fungal products is likely to test the flexibility of the current standardization algorithm and may require compromise on the part of regulators as well as manufacturers.

Conclusions

In summary, the manufacturing of allergenic extracts in the United States strives to incorporate scientific progress made in allergen standardization while ensuring the safe and efficacious use of these products in clinical practice. The US approach to standardization, which aims to provide allergy vaccines labeled in a common potency unit (BAU) was adopted to facilitate the use of common dose regimens and to reduce the uncertainty of safe and effective doses for the large number of products available for clinical use.

Some allergen extracts, particularly those derived from fungal source materials, may require creative solutions to achieve this. The major challenges for the future include how current standardized extracts can be improved as well as the targeting of nonstandardized products for standardization and the implementation of allergen standardization approach in a timely fashion.

References

1. Code of Federal Regulations, Food and Drug Administration Title 21, Vol 7, Part 610.10 General Biological Products Standards: Potency. Revised April 1, 2018.
2. Code of Federal Regulations, Food and Drug Administration Title 21, Vol 7, Part 680.3 Additional Standards for Miscellaneous Products: Tests. Revised April 1, 2018.
3. Slater JE, Esch RE. Preparation and standardization of allergen extracts. In: Adkinson NF, Bochner BS, Burks W, et al., eds. *Allergy: Principles of Practice*. 8th ed. Philadelphia: Mosby; 2014:470−481.
4. Hauck PR, Williamson S. The manufacture of allergenic extracts in North America. *Clin Rev Allergy Immunol*. 2001;21:93−110.
5. Codina R, Lockey RF. Pollen used to produce allergen extracts. *Ann Allergy Asthma Immunol*. 2017;118:148−153.
6. Esch RE, Codina R. Fungal raw materials used to produce allergen extracts. *Ann Allergy Asthma Immunol*. 2017;118:399−405.
7. Carnes J, Iraola V, Cho SH, Esch RE. Mite allergen extracts and clinical practice. *Ann Allergy Asthma Immunol*. 2017;118:249−256.
7a. Weghofer, Margit. Identification of Der P 23, a Peritrophin-Like Protein, as a New Major Dermatophagoides Pteronyssinus Allergen Associated with the Peritrophic Matrix of Mite Fecal Pellets. *The Journal of Immunology*. 2013;190(7):3059−3067.
8. Benton AW, Morse RA, Stewart JD. Venom collection from honeybees. *Science*. 1963; 142:228−230.
9. Plunkett G, Jacobson RS, Golden DBK. Hymenoptera venoms used to produce allergen extracts. *Ann Allergy Asthma Immunol*. 2017;118:649−654.
10. Instructions and Dosage Schedule for Allergen Extracts: Hymenoptera venom products (Honey Bee, Yellow Jacket, Yellow Hornet, White-faced Hornet, Wasp, and Mixed Vespid) VENOMIL®. http://www.hsallergy.com/wp-content/uploads/2018/06/Hymenoptera-Venom-Venomil-5-Mannitol-355205-H04-WEB.pdf.
11. Khurana T, Bridgewater JL, Rabin RL. Allergenic extracts to diagnose and treat sensitivity to insect venoms and inhaled allergens. *Ann Allergy Asthma Immunol*. 2017;118: 531−536.
12. Freeman TM, Hylander R, Ortiz A, Martin ME. Imported fire ant immunotherapy: effectiveness of whole body extracts. *J Allergy Clin Immunol*. 1992;90:210−215.
13. Banks WA, Lofgren CS, Jouvenaz DP, et al. *Techniques for Collecting, Rearing and Handling Imported Fire Ants*. U.S. Dept Agric Tech. AAT-S-21; 1981.
14. Peng Z, Li H, Simons ER. Immunoblot analysis of salivary allergens in 10 mosquito species with worldwide distribution and the human IgE responses to these allergens. *J Allergy Clin Immunol*. 1998;101:498−505.

15. Fernandez-Caldas E, Cases B, El-Qutob D, Cantillo JF. Mammalian raw materials used to produce allergen extracts. *Ann Allergy Asthma Immunol*. 2017;119:1−8.

16. Esch RE. Allergen source materials and quality control of allergenic extracts. *Methods Enzymol*. 1997;13:2−13.

17. David NA, Penumarti A, Burks AW, Slater JA. Food allergen extracts to diagnose food-induced allergic diseases. *Ann Allergy Asthma Immunol*. 2017;119:101−107.

18. Rabin RL, Slater JE. Standardized allergen vaccines in the United States. In Allergens and Allergen Immunotherapy: Subcutaneous, Sublingual and Oral. 5th ed. Lockey RF, Leford DK (eds) CRC Press, Boca Raton, pp.281-287.

19. Larsen JN, Houghton, Vega ML. Manufacturing and standardizing allergen extracts in Europe. In Allergens and Allergen Immunotherapy: Subcutaneous, Sublingual and Oral. 5th ed. Lockey RF, Leford DK (eds) CRC Press, Boca Raton, pp.289-305.

20. Slater JE, Pastor RW. The determination of equivalent doses of standardized allergen vaccines. *J Allergy Clin Immunol*. 2000;105:468−474.

21. Turkeltaub PC. Biological standardization. *Arb Paul Ehrlich Institut*. 1997;91:145−156.

22. Grier TJ. Laboratory methods for allergen extract analysis and quality control. *Clin Rev Allergy Immunol*. 2001;21:111−140.

23. Guidance for Reviewers: Potency limits for standardized dust mite and grass allergen vaccines: A revised protocol. https://www.fda.gov/downloads/BiologicsBloodVaccines/GuidanceComplianceRegulatoryInformation/Guidances/Allergenics/UCM078624.pdf.

24. Greer ® Allergenic Extracts Package Inserts: Standardized Grass Pollen Extracts. https://stagrallergy.com/wp-content/uploads/2017/08/Grass-Pollen-PI.pdf.

25. Slater JE, Pastor RW. Allergenic Products Advisory Committee Meeting. February 10, 2000; https://wayback.archive-it.org/7993/20170404105247/https://www.fda.gov/ohrms/dockets/ac/00/transcripts/3589t1a.pdf.

26. Patterson ML, Slater JE. Characterization and comparison of commercially available German and American cockroach allergen extracts. *Clin Exp Allergy*. 2002;32:721−727.

Further reading

1. Cox L, et al. Allergen immunotherapy: a practice parameter third update. *J Allergy Clin Immunol*. 2011;127(1 Suppl):S1−S55.

2. Grier, 2002.

3. Grier TJ, et al. Stability and mixing compatibility of dog epithelia and dog dander allergens. *Ann Allergy Asthma Immunol*. 2009;103(5):411−417.

Allergic diseases

Atopic dermatitis

Marcella Aquino, MD [1], **Stephanie Lynn Mawhirt, DO** [2], **Luz Fonacier, MD** [3,4,5]

[1]*Hasbro Children's Hospital, Department of Pediatrics, Division of Allergy & Immunology, Associate Professor of Pediatrics, Warren Alpert Medical School of Brown University, 593 Eddy Street, Providence, Rhode Island, United States;* [2]*Professor of Clinical Medicine, NYU Langone Long Island School of Medicine, NYU Winthrop Rheumatology, Allergy & Immunology, Mineola, NY, United States;* [3]*Professor of Medicine, NYU Long Island School of Medicine, Mineola, NY, United States;* [4]*Head of Allergy, Internal Medicine, NYU Langone Health, NYU Winthrop Hospital, Mineola, NY, United States;* [5]*Training Program Director, Allergy and Immunology, NYU Winthrop Hospital, Mineola, NY, United States*

LIST OF ABBREVIATIONS

AD	atopic dermatitis
APT	atopy patch test
CS	corticosteroids
DBPC	double-blinded, placebo-controlled
Der f	*Dermatophagoides farinae*
Der p	*Dermatophagoides pteronyssinus*
DLQI	dermatology life quality index
DM	dust mite
EASI	eczema area and severity index
IGA	Investigator's Global Assessment
IT	immunotherapy
mAb	monoclonal antibody
mg	milligrams
POEM	patient-oriented eczema measure
QoLIAD	Quality of Life Index of Atopic Dermatitis
SCIT	subcutaneous immunotherapy
SCORAD	SCORing Atopic Dermatitis
SLIT	sublingual immunotherapy
TCI	topical calcineurin inhibitor
TCS	topical corticosteroid
VAS	visual analogue scale

Background

Atopic dermatitis (AD) is a skin disease that results from a complex interplay of genetic abnormalities (filaggrin mutation), skin barrier defects, immune dysfunction, exposure, and susceptibility to infectious agents and environmental factors (microbiome, allergens).[1,2] Aeroallergens including dust mite (DM) and pollen can be triggers for AD.[3,4] Current strategies for treatment of DM allergy include allergen avoidance measures (encasing for mattress, pillow, and box spring), maintaining a relative humidity of 35%–50% in the home, use of vacuums with high-efficiency particulate air filtration, and immunotherapy.[5] However, the evidence for these measures as treatment for AD is not strong.[6] Patients are exposed to DM via skin and respiratory tract.[7] Sensitivity to DM is assessed via allergen skin prick testing and/or specific IgE to DM in the blood. The atopy patch test (APT) is another method of evaluation for sensitivity to DM in AD patients[8] although in clinical practice its use is limited due to variability in methods and interpretation among practitioners and until recently commercially available products. It can be considered when there is a high suspicion of aeroallergen-related symptoms or if there is severe and/or persistent AD with unknown triggering factors[9] particularly in adolescent or adult patients.[10] It involves epicutaneous application of aeroallergens on uninvolved atopic skin with readings at day 2 and day 3 or 4. Positive eczematoid reactions have been observed in 30%–50% of patients with AD but are rarely positive in patients with respiratory allergy alone or healthy controls.[11]

Current treatment for AD is focused on emollient therapy, bathing with or without bleach, use of topical corticosteroids (TCSs) and topical calcineurin inhibitors (TCIs), systemic agents (cyclosporine, corticosteroids, methotrexate, mycophenolate mofetil), and phototherapy.[1,12,13] Recently approved therapies include a topical phosphodiesterase (PDE-4) inhibitor[14] and dupilumab (a human monoclonal antibody to the IL-4α receptor inhibiting downstream effects of IL-4 and IL-13).[15] New expert consensus have addressed the changing landscape of treatment for AD and started to incorporate these new treatment modalities.[16,17] The use of immunotherapy for treatment of AD is controversial, as there is a limited body of evidence with conflicting results. Our limited evidence for the use of subcutaneous immunotherapy (SCIT) or sublingual immunotherapy (SLIT) for AD involves mostly studies with DM but a few also involve pollen.

Prospective studies with favorable results of SCIT for AD

A recent observational cohort study in Korea[18] evaluated 251 pediatric and adult patients with AD who were treated with SCIT to DM. Diagnosis of AD was made clinically by Hanifin and Rajka criteria[19] and patients had positive specific IgE to either *Dermatophagoides pteronyssinus (Der p)* and/or *Dermatophagoides farinae (Der f)*.

Treatment outcome was determined by a decrease of the severity scoring of atopic dermatitis (SCORAD) score greater than 50% after 12 months of therapy in comparison to baseline values. Overall, SCIT produced a favorable outcome in most patients (73.6%) but was higher in patients with severe AD (90.6%) as opposed to mild-to-moderate AD (63.7%).

In a multisite German study,[7] 168 adult patients with moderate-to-severe AD diagnosed via Hanifin and Rajka criteria[19] were randomized (2−1) into a double-blinded, placebo-controlled (DBPC) phase III study with depigmented polymerized mite extract. These patients had AD of at least 2 years duration, persistent skin lesions or flare within 2 months of screening, aggravation of AD lesions by DM during September to February months, and positive skin prick and specific IgE to dust mite (*Der p, Der f*). Patients were treated with SCIT for an average of 18 months. Outcome measures included SCORAD scores and use of medications (TCIs, TCS, oral antihistamines, and oral corticosteroids [CS]). There was no statistically significant difference in the placebo and treated groups with respect to area under the curve for medications and SCORAD scores. However, analysis of the severe AD patients with baseline SCORAD scores above 50, displayed a significant improvement in SCORAD area under the curve in patients on immunotherapy (IT) therapy versus placebo. Adverse reactions were similar in both the treatment and placebo groups.

A European study from 2007[20] studied the change in baseline physician and patient SCORAD values and laboratory parameters (IgE and IgG4 to DM, CCL 17, CCL 22, IL-16, IL-4, IFN-γ, Il-10, TGF-β1) in 25 patients with AD treated with SCIT. Patients ranged in age from 5 to 65 years old, with diagnosis of AD according to Hanifin and Rajka criteria[19] with elevated IgE to DM; 44% of AD patients also had a positive APT to DM. Patients with FEV1 <70%, previous SCIT within 5 years, pregnancy, immunodeficiency, and/or serious psychiatric or psychological diseases were not included. Both the physician diagnosed and patient submitted SCORAD values showed significant improvement. Patients with a positive APT had more pronounced improvement. IL-8, IL-4, TGF-β1, and IFN-γ levels remained unchanged or did not change significantly. Levels of CCL 17 and IL-16 were reduced while IL-10 DM and DM specific IgE increased. Two patients dropped out; one due to flare of AD and the other due to asthma symptoms.

Prospective studies with favorable results of SLIT for AD

An open, nonrandomized Italian study[21] evaluated SCORAD values at baseline in 86 patients with mild-to-moderate AD after therapy for at least 12 months of SLIT to DM (SLITone, ALK Abello©). Patients ranged in age from 3 to 54 years old, with diagnosis of AD from Hanifin and Rajka criteria[19] and elevated IgE to DM. SCORAD values significantly decreased by 46% in comparison to initial values. Of the 86 patients, 51 had a 30% or higher reduction in SCORAD, 30 patients had less than 30% reduction in SCORAD and 5 patients did not show any change. There was a trend noted in decreased use of TCS and TCIs in the study, and there were no severe adverse effects observed.

A randomized, DBPC study[22] in 56 pediatric AD patients treated with SLIT to DM for 18 months displayed a significant reduction in SCORAD values in the mild–to-moderate AD group. A significant reduction in medication use and trend to lower visual analogue scale (VAS) was also seen. Patients in this study had chronic AD, IgE sensitization to house DM via skin prick and specific IgE, SCORAD of 8 or above, and FEV1 >80%. Patients with food allergy, persistent asthma, previous IT, or severe systemic disorders were excluded. Patients received SLIT via dropper vial three times (3.3 µg Der p 1; 2.7 µg Der f 1) weekly for 18 months. Two patients in therapy group discontinued study due to flare of their AD.

Negative studies of IT for AD

A small, randomized DBPC study[23] of 13 children aged 5–16 years who received SCIT to DM and 11 to placebo found no statistical difference in eczema severity at the end of the initial study period. Patients had a clinician diagnosis of severe eczema, positive skin prick to *Der p*, and the primary outcome was clinician assessed eczema severity (erythema, surface damage and lichenification) and body surface area (BSA) affected.

A study with oral IT to DM[24] given to 60 children with specific IgE or skin prick positive to DM with AD only versus AD patients with concomitant asthma and/or rhinitis versus control group (AD without oral IT therapy) did not find any significant difference in skin lesions at the end of the study period between the three groups.

Published reviews of IT for AD

A meta-analysis that focused on 8 randomized controlled trials by Bae et al.,[25] using the GRADE (Grading of Recommendations Assessment, Development and Evaluation) model found a moderate quality of evidence to support the use of IT for AD citing a significant positive effect on AD via random effects model of data pooling. Studies were from the United States and Europe and included 385 pediatric and adult patients. Subgroup analysis displayed significant efficacy for long-term treatment of AD with SCIT and severe AD but not in children and patients receiving SLIT therapy. No fatal or near fatal events were reported but exacerbation of AD was noted in IT and control groups alike.

Published in 2016, a systemic review of IT for pediatric and adult AD patients[26] included 12 studies with a total of 733 patients from the United States, Europe, South America, and Asia. All 8 of the studies mentioned in the previous meta-analysis were included. Patients were treated with a combination of SCIT ($n = 6$ studies), SLIT ($n = 4$ studies), intradermal IT ($n = 1$ study), and oral IT ($n = 1$

study) to inhalant (DM only or DM and grass) allergens. Primary outcomes included patient assessment of disease severity or AD symptoms and adverse events; secondary outcomes included investigator assessment of disease severity or validated eczema quality of life measures or use of other AD medications for therapy. The authors felt bias risk was moderate. For the primary outcomes, three studies reported no significant difference in patient reported global disease severity and eczema symptoms while two studies reported improved global disease severity. The secondary measure of investigator assessment of disease severity showed benefit for IT for AD. Four studies reported a reduction in medication use for AD and four found no difference. They concluded that the quality of evidence was low, and thus they could not provide a definitive role for IT for AD.

A systematic review[27] was published that focused on SLIT for AD also utilizing the GRADE model. Five studies were included in the review[21,22] but only one was a randomized double-blind study. Based on the review, one study was considered moderate quality, two studies low quality, and the remaining two were of very low quality. Four out of the five studies assessed SLIT to DM only. The primary outcome was an objective measure of AD severity with three studies using SCORAD. Four of the five studies displayed significant improvement in AD severity. No severe events were reported in any of the five studies; however, three patients had worsening of their AD, and an additional three patients stopped SLIT due to flare of their AD.

Practice guidelines

As for practice guidelines, the Joint Task Force Practice Parameters[1] for AD and for IT[28] support that the clinician should consider allergen IT in selected patients with AD with aeroallergen sensitivity. However, the guidelines from the American Academy of Dermatology[13] do not feel that there is sufficient evidence to endorse IT. A recent expert consensus group of allergists and dermatologists[16] recommends that SCIT be considered in select patients with AD with documented environmental allergies with close monitoring of skin exam and discontinuation of SCIT if the skin flares/worsens. The Italian consensus report[29] on clinical practice recommendations for allergen-specific IT states the efficacy of IT in AD patients is still controversial, and no clear recommendation could be made. A pro/con article published recently[30] discussed the above points and also focused on the adverse effects of IT in AD patients specifically, cost effectiveness of IT for AD, and lack of evidence for long-term efficacy of IT for AD. The authors reiterate the need for well-designed randomized control trials utilizing a uniform method for assessing efficacy and addressing whether or not specific allergens (DM vs. other aeroallergens) are efficacious, and whether disease severity or disease duration would impact which AD patient will benefit from IT.[30]

To summarize, studies that evaluated the use of IT for AD therapy mostly displayed improvement with some studies showing improvement in severe AD patients[7,18,31] while others had improvement in only mild-to-moderate patients.[22] Worsening or flare of eczema was noted in some studies as adverse effects although discontinuation was rarely required.[21,22] Almost all studies focused on IT to DM with data on other allergens lacking. However, studies varied in methodology including treatment type (SCIT vs. SLIT), intervention time frames, primary and secondary outcome measures, and statistical analysis (intention to treat analysis) and thus must be interpreted with caution as advised by practice guidelines and meta-analyses (Table 4.1).

Small molecules: phosphodiesterase inhibitors

Phosphodiesterase (PDE) is an intracellular enzyme that inactivates cyclic adenosine monophosphate. In 1996, a study reported increased PDE activity levels in peripheral leukocytes of patients with AD[37] Introduction of an in vitro PDE-4 inhibitor reduced levels of proinflammatory cytokines (IL-4) produced by Th2 cells in lesional skin of AD patients.[37] Crisaborole is a topical PDE-4 inhibitor approved for patients with mild-to-moderate AD ages 2 and above. Two multicenter, randomized, double-blind, parallel-group, vehicle-controlled trials treated a total of 1522 mild-to-moderate AD subjects (diagnosed via Hanifin and Rajka[19]) 2−79 years old with crisaborole twice daily for 28 days.[14] At baseline, 38.5% of the subjects had an Investigator Global Assessment (IGA) score of mild, and 61.5% had an IGA score of moderate. Subjects were randomized 2:1 to receive drug applied twice daily for 28 days with the primary endpoint the proportion of subjects at day 29 with clear or almost clear skin with a 2-grade or greater improvement from baseline. Significantly more crisaborole-treated patients achieved success in IGA endpoint than placebo, achieved success in IGA endpoint score earlier than placebo patients and achieved improvement in itch earlier than placebo patients. The most common adverse effect was site pain in 4% patients on drug versus 1% on placebo vehicle. In a long-term extension study, 517 patients were treated with an additional 48 weeks of crisaborole[38] and site pain dropped to around 2.3%. Another phosphodiesterase inhibitor (OPA-15,406) published phase II clinical trial data for mild-to-moderate treatment of AD.[39] In this randomized, double-blind, vehicle-controlled, parallel-group trial, 121 patients aged 10−70 years with mild-to-moderate AD (diagnosed by Hanifin and Rajka criteria) were treated with OPA15406 0.3% ($n = 41$), versus 1% ($n = 43$) versus vehicle placebo ($n = 37$) for 8 weeks. The primary end point was IGA score of 0 or 1 with a greater than or equal to 2 point reduction from baseline at 4 weeks. Patients on the OPA 15406 1% dose achieved the primary endpoint ($P = .165$ vs. placebo); they also demonstrated improvement in eczema area and severity index (EASI) at week 1 and had improvement in VAS for itch. There was a drop out of 27 patients in similar distribution among all three groups. A distinct advantage of this therapy is that it is a steroid sparing agent and can be used for areas of the skin where steroid atrophy is a concern particularly for the face.

Table 4.1 Summary of literature for IT for AD.

Study	Number of patients	Age range	AD diagnosed by	Sensitization diagnosed via	Type of IT	Type of study	Outcome measures	Results
Bussman, C. et al.[20]	25	5–65 y	Hanifin and Rajka	Prick positive and class 3 or higher IgE to DM	SCIT to DM	Open	Primary: SCORAD scores	Significant ↓ in SCORAD
Cadario, G. et al.[21]	86	3–54 y	Hanifin and Rajka	IgE > class 2 to DM	SLIT to DM	Open, nonrandomized	Primary: SCORAD scores Secondary: Total and DM-specific IgE	46% reduction in SCORAD scores; ↓ in total and DM-specific IgE
Galli, E. et al.[24]	60 patients Group A: 26 Group B: 16 Group C:18 Group A patients with AD, asthma and/or rhinitis. Groups B and C had AD	5 months to 12 y	Hanifin and Rajka	Prick positive and/or RAST to *Der p*	Oral IT to *Der p* to groups A and B only. Group C was a control group.	Groups B and C randomized; not blinded	Primary: Physician score (erythema, vesicles, fissures, lichenification, itch) of 0–3 based on severity	No significant difference of skin lesions at the end of the study between the three groups
Glover, M.T. et al.[23]	24—13 patients received SCIT and 11 placebo	5–16 y	Clinician diagnosis of severe eczema	Positive skin prick to Dp	SCIT to DM	Randomized, DBPC	Clinician assessed eczema severity (erythema, surface damage, and lichenification)	No statistical difference in eczema severity at the end of the initial study period

Continued

Table 4.1 Summary of literature for IT for AD.—*cont'd*

Study	Number of patients	Age range	AD diagnosed by	Sensitization diagnosed via	Type of IT	Type of study	Outcome measures	Results
Kaufman, H.S. et al.[32]	52 patients enrolled but only 26 completed 2 years (16 on treatment, 10 on placebo)	2–47 y	AD diagnosis by allergist and dermatologist	Positive skin prick to ≥ 3 allergens (DM, animal dander, grass pollen and/or foods)	SCIT to DM, animal dander, pollens and mold	Blinded, placebo controlled	Skin severity (improved, no change, or worse) before and after therapy based on 24 clinical characteristics and BSA affected	Significant improvement in therapy patients (13/16) versus placebo (4/10)
Lee, J et al.[31]	217	21.16 ± 8.46 y	Investigator global assessment (IGA)	Specific IgE or prick test to DM	SCIT to DM	Retrospective	IGA scores, itch score, loss of sleep via visual analogue	Significant ↓ in IGA score, itch, loss of sleep; better outcomes in moderate-to-severe AD
Leroy, B.P. et al.[33]	23 patients (12 in active therapy and 11 placebo)	15–64 y	Hanifin and Rajka	Positive skin test to *Dp* and specific IgE to *Dp*	SCIT to DM along with autologous specific Abs	Randomized DBPC	Primary: Mean score of clinical symptoms (erythema, edema, papules, excoriations, lichenification, desquamation) with BSA Secondary: VAS	Significant ↓ in score in treated patients at 4 month mark. After 1 y, 82% patients had a mean improvement of 83%. VAS significantly lower in active group at 4 months.
Nahm, D-H. et al.[18]	251	5–55 y	Hanifin and Rajka	Positive IgE to DM	SCIT to DM	Observational cohort study	Primary: SCORAD scores	Significant ↓ in SCORAD (higher in patients with severe AD)

Study	Number/Therapy	Age	Diagnosis	Treatment	Design	Outcomes	Results
Novak, N. et al.[7]	112 received SCIT and 56 placebo	18–66 y	Hanifin and Rajka	SCIT to DM	Randomized, DBPC	Primary: SCORAD scores and medication use	Significant ↓ in SCORAD in only severe AD group but overall efficacy showed no difference between treatment and placebo groups
Pajno, G.B. et al.[22]	28 received SLIT and 28 received placebo	5–16 y	Clinical history of AD	SLIT to DM	Randomized, DBPC	Primary: SCORAD Secondary: VAS, rescue medication	Significant ↓ in SCORAD in mild-to-moderate AD group only. Significant ↓ in medication use in treatment group. VAS not significantly different between groups.
Silny, W. et al.[34]	20	5–40 y	Article in Polish; abstract does not mention how AD was diagnosed	SCIT to DM or grass pollen	Randomized, DBPC	Clinical score (W-AZS); total IgE, allergen specific IgE, Il-4, Il-5, Il-10	Significant ↓ in W-AZS index after 12 months. Il-4, Il-5, Il-10 not significantly different.
Qin, Y.E. et al.[35]	58 received SLIT plus therapy and 49 received only therapy (Xyzal® and topical CS)	18–46 y	Hanifin and Rajka	SLIT to *Df*	Randomized	Primary: SCORAD score change, VAS scale, medication scores	Treatment group: Efficacy rate significantly ↑; medication scores ↓ at 6 mos/12 mos;

Continued

Table 4.1 Summary of literature for IT for AD.—cont'd

Study	Number of patients	Age range	AD diagnosed by	Sensitization diagnosed via	Type of IT	Type of study	Outcome measures	Results
Werfel, T. et al.[36]	89 (differing doses); 51 completed 1 year study	18–55 y	Chronic AD with SCORAD ≥ 40	Specific IgE to DM (≥class 3)	SCIT to DM (20 U, 2000 U, 20,000 U)	Randomized, double blind	Primary: SCORAD score after therapy in comparison to baseline at 9 and 12 months Secondary: Medication use	VAS scores significantly ↓ SCORAD ↓ in all three groups in dose response, significantly in 2000 and 20,000 versus 20 unit groups: Drop in topical CS medication use

Abs—antibodies; BSA—body surface area; Df— Dermatophagoides farinae; Dp— Dermatophagoides pteronyssinus; DM—dust mite; SCIT—subcutaneous immunotherapy; SCORAD— scoring of atopic dermatitis; SLIT—sublingual immunotherapy; VAS—visual analogue scale; y—years

Small molecules: Janus Kinase/signal transducer and activator of transcription (JAK/STAT pathway)

This pathway is utilized by cytokines in AD in particular those that augment the Th2 response, activate eosinophils and suppress T regulatory cells.[40,41] Tofacitinib, a drug already approved for use in rheumatoid and psoriatic arthritis patients, inhibits JAK1 and JAK3.[40] There is one published double-blind, randomized phase IIa study of topical tofacitinib in patients with AD.[42] In this 4 week study, 69 mild-to-moderate adult AD patients diagnosed via Hanifin and Rajka criteria were randomized in a 1:1 fashion to either topical tofacitinib versus vehicle placebo ointment twice daily. The primary end point was percent change in baseline EASI score at week 4, which was significantly lower in those treated with tofacitinib than placebo ($P < .01$). Additionally, tofacitinib also showed significant improvement in comparison to vehicle with respect to secondary endpoints (EASI Severity Sum Score, Physician's Global Assessment) and itch with changes noted as early as week 1. In safety, four patients withdrew from the study; two of these patients were on vehicle and had developed contact dermatitis, one was lost to follow-up and one declined to further participate. Most adverse effects were mild and occurred at a higher rate in vehicle patients; there were no deaths or severe adverse effects. There are two ongoing studies for the use of ruxolitinib (another JAK/STAT inhibitor) topically for pediatric AD patients (NCT03257644 that is recruiting) and adult AD patients (NCT03011892 that is active but not currently recruiting). A small study of six patients with moderate-to-severe AD (>10% body surface area involvement and SCORAD of >20) were treated with oral tofacitinib 10 mg daily (5/6 patients) and 5 mg (1/6 patients) daily.[43] Response to therapy was measured via SCORAD score at baseline in comparison to score at the two follow-up visits (4–14 weeks and at 8–29 weeks). There was a noted decrease in SCORAD along with no noted adverse effects of infections, no cytopenias, and no elevations in liver and kidney functions or lipid levels. However, as this is a small study without randomization or blinding and variable evaluation time points, further studies are required.

Current monoclonal therapies: dupilumab

Dupilumab was approved in 2017, as the first biologic immunotherapy for adult patients and children aged 12 years and older with moderate-to-severe AD. It is a humanized mAb directed against the alpha subunit of the IL-4 cytokine receptor, thus blocking the downstream effects of IL-4 and IL-13, which play a prominent role in the Th2 cell-mediated inflammation in AD. At the molecular level, dupilumab decreases thymus and activation-regulated chemokine (TARC) levels (chemokine CCL17), which correlate with AD severity and reduce total IgE levels.[44–46] Transcriptomic analyses of AD skin biopsies pre- and postdupilumab treatment revealed that dupilumab improves the AD genetic signature in a dose-dependent manner.[47]

Dupilumab treatment is linked with significant reductions in AD markers, including mRNA expression of Th2-associated chemokines (CCL17, CCL18, CCL22, CCL26) and genes involved in epidermal hyperplasia (K16, MKI67), as well as IL-17 and IL-22 that facilitate Th17 and Th22 cell-mediated immune pathways.[46,47] As standard therapy, dupilumab is administered as a subcutaneous injection at an initial dose of 400−600 mg depending on age and weight followed by subsequent doses of 200−300 mg every 2 weeks thereafter. A steering committee of AD experts recently recommended that dupilumab be used as first-line systemic therapy in adolescence 12 and above and adults with moderate-to-severe AD who are not controlled with topical therapies.[16] Several clinical trials evaluated the treatment efficacy and safety of dupilumab for moderate-to-severe AD. Published and ongoing studies are described in the following sections.

Clinical efficacy and safety

Two randomized, placebo-controlled, phase III, international clinical trials (known as SOLO1 and SOLO2) evaluated dupilumab in adult AD patients who had been inadequately controlled with topical therapies.[15] SOLO1 included 447 patients receiving dupilumab 300 mg weekly ($n = 223$) or every 2 weeks ($n = 224$) for 16 weeks compared to 224 patients who received placebo. Similarly, SOLO2 included 472 who received the same dupilumab dosing schedule ($n = 239$ and $n = 233$, respectively) compared to 236 who received placebo. The primary outcome was an IGA score of either 0 or 1 and a decrease in IGA score of at least 2 points from baseline at week-16 of therapy. In SOLO1, 37% of patients who received dupilumab weekly and 38% of patients who received dupilumab every 2 weeks achieved the primary end point, compared to 10% of placebo-receiving patients ($P < .001$ for both comparisons). Similar results were reported in SOLO2 with 36% of dupilumab weekly and 36% of dupilumab every 2 week-receiving patients attaining an IGA score of 0 or 1, compared to 8% of patients in the placebo group ($P < .001$ for both comparisons). There were also significant reductions in EASI scores by at least 75% from baseline at week-16 in the intervention group patients compared to patients who received placebo ($P < .001$). The LIBERTY AD CHRONOS study was a large ($n = 740$) multinational, randomized, DBPC phase III clinical trial of 1-year duration assessing the long-term management of adults with moderate-to-severe AD with dupilumab and concomitant low-to-mid potency TCS (with or without TCI for involvement of the face, groin, and intertriginous regions).[48] Patients in the intervention groups received an initial dose of dupilumab 600 mg and then either 300 mg weekly ($n = 319$) or every 2 weeks ($n = 106$) thereafter. At week 16 and week 52, both dupilumab groups had greater proportions of patients who achieved 75% reduction in EASI score and IGA scores of 0 or 1 compared to placebo (all $P < .0001$). At week 52, intervention group patients also exhibited significant improvements in pruritus numerical rating scale scores, percent BSA affected with AD, and SCORAD score (all $P < .0001$). Most recently, a randomized, placebo-controlled phase III trial (LIBERTY AD CAFÉ) assessed dupilumab treatment efficacy with concomitant midpotency TCS in adults with AD not controlled and/or intolerant of cyclosporine A treatment.[49] In this study, significantly more patients who received dupilumab 300 mg weekly (59%) or every 2 weeks (63%), in conjunction with TCS, achieved 75% or more improvement in EASI scores at 16 weeks of treatment compared to placebo (30%) ($P < .0001$).

Moreover, a 2017 meta-analysis by Han et al. included seven randomized, DBPC clinical trials with a total of 1965 patients evaluated ($n = 1364$ receiving dupilumab; $n = 601$ receiving placebo).[50] All studies were deemed to be of high quality with low risk of bias. Compared to placebo, dupilumab exhibited significant clinical efficacy for the treatment of AD among multiple parameters including reduction in EASI score, IGA response (score of 0 or 1), and decrease in percent BSA involvement, as well as mean difference in the pruritus numerical rating scale score (all $P < .001$). The most effective dosing regimens were 300 mg weekly or every 2 weeks. A separate 2017 meta-analysis performed by Xu and colleagues included all of the studies in the analysis conducted by Han et al. plus one other randomized controlled trial (Blauvelt et al.), totaling 2705 patients.[51] These authors also found that significantly more dupilumab-receiving patients achieved an IGA response of 0 or 1 and an improvement of 2 points or more from baseline score and also had significantly greater reductions in EASI scores compared to placebo. The authors also stated that dosing regimens of 300 mg weekly or every other week were comparable in regard to clinical outcomes and that treatment duration of 12 weeks achieved the best outcomes for IGA response. Dupilumab has since been approved by the FDA for every other week dosing.

Quality of life outcomes

There are a few studies that aimed to directly investigate quality-of-life outcomes related to dupilumab therapy. A randomized, DBPC multicenter European clinical trial conducted from 2012 to 2013 showed significant improvements, compared to placebo-receiving patients ($n = 32$), in the Quality of Life Index of Atopic Dermatitis (QoLIAD) score in 32 adult patients with moderate-to-severe AD who received dupilumab 300 mg weekly over a period of 12 weeks.[52] QoLIAD scores were also significantly correlated with changes in clinical efficacy outcomes including EASI, SCORAD, and SCORAD VAS scores for sleep. Patients in the SOLO1 and SOLO2 studies experienced significant and clinically meaningful improvements in their health-related quality of life as measured by the 5-dimension, 3-level EuroQol (EQ-5D).[53] Patients also reported decreases on the effect of AD on their sleep, anxiety and/or depression, and quality of life in the SOLO1 and SOLO2 studies at week 16, as indicated by changes in dermatology life quality index (DLQI), patient-oriented eczema measure (POEM), and HADS-A and HADS-D scores.[15] In the LIBERTY AD CHRONOS study, there were significant reductions in the DLQI and POEM scores in both dupilumab arms compared to placebo at week 16 and week 52.[48] The meta-analysis by Xu and colleagues found that dupilumab significantly improved DLQI scores compared to placebo among four studies for a total of

2498 patients; improvements in sleep quality (measured by POEM) and alleviation of anxiety or depression (measured by HADS) were also more pronounced among the pooled dupilumab treatment groups among[3] studies including 2119 patients.[51]

Adverse effects and safety profile

Dupilumab has demonstrated an overall favorable safety profile. Previously described adverse effects of dupilumab include local injection site reactions, nasopharyngitis, and headache as well as ocular manifestations (i.e., conjunctivitis, keratitis, blepharitis).[46,54] In several clinical trials, conjunctivitis was reported to occur more often in patients receiving dupilumab (5%−28%) compared to those who had received placebo (<1−11%).[15,48,49,54] The development of alopecia areata corresponding with the start of dupilumab treatment has also been reported.[55] Herpes viral infection or reactivation is another potential adverse event that was identified in early clinical trials.[54] However, a meta-analysis by Fleming et al. including 2706 patients from 8 randomized controlled trials found that adult patients with moderate-to-severe AD receiving treatment with dupilumab exhibited a decreased incidence of skin infections compared to patients who had received placebo (RR 0.54; 95% CI 0.42−0.70).[56] In addition, there was no association of dupilumab therapy with herpes infections (RR 1.16; 95% CI 0.78−1.74), and there was decreased odds of eczema herpeticum in patients receiving therapy (OR 0.34; 95% CI 0.14−0.84). The meta-analysis by Han et al. concluded that overall adverse events occurred at similar rates among the different studies and that dupilumab treatment was associated with a lower risk of severe adverse events (defined as skin infection, inflammatory lesions, impetigo, eczema herpeticum) compared to placebo (RR 0.44; 95% CI, 0.30−0.65, $P < .001$).[50] It has been suggested that the decrease in skin infections may be attributed to overall improvements in AD disease severity and skin barrier function. The LIBERTY AD CHRONOS study evaluated the long-term (52 weeks) use of dupilumab among adult patients.[48] Rates of serious adverse events occurred in 4% of patients who received dupilumab every other week along with concomitant TCS therapy and in 5% of the placebo plus TCS group.

Dupilumab current and ongoing studies

There are several ongoing clinical trials investigating other outcomes in patients with AD receiving dupilumab treatment. An open-label extension study is following patients (estimated enrollment of 2000 adults) who participated in the placebo-controlled/dupilumab AD clinical trials to assess the long-term safety of dupilumab through identification of treatment-related adverse event rates.[57] There is also a separate phase IV observational study in the United States monitoring the efficacy and safety of dupilumab in adults with moderate-to-severe AD to address the potential of dupilumab for long-term control of AD disease.[58] Given the substantial efficacy of dupilumab in adult patients, there has been great interest regarding its potential effectiveness and safety in pediatric populations. A phase III, open-label, multinational study aims to assess the long-term safety and efficacy of dupilumab in pediatric patients (two separate cohorts: age 6 months to <6 years and age 6 years to <18 years) with AD and is estimated to be completed in 2023.[59] Furthermore, there is a phase III randomized, DBPC trial (known as Liberty AD PRESCHOOL in the United States), which plans to evaluate the safety and efficacy of dupilumab with concomitant TCS therapy in patients age 6 months to less than 6 years with severe AD.[60] Similarly, a randomized DBPC study to investigate the efficacy and safety of dupilumab with contemporaneous TCS therapy in pediatric patients age 6 years to less than 12 years, also with severe AD is underway.[61]

Other biologic immunotherapies under investigation

AD represents a complex immunopathologic disease encompassing an intricate interplay of several cell-mediated pathways and their respective chemokines and cytokines of inflammation and immune dysregulation. There are several new and emerging biologic immunotherapies being investigated that target other markers involved in the pathogenesis of AD. There are also mAb therapies, currently approved for other atopic or inflammatory/autoimmune diseases that have not demonstrated such robust treatment efficacy as dupilumab; however, there are no head-to-head comparative studies. Table 4.2 summarizes the emerging biologic monoclonal antibody immunotherapies for AD with promising preliminary results.

Potentially promising and emerging biologic therapies
Tralokinumab and Lebrikizumab (anti-IL-13)

Tralokinumab and lebrikizumab are both mAbs, administered as subcutaneous injections, which target the cytokine IL-13. Lebrikizumab is a humanized mAb against IL-13, which had been previously studied in adult asthma with conflicting outcomes. Results of a phase II, randomized, DBPC study comparing single dose lebrikizumab with TCS therapy, lebrikizumab administered every 4 weeks with TCS therapy, and placebo drug with TCS[62] known as TREBLE were recently published.[63] A total of 209 patients were randomized to (1) single-dose lebrikizumab 125 mg, (2) single-dose lebrikizumab 250 mg, (3) lebrikizumab 125 mg every 4 weeks for 12 weeks, or (4) placebo every 4 weeks for 12 weeks, all after a 2-week run in period with topical 0.1% triamcinolone acetonide therapy that continued during the study. At week 12, more patients who had received lebrikizumab 125 mg every 4 weeks achieved >50% reduction in EASI score (82.4%) compared to placebo (62.3%), ($P = .026$). Furthermore, compared to placebo, there were statistically significant differences in the proportion of patients who achieved >75% reductions in EASI score (54.9% vs. 34.0%, $P = .036$) and 50% reduction in SCORAD score (51.0% vs. 26.4%, $P = .012$); the greatest reduction in percent BSA affected by AD

Table 4.2 Potentially promising and emerging biologic therapies.

Medication	Target	Published data	Type of study	Population	Primary outcome	Result	Current study phase	Ongoing studies
Tralokinumab	IL-13	–	Phase II, randomized DBPC	Adults, moderate-to-severe AD	EASI score reduction at week 12	Reductions for all study arms observed (unspecified dosages)	III	NCT03131648[67] NCT03160885[68] NCT03363854[69] NCT03443024[64]
Lebrikizumab	IL-13	Simpson et al.[63] (TREBLE)	Phase II, randomizedDBPC	Adults, moderate-to-severe AD with concomitant TCS therapy	EASI-50 at week-12	125 mg every 4 weeks versus placebo (82.4% vs. 62.3%, $P = .026$)	II	
Fezakinumab	IL-22	Guttman-Yassky et al.[70]	Phase II, randomized DBPC	Adults, moderate-to-severe AD	SCORAD score reduction at week-12	Initial dose 600 mg followed by 300 mg every 2 weeks for 10 weeks versus placebo (-21.6% vs. -9.6%, $P = .029$)	II	–
Nemolizumab	IL-31	Ruzicka et al.[75] Silverberg et al.[76]	Phase II, randomized DBPC	Adults, moderate-to-severe AD	Pruritus VAS score at week 12	All dosages (0.1 mg/kg, 0.5 mg/kg, 2.0 mg/kg) versus placebo (-43.7%, -59.8%, -63.1% vs. -20.9%, all $P < .01$)	II	[76]
GBR 830	OX40	Guttman-Yassky et al.[71]	Phase II, randomized DBPC	Adults, moderate-to-severe AD	Incidence of treatment emergent adverse events and improvements in epidermal pathology (coprimary outcomes)	Distribution of treatment emergent adverse events: GBR 830, 63% (n=29/46) and placebo, 63% (10/16). GBR 830 led to reductions in Th1, Th2, and Th17/Th22 cytokine and chemokine mRNA expression in lesional skin.	II	–

(57.7%) was also observed in this intervention group at week 12. There was no significant difference in the proportion of patients who achieved an IGA score of 0 or 1. The authors also reported quality-of-life improvements (both statistically significant and comparable to placebo) among various parameters and no differences in adverse event rate compared to placebo. Another phase II study with an estimated enrollment of 275 patients with moderate-to-severe AD investigating the safety and efficacy of lebrikizumab in a randomized, DBPC trial was completed in May 2019 but results are not yet published.[64] The primary outcome is EASI score reduction compared to baseline at week 16.

Tralokinumab is a human recombinant IgG_4 mAb that blocks the IL-13 receptor via $R\alpha 1$ and $R\alpha 2$ and also binds to the A and D helices of the cytokine IL-13 itself, thus preventing cytokine-receptor binding.[65] Tralokinumab is currently in development as a treatment option for adults with moderate-to-severe AD. A multinational, phase IIb, randomized DBPC study to evaluate the efficacy and safety of tralokinumab in adults with moderate-to-severe AD was completed in February 2016.[66] Study results available on https://www.clinicaltrials.gov and recently published[66a] report that mean absolute changes in EASI scores at week 12 for the Intention to treat population compared to baseline were -13.67, -15.14, and -15.72 for tralokinumab (3 different dosages—45 mg, 150 mg, 300 mg every two weeks) and -10.78 for placebo. The 300 mg group of tralokinumab had a significant change from baseline EASI score versus placebo (adjusted mean difference, -4.94; 95% CI, -8.76 to -1.13; $P = .01$): a greater number of these patients also achieved an IGA response (grade of 0 or 1 with a 2 point change from baseline), displayed improvements in SCORAD, Dermatology Life Quality Index, and pruritus numeric rating scale. There are currently three phase III DBPC clinical trials that set out to investigate tralokinumab efficacy in moderate-to-severe adult AD: as monotherapy for up to 52 weeks (ECZTRA1 and ECZTRA2; currently recruiting and completed August 2019, respectively)[67,68] or in combination with TCS (ECZTRA3; not yet recruiting).[69] Given that dupilumab has proven successful for the treatment of AD with its effects on IL-4 and IL-13, it will be interesting to discover whether tralokinumab and lebrikizumab as anti-IL-13 therapies alone will produce comparable efficacies.

Fezakinumab

Fezakinumab is a mAb, administered intravenously, blocking IL-22, thus inhibiting Th22 cell-mediated immune pathways. Results of a phase IIa, randomized, DBPC trial have just been published.[70] Guttman-Yassky et al. reported on 40 adults with moderate-to-severe AD who received fezakinumab (loading dose of 600 mg followed by 300 mg every 2 weeks for 10 weeks). Compared to the placebo group ($n = 20$) the mean decrease in SCORAD for the entire study population was not significant, however those, patients with severe AD (defined as SCORAD >50) receiving fezakinumab demonstrated a significant reduction in SCORAD score compared to baseline at week 12 (21.6 vs. 9.6, $P = .029$); this effect persisted at week 20 during the follow-up period (27.4 vs. 11.5, $P = .010$). There were also statistically significant improvements in BSA involvement (moderate-to-severe AD patients) and in IGA score reduction (severe AD patients) compared to placebo at week 12. All scores continued to show improvement after the last dose (week 10) up to week 20 of the study. Upper respiratory tract infections occurred in 10% of patients who received fezakinumab ($n = 4$). The authors overall concluded that fezakinumab was well tolerated and clinically efficacious with sustained effects after a last-administered dose. They also suggested that fezakinumab could be a potential therapeutic option for patients with severe AD who may not respond to other approved biologic immunotherapies, including dupilumab.

GBR 830 monoclonal antibody (anti-OX40 (CD134))

The investigational intravenous mAb known as GBR 830 blocks the binding of OX40 and in turn, prevents downstream coreceptor signaling required for Th2 cell-mediated activation pathways. A phase IIa, randomized, DBPC study investigated the safety and tolerability of this immunologic agent in patients with moderate-to-severe AD (characterized by >10% affected body surface area; EASI >12; and inadequate response to topical treatments); patients were randomized 3:1 to 10 mg/kg intravenous GBR 830 or placebo on day 1 (baseline) and day 29.[71] The study included 64 adult subjects; coprimary outcomes were defined as the incidence of treatment emergent adverse events and improvements in epidermal pathology, while secondary outcomes assessed the effect on EASI and IGA scores. The sponsoring pharmaceutical company announced in August 2017 that patients who had received GBR 830 infusions ($n = 48$) on day 1 and 29 of the study exhibited clinical improvement in EASI scores and displayed an effect on AD-related biomarkers within skin biopsies; they also stated that the drug was safe and well tolerated.[72] At day 71 (42 days after the last dose), the proportion of intent-to-treat subjects achieving 50% or greater improvement in EASI score was greater with GBR 830 (76.9% [20/26]) versus placebo (37.5% [3/8]). $< .001$.[71]

Nemolizumab (anti-IL-31)

Cytokine IL-31 is known to be upregulated in AD and is implicated as a major culprit in the debilitating, disease-related pruritus.[73] Nemolizumab is a humanized mAb, administered subcutaneously, against the IL-31 receptor A and thus inhibits IL-31 signaling pathways. A phase I/Ib study conducted in Japan concluded that nemolizumab (called as CIM331) decreased pruritus VAS scores by about 50%, reduced sleep disturbances, and decreased the use of TCS therapy.[74] A phase II, randomized DBPC trial of 264 adults with moderate-to-severe AD were administered different weight-based dosing regimens of nemolizumab (0.1 mg/kg, 0.5 mg/kg, 2.0 mg/kg) for 12 weeks.[75] Nemolizumab treatments led to significant improvements in pruritus VAS scores compared to placebo (all $P < .01$). As secondary outcomes, there were improvements in EASI, SCORAD, and IGA scores at week 12, but no statistical analyses to placebo were performed. The authors concluded that nemolizumab 0.5 mg/kg every 4 weeks afforded the greatest reduction in pruritus scores and had the best benefit-risk profile. Another phase II randomized DBPC study assessed the efficacy of different dosing regimens of nemolizumab in adults with moderate-to-severe AD and reported that 30 mg every 4 weeks achieved safe, rapid improvements in inflammation and pruritus.[76] Based on the available but limited data thus far, it seems that nemolizumab may become a promising immunotherapy agent to alleviate pruritus in patients with AD.

Other historical and investigatory biologic immunotherapies
Secukinumab (anti-IL-17)

A mAb directed against IL-17, secukinumab is currently approved for the treatment of psoriatic arthritis, moderate-to-severe plaque psoriasis, and ankylosing spondylitis. There is a phase II, randomized, double-blind pilot study to assess secukinumab 300 mg subcutaneous injection over a 12-week period compared to placebo administration in adults with moderate-to-severe AD.[77] The primary outcome intends to measure the change in epidermal thickness of lesional skin. No results have been posted to date (accessed March 2018).

Tezepelumab (anti-TSLP)

Thymic stromal lymphopoietin (TSLP) has been shown to induce Th2 cell-mediated responses implicated in AD. Tezepelumab is a subcutaneous injectable mAb directed against TSLP. A single phase IIa randomized, DBPC study investigated the efficacy and safety of tezepelumab (known as MEDI9929) in adults with moderate-to-severe AD.[78] Results have not been published, but those available on https://www.clinicaltrials.gov report that 64.7% of patients who received MEDI9929 ($n = 55$) achieved >50% in EASI score compared to 48.2% of patients who received placebo ($n = 56$), (OR 1.97; 95% CI 0.90–4.33), without reported statistical significance.

Rituximab (anti-CD20)

Rituximab is a chimeric mAb directed against the CD20 marker on B lymphocytes. It was first approved for the treatment of non-Hodgkin lymphoma and works by antibody-dependent, cell-mediated cytotoxicity, resulting in apoptosis of B lymphocytes. Overall, there are limited data on the efficacy and safety of rituximab for the treatment of AD.

A 2008 published open-label, pilot study of six adult patients with severe AD who received 2 doses of rituximab 1000 mg, 2 weeks apart, experienced significant improvement in EASI scores at week 4 after therapy initiation, and this effect was sustained at week 24.[79] There were also observed decreases in subjective pruritus scores as well as in the amount and frequency of TCS application among these patients. The histopathological features on repeat skin biopsy of AD lesions posttherapy yielded significantly less hyperkeratosis, spongiosis, and dermal infiltrates. Interestingly, decreased IL-5 and IL-13 expression was also noted in the skin after rituximab treatment. All patients tolerated rituximab without severe adverse events. B lymphocyte depletion was observed within 3 days of therapy, and recovery of CD20+ B lymphocytes was noted in three patients at week 24.

In one case report, rituximab was administered at a dose of 1000 mg to a first trimester pregnant woman with AD previously refractory to treatment with TCS and tacrolimus, as well as systemic corticosteroids, cyclosporine, and mycophenolate mofetil.[80] Pregnancy testing became positive after the infusion, and the gestational age of the embryo at the time of rituximab administration was estimated to be about 13 days. The patient experienced significant response after one dose of rituximab as her total BSA affected by AD decreased from approximately 80% to 5%, and she experienced no subsequent exacerbations or adverse effects. There were also no reported adverse effects noted in the twin infants, up to age 8 months during the follow-up period. In contrast, there is a published report of 2 patients with severe AD who failed to respond to rituximab therapy at a lower dose of 500 mg, administered 2 weeks apart.[81] Additionally, a Spanish group described their experience of six patients who had received sequential therapy with omalizumab and rituximab or vice versa.[82] Three patients experienced clinical improvement after rituximab therapy had been administered for AD disease recurrence. However, one patient had an anaphylactic reaction to rituximab, and another developed severe neutropenia, requiring granulocyte colony stimulating factor administration.

Omalizumab (anti-IgE)

Omalizumab is a recombinant humanized mAb that binds freely circulating IgE, thus blocking IgE binding to the high-affinity IgE receptor on basophils and mast cells, preventing their activation and degranulation. The therapeutic efficacy of omalizumab in moderate-to-severe, persistent allergic asthma and in chronic idiopathic/autoimmune urticaria is well established. However, data regarding the use of omalizumab for AD has been less promising.

There are 2 published randomized, placebo-controlled clinical trials both of which have demonstrated no beneficial clinical effects of omalizumab on disease activity in AD. A study by Iyengar et al. included a total of 8 pediatric patients (mean age 11.6

years) with severe, refractory AD.[83] In the four patients who received omalizumab at a dose of 150—375 mg every 2—4 weeks for 24 weeks, there were markedly decreased plasma levels of TSLP, OX40L, TARC, and IL-9 posttreatment compared to the control group ($n = 4$). Despite reductions in these Th2-associated markers, clinical outcomes between the two groups in regard to SCORAD reduction pre- versus posttreatment were comparable. The other study conducted by Heil and colleagues compared the outcomes of 13 patients receiving omalizumab at a weight-based, IgE level-determined dose every 4 weeks for 16 weeks to a placebo group ($n = 7$).[84] Patients who received omalizumab demonstrated reductions in serum free IgE and surface expression of IgE on peripheral mononuclear cells; however, there were no significant changes observed in clinical parameters among the intervention group.

Furthermore, a 2016 systematic review and meta-analysis comprising 103 pediatric and adult patients (mean age 30.2 ± 15.1 years) from 1 randomized controlled trial (Iyengar et al.) and 12 case series investigated the efficacy of omalizumab in AD.[85] Approximately 60% of patients were classified as having severe AD with a mean baseline serum IgE level of 6838 ($n = 83$). Most patients were treated at a dose of >600 mg every month (range 150—900 mg/month); 43% attained excellent clinical response while 30% had no change or worsened AD disease severity. Patients with total serum IgE levels less than 700 IU/mL were significantly associated with more favorable clinical responses. It was theorized that this correlation may be attributed to the effectiveness of omalizumab at neutralizing freely circulating IgE at comparatively lower serum concentrations with the dosage administered in these studies. The authors concluded overall from the meta-analysis that there was a lack of substantial evidence for omalizumab treatment effectiveness in AD.

It is interesting to note that one study found that patients ($n = 8$) who showed very good clinical response or responded with satisfying results (defined as SCORAD reductions >50% and 25%—50%, respectively) with omalizumab did not possess genetic alterations in the filaggrin gene. Correspondingly, no patients ($n = 7$) with filaggrin mutations responded to omalizumab.[86] The authors suggested that patients with skin barrier defects due to filaggrin mutations were less likely to benefit from anti-IgE therapy. Additional studies would help to confirm or dispute this observation.

The ADAPT (Atopic Dermatitis Anti-IgE Pediatric Trial) is an active study in the United Kingdom involving pediatric patients (age range 4—19 years) with severe atopic dermatitis (SCORAD >40) and IgE level >300 kU/L in a randomized, DBPC study to assess the role of omalizumab in the management of severe AD.[87] The primary outcome measures objective SCORAD scores at 24 weeks of omalizumab therapy. The study is anticipated for completion in August 2018.

Although there has been reported treatment success in several case series, the two relatively small, randomized, placebo-controlled, clinical trials and single meta-analysis regarding the use of omalizumab for AD suggest that this particular anti-IgE therapy lacks definitive therapeutic efficacy for moderate-to-severe AD. A particular patient subtype without filaggrin genetic mutations may derive greater benefit from omalizumab treatment. Other insights on omalizumab in pediatric AD may eventually be gleaned from the ongoing ADAPT study.

Mepolizumab (anti-IL-5)

A mAb against cytokine IL-5, mepolizumab primarily targets eosinophil growth and differentiation. Despite its success in the treatment of allergic asthma with an eosinophilic phenotype, mepolizumab has failed to demonstrate treatment effectiveness for moderate-to-severe AD. In a randomized, placebo-controlled parallel-group study, 18 patients treated with two doses of mepolizumab 750 mg administered 1 week apart demonstrated significant reductions in peripheral eosinophil counts; however, clinical outcomes measured via the Physician's Global Assessment score, SCORAD, and pruritus scoring were comparable to placebo.[88] Additionally, a randomized, DBPC clinical trial investigating the efficacy and safety of mepolizumab for adults with moderate-to-severe AD was terminated in 2017 due to predetermined clinical trial futility.[89]

Ustekinumab (anti-p40 subunit)

Ustekinumab, a mAb that binds to the p40 subunit of cytokines IL-12 and IL-23 suppresses the activation of Th17 and Th22 cell-mediated pathways. Despite its mechanism of action, ustekinumab has demonstrated no clinically meaningful outcomes for the treatment of AD. One phase II, randomized DBPC study from Japan reported no significant improvements in change in EASI score at week 12 compared to baseline in patients receiving ustekinumab 45 mg or 90 mg compared to placebo in adults with severe AD.[90] Another phase II, DBPC study including 33 patients with moderate-to-severe AD found that ustekinumab did not lead to clinical improvements despite significant changes in the genetic profile of biopsied tissue specimens.[91] Overall, the available data suggest that ustekinumab does not constitute an effective AD therapy, and there are no current ongoing studies investigating its utility for AD treatment.

Summary of biologic immunotherapies for atopic dermatitis

In summary, dupilumab has demonstrated significant clinical efficacy and positive effects on patient-reported quality of life outcomes in several randomized, DBPC clinical trials of adult patients with moderate-to-severe AD. Hopefully, the ongoing studies involving pediatric patients will demonstrate comparative safety and efficacy. Upon the completion and publication of postmarketing phase IV studies, it will be interesting to note the clinical outcomes and potential adverse effects of long-term dupilumab therapy. Although the immune pathology of AD involves a complex interplay of several inflammatory markers, the available data thus far suggest that the cytokines IL-4 and IL-13, as well as IL-22 and IL-31 harbor clinical significance as immunotherapy targets for AD. The investigatory monoclonal antibodies with promising preliminary results currently in phase II to phase III clinical studies include tralokinumab, lebrikizumab, and fezakinumab, as well as nemolizumab specifically for the relief of pruritus. Dupilumab and these emerging biologic immunotherapies that target varied Th2-associated pathways represent an expanding armamentarium of systemic treatment options for patients afflicted with moderate-to-severe, chronic AD.

References

1. Schneider L, Tilles S, Lio P, et al. Atopic dermatitis: a practice parameter update 2012. *J Allergy Clin Immunol.* 2013;131(2). https://doi.org/10.1016/j.jaci.2012.12.672, 295-299 e1-27.

2. Bieber T. Atopic dermatitis. *Ann Dermatol.* 2010;22(2):125–137. https://doi.org/10.5021/ad.2010.22.2.125.

3. Tupker RA, De Monchy JG, Coenraads PJ, Homan A, van der Meer JB. Induction of atopic dermatitis by inhalation of house dust mite. *J Allergy Clin Immunol.* 1996;97(5):1064–1070.

4. Novak N, Simon D. Atopic dermatitis — from new pathophysiologic insights to individualized therapy. *Allergy.* 2011;66(7):830–839. https://doi.org/10.1111/j.1398-9995.2011.02571.x.

5. Portnoy J, Miller JD, Williams PB, et al. Environmental assessment and exposure control of dust mites: a practice parameter. *Ann Allergy Asthma Immunol.* 2013;111(6):465–507. https://doi.org/10.1016/j.anai.2013.09.018.

6. Nankervis H, Pynn EV, Boyle RJ, et al. House dust mite reduction and avoidance measures for treating eczema. *Cochrane Database Syst Rev.* 2015;1:CD008426. https://doi.org/10.1002/14651858.CD008426.

7. Novak N, Bieber T, Hoffmann M, et al. Efficacy and safety of subcutaneous allergen-specific immunotherapy with depigmented polymerized mite extract in atopic dermatitis. *J Allergy Clin Immunol.* 2012;130(4):925–931.e4. https://doi.org/10.1016/j.jaci.2012.08.004.

8. Liu Y, Peng J, Zhou Y, Cui Y. Comparison of atopy patch testing to skin prick testing for diagnosing mite-induced atopic dermatitis: a systematic review and meta-analysis. *Clin Transl Allergy.* 2017;7:41. https://doi.org/10.1186/s13601-017-0178-3.

9. Turjanmaa K, Darsow U, Niggemann B, Rance F, Vanto T, Werfel T. EAACI/GA2LEN position paper: present status of the atopy patch test. *Allergy.* 2006;61(12):1377–1384. https://doi.org/10.1111/j.1398-9995.2006.01136.x.

10. Dou X, Kim J, Ni CY, Shao Y, Zhang J. Atopy patch test with house dust mite in Chinese patients with atopic dermatitis. *J Eur Acad Dermatol Venereol.* 2016;30(9):1522–1526. https://doi.org/10.1111/jdv.13655.

11. Seidenari S, Giusti F, Pellacani G, Bertoni L. Frequency and intensity of responses to mite patch tests are lower in nonatopic subjects with respect to patients with atopic dermatitis. *Allergy.* 2003;58(5):426–429.

12. Sidbury R, Davis DM, Cohen DE, et al. Guidelines of care for the management of atopic dermatitis: section 3. Management and treatment with phototherapy and systemic agents. *J Am Acad Dermatol.* 2014;71(2):327–349. https://doi.org/10.1016/j.jaad.2014.03.030.

13. Sidbury R, Tom WL, Bergman JN, et al. Guidelines of care for the management of atopic dermatitis: section 4. Prevention of disease flares and use of adjunctive therapies and approaches. *J Am Acad Dermatol*. 2014;71(6):1218−1233. https://doi.org/10.1016/j.jaad.2014.08.038.

14. Paller AS, Tom WL, Lebwohl MG, et al. Efficacy and safety of crisaborole ointment, a novel, nonsteroidal phosphodiesterase 4 (PDE4) inhibitor for the topical treatment of atopic dermatitis (AD) in children and adults. *J Am Acad Dermatol*. 2016;75(3). https://doi.org/10.1016/j.jaad.2016.05.046, 494-503 e6.

15. Simpson EL, Bieber T, Guttman-Yassky E, et al. Two phase 3 trials of dupilumab versus placebo in atopic dermatitis. *N Engl J Med*. 2016;375(24):2335−2348. https://doi.org/10.1056/NEJMoa1610020.

16. Boguniewicz M, Alexis AF, Beck LA, et al. Expert perspectives on management of moderate-to-severe atopic dermatitis: a multidisciplinary consensus addressing current and emerging therapies. *J Allergy Clin Immunol Pract*. 2017;5(6):1519−1531. https://doi.org/10.1016/j.jaip.2017.08.005.

17. Boguniewicz M, Fonacier L, Guttman-Yassky E, Ong PY, Silverberg J, Farrar JR. Atopic dermatitis yardstick: practical recommendations for an evolving therapeutic landscape. *Ann Allergy Asthma Immunol*. 2018;120(1). https://doi.org/10.1016/j.anai.2017.10.039, 10−22 e2.

18. Nahm DH, Kim ME, Kwon B, Cho SM, Ahn A. Clinical efficacy of subcutaneous allergen immunotherapy in patients with atopic dermatitis. *Yonsei Med J*. 2016;57(6):1420−1426. https://doi.org/10.3349/ymj.2016.57.6.1420.

19. Hanifin JM, Rajka G. Diagnostic features of atopic dermatitis. *Acta Derm Venereol*. 1980;92:44−47.

20. Bussmann C, Maintz L, Hart J, et al. Clinical improvement and immunological changes in atopic dermatitis patients undergoing subcutaneous immunotherapy with a house dust mite allergoid: a pilot study. *Clin Exp Allergy*. 2007;37(9):1277−1285. https://doi.org/10.1111/j.1365-2222.2007.02783.x.

21. Cadario G, Galluccio AG, Pezza M, et al. Sublingual immunotherapy efficacy in patients with atopic dermatitis and house dust mites sensitivity: a prospective pilot study. *Curr Med Res Opin*. 2007;23(10):2503−2506. https://doi.org/10.1185/030079907X226096.

22. Pajno GB, Caminiti L, Vita D, et al. Sublingual immunotherapy in mite-sensitized children with atopic dermatitis: a randomized, double-blind, placebo-controlled study. *J Allergy Clin Immunol*. 2007;120(1):164−170. https://doi.org/10.1016/j.jaci.2007.04.008.

23. Glover MT, Atherton DJ. A double-blind controlled trial of hyposensitization to Dermatophagoides pteronyssinus in children with atopic eczema. *Clin Exp Allergy*. 1992;22(4):440−446.

24. Galli E, Chini L, Nardi S, et al. Use of a specific oral hyposensitization therapy to Dermatophagoides pteronyssinus in children with atopic dermatitis. *Allergol Immunopathol*. 1994;22(1):18−22.

25. Bae JM, Choi YY, Park CO, Chung KY, Lee KH. Efficacy of allergen-specific immunotherapy for atopic dermatitis: a systematic review and meta-analysis of randomized controlled trials. *J Allergy Clin Immunol*. 2013;132(1):110−117. https://doi.org/10.1016/j.jaci.2013.02.044.

26. Tam HH, Calderon MA, Manikam L, et al. Specific allergen immunotherapy for the treatment of atopic eczema: a Cochrane systematic review. *Allergy*. 2016;71(9):1345−1356. https://doi.org/10.1111/all.12932.

27. Gendelman SR, Lang DM. Sublingual immunotherapy in the treatment of atopic dermatitis: a systematic review using the GRADE system. *Curr Allergy Asthma Rep.* 2015; 15(2):498. https://doi.org/10.1007/s11882-014-0498-5.

28. Cox L, Nelson H, Lockey R, et al. Allergen immunotherapy: a practice parameter third update. *J Allergy Clin Immunol.* 2011;127(1 Suppl):S1−S55. https://doi.org/10.1016/j.jaci.2010.09.034.

29. Pajno GB, Bernardini R, Peroni D, et al. Clinical practice recommendations for allergen-specific immunotherapy in children: the Italian consensus report. *Ital J Pediatr.* 2017; 43(1):13. https://doi.org/10.1186/s13052-016-0315-y.

30. Cox L, Calderon MA. Allergen immunotherapy for atopic dermatitis: is there room for debate? *J Allergy Clin Immunol Pract.* 2016;4(3):435−444. https://doi.org/10.1016/j.jaip.2015.12.018.

31. Lee J, Lee H, Noh S, et al. Retrospective analysis on the effects of house dust mite specific immunotherapy for more than 3 Years in atopic dermatitis. *Yonsei Med J.* 2016; 57(2):393−398. https://doi.org/10.3349/ymj.2016.57.2.393.

32. Kaufman HS, Roth HL. Hyposensitization with alum precipitated extracts in atopic dermatitis: a placebo-controlled study. *Ann Allergy.* 1974;32(6):321−330.

33. Leroy BP, Boden G, Lachapelle JM, Jacquemin MG, Saint-Remy JM. A novel therapy for atopic dermatitis with allergen-antibody complexes: a double-blind, placebo-controlled study. *J Am Acad Dermatol.* 1993;28(2 Pt 1):232−239.

34. Silny W, Czarnecka-Operacz M. Specific immunotherapy in the treatment of patients with atopic dermatitis–results of double blind placebo controlled study. *Pol Merkur Lek.* 2006;21(126):558−565.

35. Qin YE, Mao JR, Sang YC, Li WX. Clinical efficacy and compliance of sublingual immunotherapy with dermatophagoides farinae drops in patients with atopic dermatitis. *Int J Dermatol.* 2014;53(5):650−655. https://doi.org/10.1111/ijd.12302.

36. Werfel T, Breuer K, Rueff F, et al. Usefulness of specific immunotherapy in patients with atopic dermatitis and allergic sensitization to house dust mites: a multi-centre, randomized, dose-response study. *Allergy.* 2006;61(2):202−205. https://doi.org/10.1111/j.1398-9995.2006.00974.x.

37. Hanifin JM, Chan SC, Cheng JB, et al. Type 4 phosphodiesterase inhibitors have clinical and in vitro anti-inflammatory effects in atopic dermatitis. *J Investig Dermatol.* 1996; 107(1):51−56.

38. Eichenfield LF, Call RS, Forsha DW, et al. Long-term safety of crisaborole ointment 2% in children and adults with mild to moderate atopic dermatitis. *J Am Acad Dermatol.* 2017;77(4). https://doi.org/10.1016/j.jaad.2017.06.010, 641−649 e5.

39. Hanifin JM, Ellis CN, Frieden IJ, et al. OPA-15406, a novel, topical, nonsteroidal, selective phosphodiesterase-4 (PDE4) inhibitor, in the treatment of adult and adolescent patients with mild to moderate atopic dermatitis (AD): a phase-II randomized, double-blind, placebo-controlled study. *J Am Acad Dermatol.* 2016;75(2):297−305. https://doi.org/10.1016/j.jaad.2016.04.001.

40. Ghoreschi K, Jesson MI, Li X, et al. Modulation of innate and adaptive immune responses by tofacitinib (CP-690,550). *J Immunol.* 2011;186(7):4234−4243. https://doi.org/10.4049/jimmunol.1003668.

41. O'Sullivan LA, Liongue C, Lewis RS, Stephenson SE, Ward AC. Cytokine receptor signaling through the Jak-Stat-Socs pathway in disease. *Mol Immunol.* 2007;44(10): 2497−2506. https://doi.org/10.1016/j.molimm.2006.11.025.

42. Bissonnette R, Papp KA, Poulin Y, et al. Topical tofacitinib for atopic dermatitis: a phase IIa randomized trial. *Br J Dermatol.* 2016;175(5):902−911. https://doi.org/10.1111/bjd.14871.

43. Levy LL, Urban J, King BA. Treatment of recalcitrant atopic dermatitis with the oral Janus kinase inhibitor tofacitinib citrate. *J Am Acad Dermatol.* 2015;73(3):395−399. https://doi.org/10.1016/j.jaad.2015.06.045.

44. Kakinuma T, Nakamura K, Wakugawa M, et al. Thymus and activation-regulated chemokine in atopic dermatitis: serum thymus and activation-regulated chemokine level is closely related with disease activity. *J Allergy Clin Immunol.* 2001;107(3):535−541. https://doi.org/10.1067/mai.2001.113237.

45. Hijnen D, De Bruin-Weller M, Oosting B, et al. Serum thymus and activation-regulated chemokine (TARC) and cutaneous T cell- attracting chemokine (CTACK) levels in allergic diseases: TARC and CTACK are disease-specific markers for atopic dermatitis. *J Allergy Clin Immunol.* 2004;113(2):334−340. https://doi.org/10.1016/j.jaci.2003.12.007.

46. Beck LA, Thaci D, Hamilton JD, et al. Dupilumab treatment in adults with moderate-to-severe atopic dermatitis. *N Engl J Med.* 2014;371(2):130−139. https://doi.org/10.1056/NEJMoa1314768.

47. Hamilton JD, Suarez-Farinas M, Dhingra N, et al. Dupilumab improves the molecular signature in skin of patients with moderate-to-severe atopic dermatitis. *J Allergy Clin Immunol.* 2014;134(6):1293−1300. https://doi.org/10.1016/j.jaci.2014.10.013.

48. Blauvelt A, de Bruin-Weller M, Gooderham M, et al. Long-term management of moderate-to-severe atopic dermatitis with dupilumab and concomitant topical corticosteroids (LIBERTY AD CHRONOS): a 1-year, randomised, double-blinded, placebo-controlled, phase 3 trial. *Lancet.* 2017;389(10086):2287−2303. https://doi.org/10.1016/S0140-6736(17)31191-1.

49. de Bruin-Weller M, Thaci D, Smith CH, et al. Dupilumab with concomitant topical corticosteroid treatment in adults with atopic dermatitis with an inadequate response or intolerance to ciclosporin A or when this treatment is medically inadvisable: a placebo-controlled, randomized phase III clinical trial (LIBERTY AD CAFE). *Br J Dermatol.* 2018;178(5):1083−1101. https://doi.org/10.1111/bjd.16156.

50. Han Y, Chen Y, Liu X, et al. Efficacy and safety of dupilumab for the treatment of adult atopic dermatitis: a meta-analysis of randomized clinical trials. *J Allergy Clin Immunol.* 2017;140(3). https://doi.org/10.1016/j.jaci.2017.04.015, 888−891 e6.

51. Xu X, Zheng Y, Zhang X, He Y, Li C. Efficacy and safety of dupilumab for the treatment of moderate-to-severe atopic dermatitis in adults. *Oncotarget.* 2017;8(65):108480−108491. https://doi.org/10.18632/oncotarget.22499.

52. Tsianakas A, Luger TA, Radin A. Dupilumab treatment improves quality of life in adult patients with moderate-to-severe atopic dermatitis: results from a randomized, placebo-controlled clinical trial. *Br J Dermatol.* 2018;178(2):406−414. https://doi.org/10.1111/bjd.15905.

53. Simpson EL. Dupilumab improves general health-related quality-of-life in patients with moderate-to-severe atopic dermatitis: pooled results from two randomized, controlled phase 3 clinical trials. *Dermatol Ther.* 2017;7(2):243−248. https://doi.org/10.1007/s13555-017-0181-6.

54. Thaci D, Simpson EL, Beck LA, et al. Efficacy and safety of dupilumab in adults with moderate-to-severe atopic dermatitis inadequately controlled by topical treatments: a

randomised, placebo-controlled, dose-ranging phase 2b trial. *Lancet*. 2016;387(10013): 40−52. https://doi.org/10.1016/S0140-6736(15)00388-8.

55. Mitchell K, Levitt J. Alopecia areata after dupilumab for atopic dermatitis. *JAAD Case Rep*. 2018;4(2):143−144. https://doi.org/10.1016/j.jdcr.2017.11.020.

56. Fleming P, Drucker AM. Risk of infection in patients with atopic dermatitis treated with dupilumab: a meta-analysis of randomized controlled trials. *J Am Acad Dermatol*. 2018; 78(1):62−69 e1. https://doi.org/10.1016/j.jaad.2017.09.052.

57. NCT01949311. Open-Label Study of Dupilumab (REGN668/SAR231893) in Patients with Atopic Dermatitis. Secondary Open-Label Study of Dupilumab (REGN668/ SAR231893) in Patients With Atopic Dermatitis. https://www.clinicaltrials.gov.

58. NCT03411837. Dupilumab Phase 4 Study (DRS). https://www.clinicaltrials.gov. Secondary Dupilumab Phase 4 Study (DRS). https://www.clinicaltrials.gov. https://www. clinicaltrials.gov.

59. NCT02612454. Study to Assess Long-Term Safety of Dupilumab (REGN668/ SAR231893) Administered in Participants >6 Months to <18 Years of Age With Atopic Dermatitis (AD). . Secondary Study to Assess Long-Term Safety of Dupilumab (REGN668/SAR231893) Administered in Participants >6 Months to <18 Years of Age with Atopic Dermatitis (AD). https://www.clinicaltrials.gov. .

60. NCT03346434. Safety, Pharmacokinetics and Efficacy of Dupilumab in Patients >6 Months to <6 Years With Severe Atopic Dermatitis (Liberty AD PRESCHOOL). Secondary Safety, Pharmacokinetics and Efficacy of Dupilumab in Patients >6 Months to <6 Years With Severe Atopic Dermatitis (Liberty AD PRESCHOOL). https://www. clinicaltrials.gov.

61. NCT03345914. Study to Investigate the Efficacy and Safety of Dupilumab Administered With Topical Corticosteroids (TCS) in Participants >6 to <12 Years With Severe Atopic Dermatitis (AD). Secondary Study to Investigate the Efficacy and Safety of Dupilumab Administered With Topical Corticosteroids (TCS) in Participants >6 to <12 Years With Severe Atopic Dermatitis (AD). https://www.clinicaltrials.gov.

62. NCT02340234. A Study of Lebrikizumab in Participants With Persistent Moderate to Severe Atopic Dermatitis. Secondary a Study of Lebrikizumab in Participants With Persistent Moderate to Severe Atopic Dermatitis. https://www.clinicaltrials.gov.

63. Simpson EL, Flohr C, Eichenfield LF, et al. Efficacy and safety of lebrikizumab (an anti-IL-13 monoclonal antibody) in adults with moderate-to-severe atopic dermatitis inadequately controlled by topical corticosteroids: a randomized, placebo-controlled phase II trial (TREBLE). *J Am Acad Dermatol*. 2018;78(5). https://doi.org/10.1016/ j.jaad.2018.01.017, 863-871 e11[published Online First: Epub Date]|.

64. NCT03443024. A Study of Lebrikizumab in Patients With Moderate-to-Severe Atopic Dermatitis. Secondary a Study of Lebrikizumab in Patients With Moderate-to-Severe Atopic Dermatitis. https://www.clinicaltrials.gov.

65. Popovic B, Breed J, Rees DG, et al. Structural characterisation reveals mechanism of IL-13-neutralising monoclonal antibody tralokinumab as inhibition of binding to IL-13ralpha1 and IL-13ralpha2. *J Mol Biol*. 2017;429(2):208−219. https://doi.org/ 10.1016/j.jmb.2016.12.005.

66. NCT02347176. Phase 2 Study to Evaluate the efficacy and Safety of Tralokinumab in Adults With Atopic Dermatitis (D2213C00001). Secondary Phase 2 Study to Evaluate the Efficacy and Safety of Tralokinumab in Adults With Atopic Dermatitis (D2213C00001). https://www.clinicaltrials.gov.

66a Wollenberg A, Howell MD, Guttman-Yassky E, Silverberg JI, Kell C, Ranade K, Moate R, van der Merwe R. Treatment of atopic dermatitis with tralokinumab, an anti-IL-13 mAb. *J Allergy Clin Immunol*. 2019;143(1):135−141.

67. NCT03131648. Tralokinumab Monotherapy for Moderate to Severe Atopic Dermatitis—ECZTRA 1 (ECZema TRAlokinumab Trial no. 1) (ECZTRA1). Secondary Tralokinumab Monotherapy for Moderate to Severe Atopic Dermatitis—ECZTRA 1 (ECZema TRAlokinumab Trial no. 1) (ECZTRA1). https://www.clinicaltrials.gov.

68. NCT03160885. Tralokinumab Monotherapy for Moderate to Severe Atopic Dermatitis—ECZTRA 2 (ECZema TRAlokinumab Trial no. 2) (ECZTRA 2). . Secondary Tralokinumab Monotherapy for Moderate to Severe Atopic Dermatitis—ECZTRA 2 (ECZema TRAlokinumab Trial no. 2) (ECZTRA 2). https://www.clinicaltrials.gov.

69. NCT03363854. Tralokinumab in Combination With Topical Corticosteroids for Moderate to severe Atopic Dermatitis—ECZTRA 3 (ECZema TRAlokinumab Trial no. 3). . Secondary Tralokinumab in Combination With Topical Corticosteroids for Moderate to Severe Atopic Dermatitis—ECZTRA 3 (ECZema TRAlokinumab Trial No. 3). https://www.clinicaltrials.gov.

70. Guttman-Yassky E, Brunner PM, Neumann AU, et al. Efficacy and safety of fezakinumab (an IL-22 monoclonal antibody) in adults with moderate-to-severe atopic dermatitis inadequately controlled by conventional treatments: a randomized, double-blind, phase 2a trial. *J Am Acad Dermatol*. 2018;78(5). https://doi.org/10.1016/j.jaad.2018.01.016, 872-881 e6.

71. Guttman-Yassky E, Pavel AB, Zhou L, et al. GBR 830, an anti-OX40, improves skin gene signatures and clinical scores in patients with atopic dermatitis. *J Allergy Clin Immunol*. 2019 Aug;144(2):482−493.

72. Glenmark Pharmaceuticals Presents New Data on GBR 830, a First-in-Class, Investigational, Anti-OX40 Monoclonal Antibody for the Treatment of Moderate-to-Severe Atopic Dermatitis at the 2018 American Academic of Dermatology Annual Meeting. Secondary Glenmark Pharmaceuticals Presents New Data on GBR 830, a First-in-Class, Investigational, Anti-OX40 Monoclonal Antibody for the Treatment of Moderate-to-Severe Atopic Dermatitis at the 2018 American Academic of Dermatology Annual Meeting. http://www.glenmarkpharma.com/sites/default/files/E_Glenmark_presents_data_on_GBR_830_at_ADA.pdf.

73. Bilsborough J, Leung DY, Maurer M, et al. IL-31 is associated with cutaneous lymphocyte antigen-positive skin homing T cells in patients with atopic dermatitis. *J Allergy Clin Immunol*. 2006;117(2):418−425. https://doi.org/10.1016/j.jaci.2005.10.046.

74. Nemoto O, Furue M, Nakagawa H, et al. The first trial of CIM331, a humanized anti-human interleukin-31 receptor A antibody, in healthy volunteers and patients with atopic dermatitis to evaluate safety, tolerability and pharmacokinetics of a single dose in a randomized, double-blind, placebo-controlled study. *Br J Dermatol*. 2016;174(2):296−304. https://doi.org/10.1111/bjd.14207.

75. Ruzicka T, Hanifin JM, Furue M, et al. Anti-Interleukin-31 receptor a antibody for atopic dermatitis. *N Engl J Med*. 2017;376(9):826−835. https://doi.org/10.1056/NEJMoa1606490.

76. Silverberg JI, Pinter A, Pulka G, et al. Phase 2b Randomized Study of Nemolizumab in Adults with Moderate-Severe Atopic Dermatitis and Severe Pruritus. *J Allergy Clin Immunol*. 2019 Aug 23. pii: S0091-6749(19)31099-1. doi:10.1016/j.jaci.2019.08.013. [Epub ahead of print].

77. NCT02594098. Secukinumab for Treatment of Atopic Dermatitis. Secondary Secukinumab for Treatment of Atopic Dermatitis. https://www.clinicaltrials.gov.

78. NCT02525094. Phase 2a Study to Evaluate the Efficacy and Safety o fMEDI9929 in Adults With Atopic Dermatitis (ALLEVIAD). Secondary Phase 2a Study to Evaluate the Efficacy and Safety o fMEDI9929 in Adults With Atopic Dermatitis (ALLEVIAD). https://www.clinicaltrials.gov.

79. Simon D, Hosli S, Kostylina G, Yawalkar N, Simon HU. Anti-CD20 (rituximab) treatment improves atopic eczema. *J Allergy Clin Immunol*. 2008;121(1):122−128. https://doi.org/10.1016/j.jaci.2007.11.016.

80. Ponte P, Lopes MJ. Apparent safe use of single dose rituximab for recalcitrant atopic dermatitis in the first trimester of a twin pregnancy. *J Am Acad Dermatol*. 2010;63(2):355−356. https://doi.org/10.1016/j.jaad.2009.05.015.

81. Sediva A, Kayserova J, Vernerova E, et al. Anti-CD20 (rituximab) treatment for atopic eczema. *J Allergy Clin Immunol*. 2008;121(6):1515−1516. https://doi.org/10.1016/j.jaci.2008.03.007. Author reply 16-7.

82. Sanchez-Ramon S, Eguiluz-Gracia I, Rodriguez-Mazariego ME, et al. Sequential combined therapy with omalizumab and rituximab: a new approach to severe atopic dermatitis. *J Investig Allergol Clin Immunol*. 2013;23(3):190−196.

83. Iyengar SR, Hoyte EG, Loza A, et al. Immunologic effects of omalizumab in children with severe refractory atopic dermatitis: a randomized, placebo-controlled clinical trial. *Int Arch Allergy Immunol*. 2013;162(1):89−93. https://doi.org/10.1159/000350486.

84. Heil PM, Maurer D, Klein B, Hultsch T, Stingl G. Omalizumab therapy in atopic dermatitis: depletion of IgE does not improve the clinical course - a randomized, placebo-controlled and double blind pilot study. *J Dtsch Dermatol Ges*. 2010;8(12):990−998. https://doi.org/10.1111/j.1610-0387.2010.07497.x.

85. Wang HH, Li YC, Huang YC. Efficacy of omalizumab in patients with atopic dermatitis: a systematic review and meta-analysis. *J Allergy Clin Immunol*. 2016;138(6):1719−17122 e1. https://doi.org/10.1016/j.jaci.2016.05.038.

86. Hotze M, Baurecht H, Rodriguez E, et al. Increased efficacy of omalizumab in atopic dermatitis patients with wild-type filaggrin status and higher serum levels of phosphatidylcholines. *Allergy*. 2014;69(1):132−135. https://doi.org/10.1111/all.12234.

87. NCT02300701. Role of Anti-IgE in Severe Childhood Eczema (ADAPT). Secondary Role of Anti-IgE in Severe Childhood Eczema (ADAPT). https://www.clinicaltrials.gov.

88. Oldhoff JM, Darsow U, Werfel T, et al. Anti-IL-5 recombinant humanized monoclonal antibody (mepolizumab) for the treatment of atopic dermatitis. *Allergy*. 2005;60(5):693−696. https://doi.org/10.1111/j.1398-9995.2005.00791.x.

89. NCT03055195. Efficacy and Safety Study of Mepolizumab in Subjects With Moderate to Severe Atopic Dermatitis. Secondary Efficacy and Safety Study of Mepolizumab in Subjects With Moderate to Severe Atopic Dermatitis. https://www.clinicaltrials.gov.

90. Saeki H, Kabashima K, Tokura Y, et al. Efficacy and safety of ustekinumab in Japanese patients with severe atopic dermatitis: a randomized, double-blind, placebo-controlled, phase II study. *Br J Dermatol*. 2017;177(2):419−427. https://doi.org/10.1111/bjd.15493.

91. Khattri S, Brunner PM, Garcet S, et al. Efficacy and safety of ustekinumab treatment in adults with moderate-to-severe atopic dermatitis. *Exp Dermatol*. 2017;26(1):28−35. https://doi.org/10.1111/exd.13112.

Food allergy

5

Elizabeth Feuille, MD [1], Anna Nowak-Wegrzyn, MD, PhD [2]

[1]*Assistant Professor, Division of Pediatric Pulmonology, Department of Pediatrics, Weill Cornell Medicine, New York, NY, USA;* [2]*Professor of Pediatrics, Division of Pediatric Allergy and Immunology, Department of Pediatrics, NYU Langone School of Medicine, New York, NY, United States*

ABBREVIATIONS

AE	Adverse event
AIT	Allergen-specific immunotherapy
CM	Cow's milk
DC	Dendritic cells
DS	Desensitization
DBPCFC	Double-blind placebo-controlled food challenge
EPIT	Epicutaneous immunotherapy
EAI	Epinephrine auto-injector
FA	Food allergy
LAMP	Lysosomal-associated membrane protein-I
OFC	Oral food challenge
OIT	Oral immunotherapy
PP	Peanut protein
SCIT	Subcutaneous immunotherapy
SIT	Sublingual immunotherapy
SU	Sustained unresponsiveness
Tregs	T regulatory cells

Introduction

Food allergy (FA) affects approximately 4%—6% of adults[1] and up to 8% of children in the United States.[2] Standard management involves strict food avoidance and preparedness with an epinephrine auto-injector (EAI) for treatment of anaphylaxis.[3] Increased interest in allergen-specific immunotherapy (AIT) for FA has been driven by its public health impact, risk for severe reactions, and persistence of FA beyond childhood. Despite avoidance efforts, a third of food-allergic patients report severe accidental reactions.[2,4] With a number of methods currently under study, AIT for FA will likely become commercially available in the coming years. This chapter will review AIT for FA currently under study.

Immunotherapies for Allergic Disease. https://doi.org/10.1016/B978-0-323-54427-6.00005-5

What are the protocols of AIT for food allergy?

AIT induces tolerance through frequent delivery of allergen. Food allergen-specific immunotherapies currently include oral (OIT), sublingual (SLIT), epicutaneous (EPIT), and subcutaneous (SCIT) immunotherapy with modified allergen, as well as lysosomal-associated membrane protein (LAMP)-DNA based vaccines, compared in Table 5.1.

OIT and **SLIT** utilize daily administration of incrementally increasing allergen doses until maintenance dosing is reached and continued for varying length of time. In OIT, the food is ingested in natural or modified form. In SLIT, liquid formulation of allergen is applied under the tongue. Both are initiated under physician supervision with administration of subthreshold doses in approximately 0.5 mg (OIT) and 0.0000017 mg (SLIT) range and may be increased during an initial rapid dose-escalation day up to 6 mg and 0.07 mg range, respectively. The highest tolerated dose may be repeated the following day to confirm whether it can be safely continued. This is followed by a build-up phase, during which daily doses are increased every 1 or 2 weeks under physician supervision up to maintenance doses in gram (OIT)- and mg-range (SLIT). Daily maintenance dosing is continued for months to years.

In **EPIT**, patch with 50–500 µg (usually 250 µg) of adsorbed food allergen protein is applied to skin of upper arm or interscapular space daily for years. EPIT protocols typically start with a 2 hours of patch application under clinician supervision. Thereafter, daily patch application continues at home, with duration of application increased incrementally. During maintenance, a new patch is applied daily and worn 24 hours per day for 1 or more years.[5,6]

In **SCIT**, allergen is administered by subcutaneous injection of incrementally increasing doses under clinician supervision. Current SCIT trials utilize alum-adsorbed hypoallergen that has been modified chemically or with site-directed mutagenesis to reduce IgE-binding capacity.[7]

LAMP-DNA vaccines deliver allergen via bacterial plasmid vector, which contains DNA encoding the allergen epitope as well as lysosomal-associated membrane protein-I (LAMP-I). They are administered by intramuscular or intradermal injection, every 2 weeks for a limited number of doses.

Immune mechanisms of AIT

Immunomodulation with AIT appears to hinge on altered allergen-specific T cells response, with induction of T regulatory cells (Tregs) and suppression of T_H2 immunity. Fig. 5.1 and Table 5.2 review immune mechanisms.

Clinical trials for allergen-specific immunotherapy

As practitioners review clinical trials for their own knowledge, interpretation of results will be significantly improved by an understanding of the typical features of

Table 5.1 Comparison of allergen-specific immunotherapies for food allergy currently under study in human subjects.

	OIT	SLIT	EPIT	SCIT with hypoallergen*	LAMP-DNA vaccine*
Food allergens	Peanut, CM, egg, wheat, multi-food	Peanut, CM, hazelnut, peach	Peanut, CM	Peanut, fish	Peanut
Study phase	Phase I–IV	Phase I–III	Phase I–III	Phase 1–II	Phase I
Frequency and duration	Daily, for months to years		Daily, for years	Weekly doses*	Every 2 weeks*
Observed doses	Initial dose escalation; up-dosing every Every 1–2 weeks		Initiation and periodic observation	All	All
Dosing restrictions	Take with food; avoid physical activity 2 hours; hold for illness	Avoid eating 30 minutes after	None	Period of observation following each dose	
Advantages	Efficacy superior to SLIT and EPIT; Cost efficient	Improved safety compared to OIT	Best safety profile; ease of administration	Once observed weekly dosing	Relatively few doses*
Disadvantages	Frequent office visits; frequent AE; potential for SAE; risk of EoE	Frequent oropharyngeal AEs; risk of EoE	Reduced efficacy compared to other modalities*	Frequent office visits; injection	Injection

AE, adverse event; AIT, allergen-specific immunotherapy; CM, cow's milk; EoE, eosinophilic esophagitis; EPIT, epicutaneous immunotherapy; LAMP, lysosomal-associated membrane protein; OIT, oral immunotherapy; SAE, severe adverse event; SCIT, subcutaneous immunotherapy; SLIT, sublingual immunotherapy.
* Limited data in humans.

Reprinted from Feuille E, Nowak-Wegrzyn A. Allergen-specific immunotherapies for food allergy. Allergy Asthma Immunol Res 2018;10:191, with permission from The Korean Academy of Asthma, Allergy and Clinical Immunology; and The Korean Academy of Pediatric Allergy and Respiratory Disease.

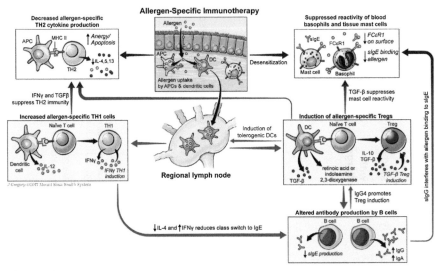

FIGURE 5.1

Putative mechanisms of tolerance induction in allergen-specific immunotherapy. In allergen-specific immunotherapy (AIT), allergen is taken up by dendritic cells that migrate to regional lymph nodes, where they induce naïve T cells to regulatory T cell phenotype, through presentation of the allergen in context of MHC, secretion of cytokines such as TGF-β, generation of retinoic acid and indoleamine 2,3-dioxygenase, and other mechanisms. Secretion of cytokines IL-10 and TGF-β suppress T_H2 immunity and mast cell reactivity, reduce sIgE synthesis, and may increase sIgG and sIgA synthesis. AIT, particularly with LAMP-DNA vaccines, may also enhance tolerance through increased T_H1 immunity: presentation of allergen by dendritic cells in context of MHC to naïve T cell may induce T_H1 commitment particularly in the presence of costimulators; and production of IFNγ by T_H1 cells suppresses T_H2 responses and reduces class switch to IgE. Other mechanisms of AIT may include increased anergy and apoptosis of T_H2 cells through persistent antigenic stimulation.

Reprinted from Feuille E, Nowak-Wegrzyn A. Allergen-specific immunotherapies for food allergy. Allergy Asthma Immunol Res 2018;10:191, with permission from The Korean Academy of Asthma, Allergy and Clinical Immunology; and The Korean Academy of Pediatric Allergy and Respiratory Disease.

rigorously designed AIT trials, including outcome measures, enrollment criteria, AIT protocols, and safety monitoring.

Goals of allergen-specific immunotherapy: Clinical trials typically use practical endpoints of desensitization and sustained unresponsiveness (SU). ***Desensitization*** is a temporary state of hyporesponsiveness to allergen, and is induced and maintained by frequent (usually daily) exposure to the offending antigen. Immune reactivity may return upon withdrawal of antigen exposure for a sufficient period of time. *SU* is a prolonged state of antigen hyporesponsiveness, which persists after a period (typically 2—12 weeks) of cessation of therapy and avoidance of allergen.

Table 5.2 Immunomodulation in allergen-specific immunotherapy.

Immune parameter	Functional correlate
↓SPT wheal diameter	Decreased mast cell reactivity
↓CD63 expression in basophil activation test	Decreased basophil reactivity
Initial ↑sIgE, followed by sustained ↓sIgE ↑sIgG, particularly ↑sIgG4 ↑sIgA (limited to OIT and SLIT)	Altered antibody isotype production by B cells
↓IL-4 and IL-13 production by PBMCs ↑IFN-γ production by production by PBMCs	Suppression of T_H2 immunity Induction of T_H1 CD4+ T cells
↑IL-10, TGF-β production by PBMCs ↑FoxP3$^+$CD25$^+$CD4$^+$ T cells	Induction of T-regulatory cells

Reprinted from Feuille E, Nowak-Wegrzyn A. Allergen-specific immunotherapies for food allergy. Allergy Asthma Immunol Res 2018;10:191, with permission from The Korean Academy of Asthma, Allergy and Clinical Immunology; and The Korean Academy of Pediatric Allergy and Respiratory Disease.

Unifying features of AIT clinical trials: Clinical trials typically require a history of food reaction with evidence of IgE-sensitization, and exclude those with life-threatening anaphylaxis, poorly controlled asthma, or other chronic medical conditions or certain medications. Rigorous studies require confirmatory double-blind placebo-controlled oral food challenge (DBPCFC) before therapy initiation. Clinical trials usually perform allergen-specific immune evaluation before AIT initiation, at various time-points during the study, and at the conclusion of therapy. Adverse events (AE) are monitored through the trial. Withdrawals may be due to AE, anxiety, nonadherence, or new medical problems or medications. Outcomes are typically evaluated with DBPCFC immediately following therapy (desensitization) or after a period of therapy cessation of 2–12 weeks (SU). A general schematic of OIT and SLIT is provided in Fig. 5.2.

Divergent features of AIT clinical trials: Direct comparison of results of AIT studies is hampered by heterogeneous design. The following frequently differ between various trials: degree of allergic sensitization, duration of initial dose-escalation, build-up, maintenance phases, as well as avoidance period before SU OFC; protein quantity administered as daily maintenance dose, and criteria defining desensitization and SU. Although all trials report moderate and severe AE as well as administration of epinephrine, reporting of minor AE may differ, with some trials reporting only what are deemed clinically relevant dose-related AE, and others reporting all minor AE.

Oral immunotherapy in research trials and clinical practice

OIT is the only therapy currently accessible to physicians and patients, as food is often delivered in native form and can be purchased and/or prepared at home. In

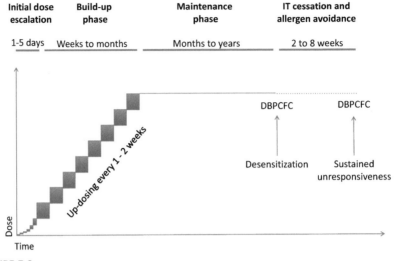

FIGURE 5.2

Typical protocol for oral and sublingual immunotherapy. Fig. 5.1. Typical protocol for oral (OIT) or sublingual (SLIT) immunotherapy. Initial dose escalation day(s) under medical supervision starting at subthreshold dose with increasing doses given every 30 minutes over several hours is more common for OIT than for SLIT. Highest tolerated dose given under observation is then continued daily at home, and increased every 1–2 weeks under supervision during the build-up phase. The dose achieved at the end of the build-up is continued daily during a maintenance phase. After months to years of maintenance, double-blind placebo-controlled food challenge (DBPCFC) to the food is performed to assess for desensitization. Daily dosing may then be discontinued for a period of 4–12 weeks and reintroduced during DBPCFC, to assess sustained unresponsiveness (SU).

Reprinted from Gernez Y, Nowak-Wegrzyn A. Immunotherapy for food allergy: are we there yet? J Allergy Clin Immunol Pract 2017;5:253, with permission from Elsevier.

the United States, several phase III clinical trials with AR101 (Aimmune Therapeutics) in subjects with peanut allergy are ongoing; pending favorable results, the FDA approval might be achieved by 2019. For these reasons, we provide a thorough discussion of evidence for and decisions around offering OIT in clinical practice.

Clinical trials for OIT: OIT remains a subject of active investigation, with most trials demonstrating efficacy limited by safety and adherence. Published studies evaluated milk, egg, peanut, and wheat OIT, with safety and efficacy varying by food allergen (Tables 5.3–5.5). In recent years, investigators evaluated OIT with modified proteins, with multiple foods, and/or combined with immunomodulatory agents (Tables 5.3 and 5.5). Direct comparison of clinical trials is often hampered by significant variations in protocol design.

Benefits of OIT: OIT induces desensitization in a majority of patients, although only a portion of those desensitized achieves SU.[8–17] For those achieving SU, long-

Table 5.3 Representative milk and egg oral immunotherapy trials.

Reference and design	Outcome (by ITT) and other significant findings
Native milk	
Meglio et al., 2004 Open-label	Desensitization to daily 200 mL dose in 71% of 21 subjects (age 5–10 y) considered to have severe cow milk allergy. 14% had dose-limiting symptoms.
Staden et al., 2007 RCT	64% of 25 subjects (14 milk, 11 egg) aged 1–12 y were able to incorporate the food into their diet after a mean of 21 months OIT with 100 mL/day milk or 1.5 g/day egg maintenance, compared to 35% of avoidance group ($P = .05$). 2 month-SU in 36% of OIT group. 4 moderate AE.
Skripak et al., 2008 RCT	Increased median eliciting dose of 5140 mg in 12 active subjects (age 6–17 y) 5140 mg, compared to 40 mg in 7 placebo subjects, after 6 months of therapy with 15 mL/day maintenance dose ($P < .001$). 1% of active doses elicit multi-system AE.
Narisety et al., 2009 Open-label follow up	Desensitization between 90 and 480 mL in 87% of 15 of the above subjects (age 6–17 y) after median 10 months OIT with 15 mL/day maintenance dose. 11% with multisystem reactions. EoE in 1 subject.
Pajno et al., 2010 RCT	Desensitization in 66% of active subjects (age 4–10 y), versus 0 of 15 placebo subjects, after 4.5 months of OIT with 200 mL maintenance dose. 3 severe AE.
Martorell et al., 2011 RCT	Desensitization to 200 mL in 90% of 30 active subjects (age 2–3 y) versus 23% of 30 placebo subjects, after 1 year OIT with 200 mL maintenance dose. 37% of patients with multisystem reaction.
Yanagida et al., 2015 Open label	Desensitization to 3 mL in 58% and to 25 mL in 33% of 12 active subjects (6–13 y) compared to 14% and 0% of 25 avoidance subjects ($P = .018$, $P = .007$, respectively), after 1 year OIT with 3 mL maintenance dose. 1 EAI after home dose.
Native egg	
Buchanan et al., 2007 Open-label	Desensitization to 8 g in 4 of 7 subjects (age 1–7 y) after 2 years OIT with 0.3 g/day maintenance dose. No severe AE.
Staden et al., 2007	See above under milk OIT
Vickery et al., 2010 Open-label	Desensitization to 3.9 g achieved in 75% of 8 subjects (age 3–13 y) after 18–40 months OIT with maximum 3.6 g/day maintenance dose. No severe AE.
Burks et al., 2012 RCT	Desensitization to 5 g in 55% of 40 active subjects (age 5–11 y) versus 0 of 15 placebo subjects after 10 months OIT with 2 g/day maintenance dose. SU in 28% of active. No severe AE.
Jones et al., 2016 Open-label follow up	4–6 week-SU to 10 g in 50% of 40 active subjects (age 5–11 y) after 4 years OIT. 1 year after study conclusion, 64% of active and 25% of placebo were consuming egg ($P = .04$). No severe AE.

Continued

Table 5.3 Representative milk and egg oral immunotherapy trials.—cont'd

Reference and design	Outcome (by ITT) and other significant findings
Caminiti et al., 2015 RCT	Desensitization to 4 g in 94% of 17 active subjects (age 4—10 y) versus 1 of 14 placebo after 4 months OIT with 4 g/day maintenance dose and 5 months egg-containing diet. 3 month-SU in 29%. 1 AE treated with EAI, 1 with SABA/steroid.
Escudero et al., 2015 RCT, open-label	Desensitization to 2.8 g in 93% and 1 month-SU to 2.8 g in 37% of 30 active subjects (age 5—17 y) after 3 months OIT with 1 egg (3.6 g), versus 1 of 31 on avoidance diet. 5 AE with respiratory distress.
Yanagida et al., 2016 RCT, open-label	2 week-SU to 0.2 g in 71% of 21 active subjects (age 6—19 y) with history of anaphylaxis or sIgE >30 kIU/L after 12 months OIT with 0.1—0.2 g maintenance dose, versus 0 of 12 on avoidance diet. SU to 1.8 g in 33% of active. No severe AE.
Perez-Rangel et al., 2017 RCT	Desensitization in 89% of 19 active subjects (mean age 10.4 y) after 5 months OIT with 3.6 g every 48 hours, versus 0 of 14 on placebo. 2 episodes anaphylaxis with build-up.
Modified egg and milk	
Goldberg et al., 2015 Open-label	20% of 15 subjects (age 6—12 y) tolerated 1.3 g/day dosing of baked milk and had increased challenge threshold after 12 months OIT. 2 episodes of anaphylaxis after home dosing.
Giavi et al., 2016 RCT	Rates of desensitization in 15 active subjects (aged 1—5 y) after 9 g hydrolyzed egg/day for 6 months compared to 14 placebo subjects. No entry OFC. No severe AE.
Bravin et al., 2016 Open-label	Desensitization to 1 boiled egg (3.6 g) in 53% of 15 subjects (aged 5—17 y) after 2—9 months OIT with 6.25 g baked egg/day. No moderate or severe AE.
Perezábad et al., 2017 Open-label	Desensitization to 200 mL cow milk in 70% of 20 subjects (age 1—11 y) after 18—36 months OIT with 25 g goat or sheep milk (30% protein). 6 subjects had severe AE or AE-related withdrawal.

AE, adverse effect; EoE, eosinophilic esophagitis; EAI, epinephrine auto-injector; ITT, intention to treat; OIT, oral immunotherapy; RCT, randomized controlled trial; SU, sustained unresponsiveness.

term follow-up studies demonstrate continued ingestion of offending food months to years after OIT completion.[10,15,18] In the first meta-analysis, Nurmatov and colleagues reported significant benefit of OIT for desensitization (RR = 0.14; 95% CI 0.08—0.24); and a nonsignificant benefit for SU (R = 0.29, 95% CI: 0.08—1.13).[19] OIT efficacy varies by food, protocol design (duration, dosing, and other aspects), and subjects (age, degree of sensitization, and concomitant allergic disease). Despite its risks and frequent adverse effects, OIT appears to improve quality of life (QoL),[20—22] food-related anxiety, social and dietary limitations. However, OIT has been associated with a worsening QoL among some patients with favorable scores before therapy.[23]

Table 5.4 Representative peanut and wheat oral immunotherapy clinical trials.

Design and reference	Outcome (by intention to treat) and other significant findings
Peanut	
Jones et al., 2009 Open-label	Desensitization to 3.9 g in 74% of 39 subjects (age 1–16 y) after 36 months OIT with 1.8 g/day maintenance. 2 EAI after home dosing.
Blumchen et al., 2010 Open-label	At 1-wk SU OFC, median highest tolerated dose among 23 subjects (age 3–14 y) was 1 g after 9 months OIT with 0.5 g/day minimum maintenance. 4 AE-related withdrawals.
Varshney et al., 2011 RCT	DS to 5 g in 84% of 19 active subjects (1–16 y) after 12 months OIT with 5 g maintenance, versus 0 on placebo ($P < .001$). No EAI after home dosing.
Anagnostou et al., 2011 Open-label	DS to 6.6 g in 64% of 22 subjects (age 4–18 y) after 9–17 months of OIT with 0.8 g/day maintenance. No EAI administrations.
Anagnostou et al., 2014 RCT	DS to 1.4 g in 50% of 49 active subjects (age 7–16 y) after 6 months OIT with 0.8 g/day maintenance, versus 0 of 46 on avoidance. 2 home EAI; dose-related wheeze in 22% of subjects
Vickery et al., 2014 Open-label, follow-up	4 week-SU to 5 g in 31% of 39 subjects (age 1–16 y) after 22 month of OIT with 4 g/day maximum daily maintenance dose. All with SU were consuming peanut 40 months post-OIT. 6 AE-related withdrawals.
Vickery et al., 2017 RCT	DS to 5 g in 81% and 1-month-SU in 78% of 37 subjects (age 9–36 months) after 29 months of OIT. No significant difference between daily maintenance with low (0.3 g, n = 20) and high dose (3 g, n = 17). No severe AE. 2 AE-related withdrawals.
Bird et al., 2017 RCT	DS to 0.443 and 1.043 g in 79% and 62% of 29 active subjects after 5–9 months OIT with 0.3 g/day maintenance, versus 19% and 0% on placebo. No severe AE. 6 AE-related withdrawals.
Wheat	
Rodriguez del Rio et al., 2014, open-label	DS to daily maintenance dose of 10.6 g in 5 or 6 subjects (age 5–11 y) with 6–7 months OIT. 2 urticarial reactions during maintenance.
Sato et al., 2015 Open-label	2 week-SU to 5.2 g in 61% of 18 subjects (age 5–14 y) considered highly sensitized, versus 9% of 11 historical controls on avoidance. 1 EAI after home dose.
Khayatzadeh et al., 2016 Open-label	DS to 5.2 g in 12 of 13 subjects (age 5–19 y) after 3 month OIT with 5.2 g/day maintenance dose. 3 patients required EAI for dose-related symptoms.

Continued

Table 5.4 Representative peanut and wheat oral immunotherapy clinical trials.—*cont'd*

Design and reference	Outcome (by intention to treat) and other significant findings
Lauener et al., 2017 Open-label	DS to 4.43 g in 4 of 9 patients (mean age 7.2 y) after 1 –6 months OIT with 10.2–35.2 g/day of hydrolyzed wheat protein maintenance dose

AE, adverse effect; DS, desensitization; EoE, eosinophilic esophagitis; EAI, epinephrine auto-injector; OFC, oral food challenge; OIT, oral immunotherapy; RCT, randomized controlled trial; SU, sustained unresponsiveness.

Table 5.5 Oral immunotherapy trials with omalizumab.

Design & reference	Outcome (by intention to treat) and other significant findings
Nadeau et al., 2011 Open-label	DS to 2 g in 82% of 11 subjects (age 7–12 y) after 6 months milk-OIT, with omalizumab for first 4 months. AE with 1.6% of doses. 2 EAI for dose-related AE after omalizumab cessation.
Wood et al., 2016 RCT	Reduced reactions (2% vs. 16%) and reduced drop-out (2 vs. 5) in 27 omalizumab-treated subjects (age 7–32 y) compared to 18 placebo, during 28 months of milk-OIT. DS rates not significantly different.
Martorell-Calatayud et al., 2016, open-label	All 14 milk or egg allergic subjects (age 3–11 y) intolerant of conventional OIT tolerated 200 mL milk or 1.8 g egg per day after 14 months OIT with omalizumab for first 2 months. Anaphylaxis 2.5–4 months after omalizumab cessation in 60% of milk and 33% of egg subjects.
Schneider et al., 2013 Open-label	92% of 13 highly sensitized subjects (age 7–15 y) completed therapy and achieved DS to 8 g peanut, with 8-month peanut-OIT with omalizumab for first 2 months. 2 grade 3 reactions.
MacGinnitie et al., 2017, RCT	Omalizumab-treated subjects (n = 29, age 6–19 y) tolerated peanut-OIT at higher doses, with 79% achieving DS to 4 g peanut, versus 1 of 8 placebo subjects ($P < .01$). AE after 8% of doses in active subjects compared to 17% in placebo subjects ($P = .15$).
Begin et al., 2014 Open-label	6 months of OIT for up to 5 foods (4 g protein/day per food) given with omalizumab for first 4 months enabled all 25 participants (age 4–15 y) to achieve doses 10-fold higher than eliciting dose at enrollment. Moderate reactions with 0.06% of doses and 1 EAI administration.

Peanut-OIT with probiotic was found to be cost-effective compared to avoidance in a long-term economic model, with incremental cost-effectiveness ratio of $2142 per quality-adjusted life year.[24]

Risks and challenges of OIT: Frequent and sometimes chronic and/or severe AE continue to limit broad application of OIT in practice. Most OIT subjects experience some symptoms with OIT; safety varies by allergen, with milk carrying increased risk of AE compared to peanut, egg, and perhaps wheat.

Dose-related symptoms are typically mild and limited to oropharyngeal pruritus, rhinitis, and abdominal discomfort. Occasionally, severe reactions occur, including vomiting, urticaria, angioedema, cough, and/or wheeze. Usually, symptoms are self-resolving; sometimes administration of antihistamine, short-acting beta agonists, or systemic steroids is required. Most OIT trials are also accompanied by a few severe reactions requiring epinephrine administrations. Although severe reactions occur most often during escalation, they can occur with home administration of previously tolerated doses. More chronic complications may include atopic dermatitis flare, chronic gastrointestinal (GI) discomfort, and eosinophilic esophagitis (EoE). Persistent, frequent, or severe symptoms often decrease adherence and result in withdrawals accompanying virtually every OIT trial.

In a meta-analysis of 25 OIT RCT, Nurmatov and colleagues reported increased risk of systemic reaction on OIT compared to controls (RR 1.16; 95% CI: 1.03−1.30).[19] In a retrospective analysis of pooled data from 104 participants in three pediatric peanut-OIT trials, Virkud and colleagues reported that 80% of OIT subjects experienced dose-related AE, with 72% and 47% reporting symptoms during build-up and maintenance, respectively. Over 90% of AEs occurred at home. Among the 104 subjects, 42% reported systemic symptoms, 49% GI symptoms; 59% received antihistamines and 12% epinephrine; 20% dropped out, with half of these drop-outs citing GI symptoms as the cause. Predictors of AEs (overall and during build-up and maintenance) included larger SPT wheal diameter (OR 1.4, $P = .005$) and allergic rhinitis (OR 2.9, $P < .001$), which were associated with increased GI AEs and systemic reactions, respectively. Asthma was associated with AE only in maintenance phase (OR 2.3, $P = .03$). Gender, age, IgE, and history of atopic dermatitis were not significantly associated with AE.[25]

Augmentation factors: Adverse reactions occurring with previously tolerated doses often occur in the setting of cofactors that lower allergic threshold, such as viral infection, febrile illness, active allergic rhinitis in the pollen season, physical exertion, or administration on an empty stomach.[26−29] To address cofactors, most OIT protocols advise dose adjustments in the setting of viral infection, avoidance of exertion in the hours following a dose, and administration after a full meal.

EoE: EoE has been reported in trials of milk-, peanut-, and egg-OIT.[9,17,28,30−32] A meta-analysis concluded that EoE may develop in up to 2.7% (95% CI: 1.7% −4.0%) of subjects, and often resolves on withdrawal of OIT.[33] It is possible more subjects develop OIT-related EoE than is reported, as some discontinue OIT for GI symptoms suspicious for EoE are not evaluated with endoscopy.[15,28,34] It is not clear whether OIT unmasks EoE or induces EoE in a way that other AIT therapy would not.

Adherence: OIT protocols require significant commitment from families and patients, including the flexibility in their schedules and access to transportation to return many times during the protocol. Initial dose escalation may require a full day (or several days depending on the protocol) in an inpatient setting. For build-up phases (which may take weeks to months), patients return every 1–2 weeks for observed dosing. Subjects take their dose every day for months to years; for patients with taste aversion, anxiety, or significant life events, this may prove challenging. Therefore, most OIT studies report withdrawals for issues not related to AE.

OIT with immunomodulatory agents: Use of omalizumab as pretreatment and during OIT build-up offers significant protection from dose-related IgE-mediated AE, allowing for safer and more rapid dose escalation. However, reactions to previously tolerated doses may occur after cessation of omalizumab.[30,35,36] Omalizumab does not alter risk of developing EoE on OIT. In addition, omalizumab does not enhance the efficacy of OIT.[17] Clinical trials of OIT with omalizumab are summarized in Table 5.5.

Another strategy to improve safety and efficacy of OIT has been concomitant administration of probiotic. Two studies published from one cohort of peanut-allergic subjects (age 1–10 years, mean 6 years; mean baseline peanut sIgE 14 kIU/L; mean SPT wheal diameter 18 mm) suggest administration of peanut OIT with probiotic (PPOIT) induces lasting tolerance in a majority. Investigators reported higher rates of desensitization (90% vs. 7%) and 2–5 week-SU (82% vs. 4%) among 31 PPOIT subjects compared to 28 placebo (placebo OIT and placebo probiotic) subjects.[13] A follow-up study published in 2017 found that after a mean of 4.2 years from PPIOT cessation, 67% of 24 PPOIT subjects were consuming peanut on a regular basis; and 58% of 12 PPIOT subjects demonstrated 8-week SU, compared to 1 of 12 placebo.[18] The impact of this RCT is significantly limited by the lack of a proper control for the effect of peanut-OIT alone, absence of blinding, and omission of confirmatory DBPCFC at baseline.

Studies of Chinese herbs have demonstrated evidence of immunomodulation without appreciable clinical benefit.[37] A clinical trial is underway evaluating combination of FAHF-2 (concentrated formulation to improve compliance), OIT, and omalizumab for multifood immunotherapy (NCT 02879006).

Offering OIT in clinical practice: The 2014 Updated Food Allergy Practice Parameter advised against performing OIT in the routine clinical practice.[3] The 2017 European Academy of Allergy and Clinical Immunology (EEACI) Task Force on Allergen Immunotherapy and the 2016 Japanese Society of Pediatric Allergy and Clinical Immunology recommended that OIT should be conducted in the medical facilities with special expertise and fully prepared to manage anaphylactic shock.[38,39] Severe reactions discussed later caution against a broad recommendation of OIT for FA.

OIT in the clinical setting continues to carry risk for severe reactions. In a retrospective chart review of 352 patients undergoing peanut-OIT in clinical practice, there were 95 severe reactions requiring EAI.[40] In Japan, an emergency audit of 287 hospitals performing clinical trials of OIT identified one child who has suffered cardiorespiratory arrest and brain damage with home dosing of milk, 3 months into the OIT treatment; 8 other children developed severe allergic symptoms during OIT or baseline OFC. The Japanese experience highlights the significant risks associated with food-OIT in clinical practice.[41]

Subjects who are highly sensitized or at risk for severe anaphylaxis are not appropriate candidates for OIT: lower threshold dose at entry challenge, higher sIgE, increased sIgE:total IgE ratio, larger SPT wheal diameter, and personal history of asthma or allergic rhinitis have been associated with worse outcomes, as measured by frequency of severe adverse event (SAE), adherence to treatment, and achievement of desensitization and SU.[10,11,15,25,34,42−44] Virtually every OIT trial excludes subjects with severe anaphylaxis, uncontrolled asthma, or other chronic conditions and medications that increase risk and severity of reactions. Risks of OIT may be unacceptable among patients and families who express hesitance in administering EAI. Adherence to therapy may be hampered by anxiety, taste aversions, and insufficient resources to ensure daily dose administration and regular follow-up.

If and when offering OIT in clinical practice, discussion should be informed by current evidence. Patients should be informed that lasting tolerance after discontinuation of therapy may not be achievable. With SLIT and EPIT becoming available in the next few years, it may be that waiting for a safer option is a better strategy for some. Alternatively, it may become clear that immunotherapies are more effective and/or safer in younger children, and should be started sooner rather than waiting for safer AIT to become available. Evidence on the safe and effective use of OIT will continue to accumulate in the coming years, with additional guidelines from experts likely to follow.

Sublingual immunotherapy trials

Efficacy: SLIT induces modest increased threshold for reactivity in a majority.[9,12] Published SLIT trials have evaluated utility in treatment hazelnut, peanut, and milk allergy.[45−48] In the first meta-analysis of SLIT studies, Nurmatov and colleagues reported significant benefit of SLIT for desensitization with RR of 0.26 (95% CI: 0.10, 0.64), which was reduced compared to OIT (RR = 0.14).[19]

Risks: AEs are common in SLIT, but are typically limited to mild and transient oropharyngeal pruritus. Moderate and severe AE occur with less frequency in SLIT compared to OIT, contributing to improved adherence over OIT.[47] In the abovementioned meta-analysis, systemic reactions did not appear to be increased compared to controls (RR = 0.98, 95% CI: 0.85, 1.14).[19] Cofactors, as described with OIT, appear to lower threshold for reactivity to SLIT.[45] Occurrence of EoE in association with aeroallergen-SLIT[49,50] suggests a theoretic risk for EoE with food-SLIT.

SLIT trials: Three RCTs have shown SLIT efficacy in inducing desensitization compared to placebo with favorable safety profile. The first, published in 2005, reported desensitization to 20 g hazelnut in 50% of 12 SLIT subjects compared to 9% of 11 placebo subjects, after 8–12 weeks of therapy. Mean eliciting dose increased significantly from 2.3 to 11.6 g in SLIT subjects ($P = .02$). Regarding safety, there were three systemic reactions, all of which occurred during build-up and responded to antihistamine. Mild reactions accompanied 7.4% of doses.[45]

In the first peanut SLIT RCT, Kim and colleagues reported that at completion of 12–18 months of SLIT, the 11 active SLIT subjects (age 1–11 years) ingested 20 times more peanut protein (PP) than seven placebo subjects ($P = .011$). Symptoms accompanied 11.5% of active and 8.6% of placebo doses; all except one home dose-related AE resolved with antihistamine alone; no EAIs were required.[47]

A 44-week SLIT protocol among older SLIT subjects (12–37 y), reported that 70% of 20 SLIT subjects responded (ingested 5 g peanut or 10-fold more than baseline), compared to 15% of 20 placebo subjects ($P < .001$). Symptoms accompanied 37% of doses; 2.9% required treatment, with 1 administration of albuterol and 1 of EAI.[48] In open-label follow-up study of this study, a small portion of SLIT subjects (11% of 37 subjects) went on to achieve 8-week SU to 10 g peanut. Twenty-five withdrew for various reasons, including 2 for dose-related AE.[46]

Two RCTs demonstrate that compared to OIT, SLIT has improved safety but reduced efficacy in inducing desensitization and SU. Narisety and colleagues reported 141-fold mean increase in highest tolerated dose among peanut-OIT subjects compared to 22-fold mean increase among SLIT subjects at the conclusion of 1 year of therapy. One-month SU was achieved by 3 of 10 OIT subjects compared to 1 of 10 SLIT. SLIT subjects experienced less severe AE, with 5 EAI administrations related to OIT versus none with SLIT.[12] In 2012, Keet and colleagues compared milk SLIT alone to therapy with SLIT for initial up-dosing followed by milk-OIT. SLIT/OIT subjects were significantly more likely to demonstrate desensitization (70% of 20) and 6 week-SU (40% of 20) compared to subjects receiving SLIT alone (1 of 10). Multisystem reactions and medical intervention (antihistamine, albuterol, and EAI) were more frequent with OIT.[9]

Epicutaneous immunotherapy trials

Efficacy: EPIT therapy for peanut and milk have been shown to increase threshold for reactivity in three published trials, with more modest efficacy compared to OIT and SLIT.[5]

Advantages: Although efficacy is less than OIT and SLIT, EPIT appears to have the most favorable side-effect profile. Most AEs are limited to local cutaneous symptoms, though occasional systemic reactions occur.[5,51] With reduced AE and fewer visits to a medical facility for up-dosing, adherence may be better with EPIT compared to OIT and SLIT.

EPIT trials: EPIT with milk and peanut is under active investigation.[6,5] In a phase IIb multicenter RCT comparing varying doses of peanut EPIT among peanut allergic subjects aged 6–55 years, investigators reported a significant response (defined as either ≥10-times increase in eliciting dose or tolerating ≥1 g PP) in subjects treated with 250 μg-patch for 12 months compared (50%) to placebo (25%, $P = .01$). When analyzed by age strata, only the 6–11-year-old group had a statistically significant response compared to placebo. There were no serious dose-related AEs and adherence was 97.6%.[52]

The press release regarding the topline results of the phase III trial (PEPITES, Peanut EPIT Efficacy and Safety) in children 4–11 years old, reported 35.3% of patients responding to VP 250 μg after 12 months, compared to 13.6% of placebo-patients (21.7% difference; 95% CI = 12.4%–29.8%; $P = .00,001$). However, the primary endpoint, defined as the 95% confidence interval (CI) in the difference in response rates between the active and placebo arms, did not reach the 15% lower bound proposed in the study's Statistical Analysis Plan. As an important secondary endpoint, investigators reported a significantly greater increase in mean eliciting dose among VP 250 subjects (from 144 to 444 mg PP) compared to placebo (no increase in mean eliciting dose) after 12 months of therapy ($P < .001$). PEPITES reported 12 SAE in 10 active-subjects (4.2%), of which 4 SAE in 3 active subjects (1.3%) were possibly related to treatment; and 6 SAE in 6 placebo-subjects (5.1%). No SAE was qualified as severe anaphylaxis. The most commonly reported AEs were mild-moderate patch application site reactions. The discontinuation rate of 10.1% was similar in active- and placebo-arms, with a 1.1% dropout due to treatment-emergent AE. Mean patient adherence exceeded 95%.

Immune mechanisms of AIT clinical trials of additional forms of AIT

Other forms of AIT studied in human subjects include SCIT with alum-adsorbed hypoallergen and LAMP-DNA-peanut-vaccine. A phase IIb clinical trial evaluating safety and efficacy of SCIT with alum-adsorbed, recombinant fish allergen parvalbumin (NCT02382718) is completed but not as yet published. Preliminary results of a clinical trial evaluating safety and immunomodulation with alum-adsorbed chemically modified peanut extract (NCT02851277)[53], have been presented in the abstract form. In this phase I study, subjects were randomized to receive 15–20 incrementally increasing weekly doses of study product (HAL-MPE, N = 17) or placebo (N = 6). Local and systemic reactions were observed more often in the active group; no late (>4 hours after therapy) systemic reactions were observed. Authors concluded that the therapy was safe and well tolerated.[53]

Two additional forms of AIT, including SCIT with native peanut allergen and rectally administered modified PP vaccine, were previously studied in humans and abandoned due to unacceptable safety profile.[54–56]

Future directions

A race to develop commercial treatment for FA is fueled by increasing prevalence and severity of FA in children, particularly peanut allergy. The large phase III clinical trials of peanut-OIT and peanut-EPIT are ongoing. There is a need for an approved, standardized protocol for food-AIT that can be safely and effectively implemented in clinical practice. We need to establish the minimum effective and safe maintenance dose, duration of AIT and frequency of maintenance dosing for long-term therapy. Considering that at least 30% of those with persistent food allergy are allergic to multiple foods, there is a need for a strategy for combining multiple foods. Approaches to mitigating side effects of AIT as well as mechanisms to enhance efficacy and development of permanent oral tolerance such as adjuvants, nanoparticles, or DNA vaccines need to be explored. Biomarkers predictive of the favorable response to AIT are highly desirable. Patients with the most severe phenotype of life-threatening anaphylaxis are currently excluded from clinical trials, yet they are in the dire need of effective treatment. The most exciting developments are within monoclonal antibodies against IL-4/IL-3 receptor, IL-33, IL-13 and possibly TSLP and IL-9. These biologic therapies alone or combined with AIT may lead to a breakthrough in FA treatment. A tremendous progress has occurred in the past decade but the permanent cure for FA remains elusive and further research into tolerance development is necessary.

References

1. Nwaru BI, Hickstein L, Panesar SS, Roberts G, Muraro A, Sheikh A. Prevalence of common food allergies in Europe: a systematic review and meta-analysis. *Allergy.* 2014; 69(8):992−1007.
2. Gupta RS, Springston EE, Warrier MR, et al. The prevalence, severity, and distribution of childhood food allergy in the United States. *Pediatrics.* 2011;128(1):e9−17.
3. Sampson HA, Aceves S, Bock SA, et al. Food allergy: a practice parameter update-2014. *J Allergy Clin Immunol.* 2014;134(5):1016−1025 e1043.
4. Savage J, Sicherer S, Wood R. The natural history of food allergy. *J Allergy Clin Immunol Pract.* 2016;4(2):196−203. quiz 204.
5. Jones SM, Sicherer SH, Burks AW, et al. Epicutaneous immunotherapy for the treatment of peanut allergy in children and young adults. *J Allergy Clin Immunol.* 2017;139(4): 1242−1252. e1249.
6. Jones SM, Agbotounou WK, Fleischer DM, et al. Safety of epicutaneous immunotherapy for the treatment of peanut allergy: a phase 1 study using the Viaskin patch. *J Allergy Clin Immunol.* 2016;137(4):1258−1261. e1251-1210.
7. Jongejan L, van Ree R, Poulsen LK. Hypoallergenic molecules for subcutaneous immunotherapy. *Expert Rev Clin Immunol.* 2016;12(1):5−7.
8. Burks AW, Jones SM, Wood RA, et al. Oral immunotherapy for treatment of egg allergy in children. *N Engl J Med.* 2012;367(3):233−243.
9. Keet CA, Frischmeyer-Guerrerio PA, Thyagarajan A, et al. The safety and efficacy of sublingual and oral immunotherapy for milk allergy. *J Allergy Clin Immunol.* 2012; 129(2):448−455, 455 e441−445.
10. Vickery BP, Scurlock AM, Kulis M, et al. Sustained unresponsiveness to peanut in subjects who have completed peanut oral immunotherapy. *J Allergy Clin Immunol.* 2014; 133(2):468−475.

11. Vickery BP, Berglund JP, Burk CM, et al. Early oral immunotherapy in peanut-allergic preschool children is safe and highly effective. *J Allergy Clin Immunol.* 2017;139(1): 173–181. e178.

12. Narisety SD, Frischmeyer-Guerrerio PA, Keet CA, et al. A randomized, double-blind, placebo-controlled pilot study of sublingual versus oral immunotherapy for the treatment of peanut allergy. *J Allergy Clin Immunol.* 2015;135(5):1275–1282. e1271-1276.

13. Tang ML, Ponsonby AL, Orsini F, et al. Administration of a probiotic with peanut oral immunotherapy: a randomized trial. *J Allergy Clin Immunol.* 2015;135(3):737–744. e738.

14. Caminiti L, Pajno GB, Crisafulli G, et al. Oral immunotherapy for egg allergy: a double-blind placebo-controlled study, with postdesensitization follow-up. *J Allergy Clin Immunol Pract.* 2015;3(4):532–539.

15. Escudero C, Rodriguez Del Rio P, Sanchez-Garcia S, et al. Early sustained unresponsiveness after short-course egg oral immunotherapy: a randomized controlled study in egg-allergic children. *Clin Exp Allergy.* 2015;45(12):1833–1843.

16. Yanagida N, Sato S, Asaumi T, Nagakura K, Ogura K, Ebisawa M. Safety and efficacy of low-dose oral immunotherapy for hen's egg allergy in children. *Int Arch Allergy Immunol.* 2016;171(3–4):265–268.

17. Wood RA, Kim JS, Lindblad R, et al. A randomized, double-blind, placebo-controlled study of omalizumab combined with oral immunotherapy for the treatment of cow's milk allergy. *J Allergy Clin Immunol.* 2016;137(4):1103–1110. e1111.

18. Hsiao KC, Ponsonby AL, Axelrad C, Pitkin S, Tang MLK, PPOIT Study Team. Long-term clinical and immunological effects of probiotic and peanut oral immunotherapy after treatment cessation: 4-year follow-up of a randomised, double-blind, placebo-controlled trial. *Lancet Child Adolesc Health.* 2017;1(2):97–105. https://doi.org/10.1016/S2352-4642(17)30041-X. Epub 2017 Aug 15. Erratum in: Lancet Child Adolesc Health 1(3), 2017, e2. PMID: 30169215.

19. Nurmatov U, Dhami S, Arasi S, et al. Allergen immunotherapy for IgE-mediated food allergy: a systematic review and meta-analysis. *Allergy.* 2017;72(8):1133–1147.

20. Anagnostou K, Islam S, King Y, et al. Assessing the efficacy of oral immunotherapy for the desensitisation of peanut allergy in children (STOP II): a phase 2 randomised controlled trial. *Lancet.* 2014;383(9925):1297–1304.

21. Factor JM, Mendelson L, Lee J, Nouman G, Lester MR. Effect of oral immunotherapy to peanut on food-specific quality of life. *Ann Allergy Asthma Immunol.* 2012;109(5): 348–352. e342.

22. Carraro S, Frigo AC, Perin M, et al. Impact of oral immunotherapy on quality of life in children with cow milk allergy: a pilot study. *Int J Immunopathol Pharmacol.* Jul-Sep 2012;25(3):793–798.

23. Rigbi NE, Goldberg MR, Levy MB, Nachshon L, Golobov K, Elizur A. Changes in patient quality of life during oral immunotherapy for food allergy. *Allergy.* May 22, 2017.

24. Shaker MS. An economic analysis of a peanut oral immunotherapy study in children. *J Allergy Clin Immunol Pract.* June 09, 2017.

25. Virkud YV, Burks AW, Steele PH, et al. Novel baseline predictors of adverse events during oral immunotherapy in children with peanut allergy. *J Allergy Clin Immunol.* 2017; 139(3):882–888. e885.

26. Skripak JM, Nash SD, Rowley H, et al. A randomized, double-blind, placebo-controlled study of milk oral immunotherapy for cow's milk allergy. *J Allergy Clin Immunol.* 2008; 122(6):1154–1160.

27. Staden U, Rolinck-Werninghaus C, Brewe F, Wahn U, Niggemann B, Beyer K. Specific oral tolerance induction in food allergy in children: efficacy and clinical patterns of reaction. *Allergy.* 2007;62(11):1261−1269.
28. MacGinnitie AJ, Rachid R, Gragg H, et al. Omalizumab facilitates rapid oral desensitization for peanut allergy. *J Allergy Clin Immunol.* 2017;139(3):873−881. e878.
29. Rodriguez del Rio P, Diaz-Perales A, Sanchez-Garcia S, et al. Oral immunotherapy in children with IgE-mediated wheat allergy: outcome and molecular changes. *J Investig Allergol Clin Immunol.* 2014;24(4):240−248.
30. Nadeau KC, Schneider LC, Hoyte L, Borras I, Umetsu DT. Rapid oral desensitization in combination with omalizumab therapy in patients with cow's milk allergy. *J Allergy Clin Immunol.* 2011;127(6):1622−1624.
31. Narisety SD, Skripak JM, Steele P, et al. Open-label maintenance after milk oral immunotherapy for IgE-mediated cow's milk allergy. *J Allergy Clin Immunol.* 2009;124(3): 610−612.
32. Garcia Rodriguez R, Mendez Diaz Y, Moreno Lozano L, Extremera Ortega A, Gomez Torrijos E. Eosinophilic esophagitis after egg oral immunotherapy in an adult with egg-allergy and egg-bird syndrome. *J Investig Allergol Clin Immunol.* 2017;27(4): 266−267.
33. Lucendo AJ, Arias A, Tenias JM. Relation between eosinophilic esophagitis and oral immunotherapy for food allergy: a systematic review with meta-analysis. *Ann Allergy Asthma Immunol.* 2014;113(6):624−629.
34. Perez-Rangel I, Rodriguez Del Rio P, Escudero C, Sanchez-Garcia S, Sanchez-Hernandez JJ, Ibanez MD. Efficacy and safety of high-dose rush oral immunotherapy in persistent egg allergic children: a randomized clinical trial. *Ann Allergy Asthma Immunol.* 2017;118(3):356, 364 e353.
35. Martorell-Calatayud C, Michavila-Gomez A, Martorell-Aragones A, et al. Anti-IgE-assisted desensitization to egg and cow's milk in patients refractory to conventional oral immunotherapy. *Pediatr Allergy Immunol.* 2016;27(5):544−546.
36. Begin P, Dominguez T, Wilson SP, et al. Phase 1 results of safety and tolerability in a rush oral immunotherapy protocol to multiple foods using Omalizumab. *Allergy Asthma Clin Immunol.* 2014;10(1):7.
37. Wang J, Jones SM, Pongracic JA, et al. Safety, clinical, and immunologic efficacy of a Chinese herbal medicine (Food Allergy Herbal Formula-2) for food allergy. *J Allergy Clin Immunol.* 2015;136(4):962−970 e961.
38. Pajno GB, Fernandez-Rivas M, Arasi S, et al. EAACI Guidelines on allergen immunotherapy: IgE-mediated food allergy. *Allergy.* September 27, 2017.
39. Ebisawa M, Ito K, Fujisawa T. Committee for Japanese pediatric guideline for food allergy TJSoPA, clinical immunology TJSoA. Japanese guidelines for food allergy 2017. *Allergol Int.* 2017;66(2):248−264.
40. Wasserman RL, Factor JM, Baker JW, et al. Oral immunotherapy for peanut allergy: multipractice experience with epinephrine-treated reactions. *J Allergy Clin Immunol Pract.* 2014;2(1):91−96.
41. Kawamura T. *Study: 9 Children Suffer Severe Symptoms in Food-Allergy Trial.* The Asahi Shimbun; 2017. http://www.asahi.com/ajw/articles/AJ201711200043.html.
42. Blumchen K, Ulbricht H, Staden U, et al. Oral peanut immunotherapy in children with peanut anaphylaxis. *J Allergy Clin Immunol.* 2010;126(1):83−91.

43. Jones SM, Burks AW, Keet C, et al. Long-term treatment with egg oral immunotherapy enhances sustained unresponsiveness that persists after cessation of therapy. *J Allergy Clin Immunol.* 2016;137(4):1117−1127. e1110.

44. Anagnostou K, Clark A, King Y, Islam S, Deighton J, Ewan P. Efficacy and safety of high-dose peanut oral immunotherapy with factors predicting outcome. *Clin Exp Allergy.* 2011;41(9):1273−1281.

45. Enrique E, Pineda F, Malek T, et al. Sublingual immunotherapy for hazelnut food allergy: a randomized, double-blind, placebo-controlled study with a standardized hazelnut extract 2. *J Allergy Clin Immunol.* 2005;116(5):1073−1079.

46. Burks AW, Wood RA, Jones SM, et al. Sublingual immunotherapy for peanut allergy: long-term follow-up of a randomized multicenter trial. *J Allergy Clin Immunol.* 2015; 135(5):1240−1248. e1241-1243.

47. Kim EH, Bird JA, Kulis M, et al. Sublingual immunotherapy for peanut allergy: clinical and immunologic evidence of desensitization. *J Allergy Clin Immunol.* 2011;127(3): 640−646. e641.

48. Fleischer DM, Burks AW, Vickery BP, et al. Sublingual immunotherapy for peanut allergy: a randomized, double-blind, placebo-controlled multicenter trial. *J Allergy Clin Immunol.* 2013;131(1):119−127. e111-117.

49. Bene J, Ley D, Roboubi R, Gottrand F, Gautier S. Eosinophilic esophagitis after desensitization to dust mites with sublingual immunotherapy. *Ann Allergy Asthma Immunol.* 2016;116(6):583−584.

50. Miehlke S, Alpan O, Schroder S, Straumann A. Induction of eosinophilic esophagitis by sublingual pollen immunotherapy. *Case Rep Gastroenterol.* 2013;7(3):363−368.

51. Dupont C, Kalach N, Soulaines P, Legoue-Morillon S, Piloquet H, Benhamou PH. Cow's milk epicutaneous immunotherapy in children: a pilot trial of safety, acceptability, and impact on allergic reactivity. *J Allergy Clin Immunol.* 2010;125(5):1165−1167.

52. Sampson HA, Shreffler WG, Yang WH, et al. Effect of varying doses of epicutaneous immunotherapy vs placebo on reaction to peanut protein exposure among patients with peanut sensitivity: a randomized clinical trial. *JAMA.* 2017;14(18):1798−1809. ;318.

53. Bindslev-Jensen C. SCIT-treatment with a chemically modified aluminum hydroxide adsorbed peanut extract (HAL-MPE1) was generally safe and well tolerated and showed immunological changes in peanut allergic patients. *J Allergy Clin Immunol.* 2017;(Suppl. S):AB191.

54. Oppenheimer JJ, Nelson HS, Bock SA, Christensen F, Leung DY. Treatment of peanut allergy with rush immunotherapy. *J Allergy Clin Immunol.* 1992;90(2):256−262.

55. Nelson HS, Lahr J, Rule R, Bock A, Leung D. Treatment of anaphylactic sensitivity to peanuts by immunotherapy with injections of aqueous peanut extract. *J Allergy Clin Immunol.* 1997;99(6 Pt 1):744−751.

56. Wood RA, Sicherer SH, Burks AW, et al. A phase 1 study of heat/phenol-killed, E. coli-encapsulated, recombinant modified peanut proteins Ara h 1, Ara h 2, and Ara h 3 (EMP-123) for the treatment of peanut allergy. *Allergy.* 2013;68(6):803−808.

57. Liu MA. DNA vaccines: an historical perspective and view to the future. *Immunol Rev.* 2011;239(1):62−84.

58. Su Y, Connolly M, Marketon A, Heiland T. CryJ-LAMP DNA vaccines for Japanese red cedar allergy induce robust Th1-type immune responses in murine model. *J Immunol Res.* 2016;2016:4857869.

59. Schofield AT. A case of egg poisoning. *Lancet.* 1908;1:716.

Venom immunotherapy

David B.K. Golden, MD

Associate Professor of Medicine, Johns Hopkins University, Baltimore, MD, United States

Background

Venom immunotherapy (VIT) may be one of the newest allergen classes introduced for immunotherapy, but it rapidly became the model for understanding and optimizing immunotherapy.[1] When they were introduced in 1979, Hymenoptera venom was the first allergen extract to be standardized and approved by the Federal Drug Administration (FDA). It is the only form of allergen immunotherapy (AIT) to be approved for the prevention of anaphylactic reactions. There are many unique things about VIT, but overall it has more similarities to, than differences from, all other types of AIT. The potential differences are related to the ways that the allergen is introduced into the "host." The route of exposure is not through the respiratory mucosa but by insect sting, i.e., injection. Thus, the reaction is systemic, not local. The exposure (insect sting) is discrete, sporadic, infrequent, and dramatic. The reaction is unpredictable and is not measured in sneezes, symptom score, medications score, air flow, or frequency of exacerbations, it is measured in near-catastrophic events. And yet the approach to immunotherapy is fundamentally the same: to reduce the mast cell response to allergen by the administration of progressively larger doses of allergen on a regular basis and induction of immune tolerance.

Patient selection

The goal of VIT is primarily to prevent anaphylaxis. Individuals who have been sensitized to a stinging insect are at risk. Therefore, the prediction of anaphylaxis is the goal of treatment. Unfortunately, there is no test that reliably predicts the outcome of a sting. There are a number of clinical and laboratory markers of the risk of sting anaphylaxis (Table 6.1).[2] Treatment should be based on the patient's clinical history and perceived risk. These can include a family history of insect sting allergy, or a general fear perhaps based on their history of other allergic problems or reactions. It could be a history of mild local reaction or severe local reaction to a sting. Or it could be a previous systemic reaction ranging from vague constitutional symptoms to mild generalized urticaria, or life-threatening anaphylactic shock. A key issue is the natural history of the condition, that is, what will happen with future

Table 6.1 Risk factors for severe reactions to stings.

Clinical markers	Laboratory markers
Very severe previous reaction	Venom skin test
Insect species	Venom-specific IgE
No urticaria/angioedema	Basal serum tryptase
Age (>45 years), Gender (male)	Basophil activation test[a]
Multiple or sequential stings	Platelet activating factor (PAF)-acetylhydrolase[a]
Medications (ACE inhibitors)	Angiotensin converting enzyme (ACE)

[a] *Not commercially available.*
Reproduced from: Golden DBK, Demain J, Freeman T et al. Stinging insect hypersensitivity: A practice parameter update 2016. Ann Allergy Asthma Immunol. 2017;118:28–54.

stings? People hear advice ranging from "the next one will kill you" to "don't worry, it was a fluke, it never happened before and won't happen again." Both are theoretically possible, and both are quite unlikely. The stratification of risk has become the focus of the diagnosis and management of insect sting allergy, and determines how we counsel our patients, whether we prescribe epinephrine autoinjectors, whether we recommend VIT, and when we recommend to discontinue VIT.

As in most other types of AIT, treatment is generally recommended mainly for patients with the most severe symptoms, or in the case of VIT, the greatest risk of future sting anaphylaxis.[2] This primarily applies to those with previous moderate to severe anaphylactic reactions to stings and positive diagnostic tests for venom-specific IgE. There are many permutations to the history, including the passage of decades without a sting, uneventful intervening stings, additive factors (exercise/heat, alcohol, medications, number or sequence of stings), the subjective or objective pattern of symptoms and signs, and response to treatment. The product package insert for commercial Hymenoptera venom extracts recommends VIT for all systemic reactions (including mild cutaneous systemic reactions) in all age groups for an indefinite period of time.

Who does not need VIT?

Patients with a history of systemic reactions limited to cutaneous signs and symptoms (pruritus, urticaria, flushing, angioedema) without involvement of any other organ systems have a relatively low risk for a more severe (anaphylactic) reaction to a future sting and therefore do not require VIT. The perception of "low risk" is relative, and some patients find a 2%–3% risk of anaphylaxis to be unacceptable, so VIT may be indicated for quality-of-life reasons in some patients. The same is true for patients with allergic large local reactions to stings. As with virtually all other allergens, asymptomatic sensitization is not an indication for VIT in this case because the risk of anaphylaxis to a future sting is relatively low (5%–15%).[3,4] A personal or family history of atopy is not an indicator of risk of anaphylaxis to stings, although asymptomatic sensitization is more common in individuals with sensitization to environmental allergens.[5] Similarly, a family history of insect allergy alone is not an indication for testing or treatment. The great majority of patients with insect sting anaphylaxis do not have affected family members.[6]

High-risk patients

There are a number of clinical and laboratory markers that indicate a high risk for severe anaphylaxis to stings. The most obvious is the severity of the previous sting reaction(s). This is the same as the observation that patients with severe asthma exacerbations have the greatest risk of future severe asthma exacerbations. Patients who have had extreme or near-fatal anaphylaxis have a higher chance of systemic reaction to a future sting and are most likely to have another severe reaction.[7] They are also more likely to relapse if they stop VIT, even after 5—10 years.[8–10]

The other very strong risk factor is elevated baseline serum tryptase, with or without mastocytosis.[11,12] A very special relation has emerged between mast cell disorders and sting anaphylaxis. The baseline serum tryptase is elevated in more than 10% of patients with systemic reactions to stings, and in more than 25% of those with hypotension.[13] The highest frequency occurs in males with rapid onset hypotensive shock, but no cutaneous signs, after a sting.[14] Mastocytosis occurs in at least 2% of all patients with insect sting anaphylaxis.[15] Insect stings are the most common cause of anaphylaxis in patients with mastocytosis.[16] A recent study reported that mastocytosis patients with positive tests for venom IgE have a 93% frequency of anaphylaxis if they are stung, and a very low frequency of asymptomatic sensitization (unlike the general population).[17] It is also known that these patients have more chance of unpredictable systemic reactions to VIT injections, less reliable protection from sting reactions (75% instead of 95%), and more chance of relapse (even fatal) if they discontinue VIT.[15] It is now recommended that patients with mastocytosis should have venom IgE tests and, if positive, should be counseled on the rationale for VIT. Tryptase may not be the only mast cell mediator to prove clinically useful. Platelet activating factor (PAF) and PAF-acetylhydrolase show predictive value for fatal and near-fatal anaphylaxis to foods and insect stings.[18] In the future, patient selection for VIT may include measurement of multiple mast cell mediators.

Frequent exposure to insect stings is a relative risk factor for reaction both because of the greater number of opportunities for reaction and the potential for augmented allergic responses after sequential stings. Beekeepers, in particular, have a higher than average chance of sensitization and of allergic reactions. They also have many unique features depending on their pattern of exposure. Some will have allergic reactions initially in the spring because their unresponsiveness is not maintained during the off-season, but is rapidly restored after a couple of stings in the spring. Some can self-immunize if they get two to three stings every 2—3 weeks all year round (100–150 stings/year). And those who get large numbers of stings in the long term will show elevated venom-specific IgG4 but no specific IgE.[19]

Some medications may increase the risk of severe anaphylaxis to stings or VIT. Beta-blockers may increase the risk of severe anaphylaxis by interfering with the action of epinephrine. Angiotensin converting enzyme inhibitors (ACEIs) increase the risk of angioedema or severe anaphylaxis by their effects on kinin pathways. There are conflicting data on the degree of risk in patients with insect sting anaphylaxis who are not on VIT.[12,20] The risk may be lower in those who are on maintenance VIT. The medical risks of stopping or changing the medication may exceed the risk of continuing the medication while receiving VIT.[21] When it is not possible to change the medication with acceptable safety, VIT should be given with suitable caution.

Hymenoptera venom extracts

Hymenoptera insects are collected and identified for species specificity by trained experts. Honeybee venom can be collected when the insects sting against an electric grid. Vespid insects are collected in the wild, and the venom extracted from the venom sacs after they are manually dissected from the bodies. The venoms are purified, solubilized, stabilized, and lyophilized for commercial use. In the United States, FDA-approved Hymenoptera venom extracts are currently manufactured only by HollisterStier Lab (Spokane, WA). The characteristics of these products have been reviewed elsewhere.[22] When products were available from other laboratories, they were considered interchangeable, even though there are known, and potentially unknown, differences that exist.[23] There are five Hymenoptera venom extracts on the market: honeybee, yellow jacket, yellow hornet, white-faced hornet, and Polistes, wasp venoms. Both the yellow jacket and Polistes venoms are mixtures of several common species. There is also a "mixed vespid venom" containing equal parts of yellow jacket, yellow hornet, and white-faced hornet venoms. All the Hymenoptera venom extracts require reconstitution with albumin-saline diluent to a concentration of 100 mcg/mL (300 mcg/mL for mixed vespid venom).

Imported fire ant venom is quite different from the other Hymenoptera venoms. A purified venom product is not commercially available. The venom is only a small proportion of the total weight in whole body extracts. Although purified fire ant venom is superior for diagnostic skin testing, and presumably for VIT, and despite the lack of a controlled trial of fire ant whole body extract immunotherapy, there is evidence that this treatment is clinically effective.[24] There are two species of IFA, *Solenopsis invicta* and *Solenopsis richterii*. Their venoms (and whole body extracts) are very similar but not antigenically identical.

Initiation of VIT

To begin VIT, one must select the venoms to be used, a target dose for maintenance treatment, and an updosing regimen for initial treatment. There is disagreement about whether it is best to treat with all venoms giving positive tests for venom IgE, or whether to include only the insect(s) that caused known anaphylactic reactions. The most cautious approach, and that preferred in the published Practice Parameters, is to be all inclusive. However, when the only known culprit has been imported fire ants, it may not be necessary to test or treat for the other venoms.

The target maintenance dose is 100 mcg of each venom. This was originally based on the empiric observation that it is equal to two honeybee stings. Vespid stings can deliver only 2–20 mcg per sting, so the 100 mcg dose may be equivalent to about 10 stings. Children may be equally protected by a maintenance dose of 50 mcg of honeybee or yellow jacket venom.[25] This approach (using a fixed maintenance dose) is somewhat different than that used most commonly for inhalant AIT, where the "highest tolerated dose" is often considered a suitable maintenance dose. With AIT, we may be willing to accept slightly less complete control of symptoms, but for sting anaphylaxis we want to prevent the reaction not partially, but completely. This is why every patient is expected to achieve the full maintenance dose, and failure to do so justifies special measures.

The clinician must choose an initial buildup schedule. The original two FDA-approved product package inserts showed two different buildup schedules: one "conventional" (16–20 weeks to reach the maintenance dose; HollisterStier Labs) and the other "semi-rush" (8 weeks; ALK Labs). There is no difference in the safety or efficacy of these two regimens. Rush regimens (2–3 days to reach 100 mcg) also show remarkable safety with VIT, even though when used with inhalant AIT they have been shown to carry more risk of systemic reactions. Ultrarush regimens (3–6 hours) have clearly greater risk of adverse events. Rush regimens of VIT have been shown to be safe even in a variety of high-risk patients and should be considered whenever practicable.[26] However, some literature suggest rush VIT carries a significant risk. More studies are needed to determine if VIT with or without premedication is safe.

Efficacy and safety

VIT is the most efficacious form of immunotherapy yet reported. In the controlled clinical trial of VIT, 98% of patients had no systemic reaction to a sting challenge.[27] This high degree of protection is achieved with mixed vespid venoms, but not quite as well by single vespid venoms (90%–95%) or by honeybee venom (75%–85%). Some experts recommend that beekeepers should receive a maintenance dose of 200 mcg to achieve more reliable protection. The onset of protection is established as soon as the full dose is reached, regardless of the regimen.[28]

The safety of VIT, perhaps surprisingly in patients being treated for anaphylactic sensitivities, is as good or better than that of any other AIT. Large local (injection site) reactions are common but rarely interfere with the buildup schedule. Unlike inhalant AIT, we try not to reduce the dose when there are large local reactions. This is partly because the maintenance dose for VIT is not determined by the patient's tolerance but by the need for protection from anaphylaxis, which is only achieved with the full 100 mcg dose. Systemic symptoms may occur in 10% −15% of patients but are usually mild. Systemic reactions requiring epinephrine injection occur in less than 5% during buildup and are rare during maintenance treatment. Large local reactions can be reduced by taking an H1-blocker prior to the injection. One investigator reported that HI-blockers at the time of injection during buildup also lead to improved clinical protection, possibly through H1 receptors on immunoregulatory cells.[29] One study also showed that a leukotriene antagonist reduced large local reactions to VIT.[30] There have been occasional cases of serum-sickness-like reactions to VIT, but none have shown any laboratory abnormalities, and most resolved with continued VIT treatment. There is no convincing evidence that VIT (or any AIT) can cause or increase autoimmune disease. No long-term adverse effects have been reported with VIT, or with large numbers of honeybee stings in beekeepers. Like all AIT, there are no unusual concerns about giving maintenance VIT during pregnancy.

Repeated systemic reactions may occasionally interfere with the ability to achieve the maintenance dose. Sometimes this can be overcome by limiting treatment to a single venom and with premedication; sometimes treatment is more successful when restarted after a 6 month hiatus. Although it is counterintuitive, the most successful approach is not a lower dose and slower schedule, but a rush (2−3 day) regimen, usually with premedication.[31] In unusual cases, particularly some patients with mastocytosis, it becomes necessary to pretreat the patient with omalizumab in order to build up VIT to maintenance without severe reactions.[32,33] In most cases, omalizumab can be discontinued after 6 months, but occasionally the reactions recur.

Treatment failure (systemic reaction to a sting while on maintenance VIT) is uncommon but requires review and adjustment of therapy. The patient should be reevaluated for high-risk factors including elevated baseline serum tryptase, systemic reactions to VIT, beekeepers, and cardiovascular medications. The protection can be improved with increased maintenance doses, usually to 200 mcg.[34]

Maintenance/monitoring

Once the maintenance dose is achieved, it must be repeated regularly in order to maintain clinical protection. If treatment is stopped after just 1−2 years, the risk of systemic reaction returns almost to pretreatment levels (25%).[35] A common recommendation is every 4 weeks for 12−18 months, then every 6 weeks for 12−18 months, then every 8 weeks for 12−18 months, then every 12 weeks.[36] These extended intervals are another way in which VIT differs from inhalant AIT (and from the FDA-approved product package inserts). Maintenance intervals of 6 months were ineffective.[37] If a systemic reaction to venom injection occurs during maintenance treatment, the interval may be reduced back to 4 weeks and/or the dose may be increased to 200 mcg.

Annual monitoring visits focus on possible adverse reactions, any insect sting events, any changes in concomitant medications or other medical conditions, with review of the treatment plan. Patients benefit from explanation about the reliability of protection (unless they have known high-risk factors) and what to do if they get stung. If the patient is taking a beta-blocker or ACEI, there is a need to review the medical indication and the relative risk of stopping/changing the medication versus continuing VIT despite the medication (see section on high-risk factors).

Repeating venom IgE tests or skin tests should be considered after 3 years of treatment, but usually do not show any clinically significant change at that point. After a mean of 6 years of VIT (5 years or more), the venom skin tests were negative in less than 25% but showed diminished sensitivity in 75%.[38] By 9.6 years (mean), the skin tests were negative in 70% and diminished in 98%.[39] It is noteworthy that even when skin tests became negative, there was still a barely detectable level of venom-specific IgE, and still some risk of reaction if VIT is stopped[8] (see below).[40]

Duration

The product package inserts recommend, as they have since 1979, that VIT be continued every 4 weeks indefinitely. This is primarily because there is no test that reliably predicts the outcome of a sting, or the persistence of protection (sustained unresponsiveness). However, decades of clinical research and experience have helped to recognize high-risk factors that distinguish those who should feel comfortable stopping VIT from those who should probably not stop (Table 6.2).

Early reports suggested that treatment could be stopped after 3 years, but those studies included patients treated 3 years or more, usually with a mean of 4 years or more. Also, most early studies required a challenge sting during VIT and/or a decline to negative venom IgE levels, both of which do not often occur in practice. Subsequent studies showed that 5 years of VIT gives better suppression of the IgE response and more sustained unresponsiveness than 3 years.[41,42]

Overall, the chance of systemic reaction to a sting after stopping VIT of at least 5 years duration is about 10% per sting. The majority of the reactions that occur are much milder than the pre-VIT sting reaction, and these patients generally do not accept the recommendation to resume VIT.[39] Severe reactions are generally associated with underlying risk factors. There is rarely any reaction to a sting in the first year after stopping treatment, but reactions were noted in years 2 to 4 off VIT. The chance of reaction did not diminish with time over 10 years of observation post-VIT.[10,43] Because the chance is 10% for every sting, the more times the patient is stung, the more chance that one of the stings will cause a reaction. The risk is therefore cumulative, with more than 15% having a systemic reaction during 10 years of

Table 6.2 Factors for elevated risk of relapse after discontinuing venom immunotherapy.

Proven:
Very severe reaction to previous stings
Elevated basal serum tryptase
Systemic reaction during venom immunotherapy (VIT) (to injection or sting)
Less than 5 years of maintenance VIT
Honeybee anaphylaxis
Frequent exposure

Possible:
No decrease in venom IgE or skin tests
Underlying cardiovascular or respiratory disease
Use of ACE inhibitors or beta-blockers

Reproduced from Golden DBK, Demain J, Freeman T et al. Stinging insect hypersensitivity: A practice parameter update 2016. Ann Allergy Asthma Immunol. *2017;118:28—54.*

observation, sometimes before and/or after an uneventful sting. The chance of reaction to a sting was also quite unpredictable, as it is pre-VIT (due to insect-related and possibly intrinsic medical factors). One patient had no reaction to a sting after 10 years off treatment, but had a reaction the next year, and in another case there was a reaction after 12 years but not the next year. Some patients developed negative venom skin tests but still had systemic reactions to a sting 2—4 years later (and were shown to have barely detectable serum venom IgE levels).[8]

When VIT is stopped after 5 years or more in patients with no high-risk factors (almost 70% of patients on VIT), the chance of a severe systemic reaction to a subsequent sting is less than 3%, whereas it is about 45% in those with known high-risk factors (almost a third of cases). The chance of relapse is higher if the pre-VIT sting reaction was extremely severe; if there is evidence of an underlying mast cell disorder; if the patient had a systemic reaction, to a shot or a sting, during VIT; if the patient has severe honeybee allergy; or if they have frequent exposure to stinging insects. There has been anecdotal evidence that patients who do not show a significant decline in venom sensitivity after 5—7 years of treatment are at higher risk for relapse if they stop VIT.

How long is long enough? Based on the above caveats, about one-third of patents on VIT might be considered high risk for discontinuing treatment. There is no available evidence on the need for VIT of longer than 15 years duration. However, many high-risk patients prefer to continue treatment every 12 weeks because "4 shots a year is easier than taking chances." There is a need for a clinical trial of stopping VIT (i.e., placebo injections) versus continued VIT, with sting challenge after 2—4 years, in patients who have been on VIT for 15—30 years (for a variety of reasons). There is no consensus on when or if Hymenopteria hypersensitive patients can discontinue carrying an epinephrine autoinjector, but many physicians allow this after 1 year of maintenance VIT.

Mechanism of VIT

VIT has been a model for the elucidation of the mechanisms of AIT. It was evident in the 1980s that venom-specific IgG antibodies were strongly correlated with protection from sting anaphylaxis, particularly IgG4 antibodies.[44] However, after more than 3 years of treatment, even patients with low IgG levels can have no reaction to a sting. Patients who stop VIT after 1–2 years have a moderately high chance of relapse, whereas those who stop after 5 years have very little risk of relapse. All of these observations suggest that a more sustained unresponsiveness is present only after more than 4 years of treatment.

Immune responses to VIT include increased production of IL-10 (also an upstream marker of IgG production) and induction of T_{reg} cells.[45,46] Although these have been described as the mechanism of tolerance with VIT, this is not strictly true. Although these response peak during the early months of treatment, the clinical protection disappears if VIT is stopped after 1–2 years, proving that these responses did not represent true sustained unresponsiveness. The true mechanism of the tolerance observed even after VIT is stopped (after 5 years or more) is not yet fully understood. The IgE response decreases slowly over many years, but can still be detected in many patients after 7–10 years off VIT. There are no reports of the fate of the venom IgE response 15–30 years after initial diagnosis. The role of IgG4 antibodies has been reexamined due to their regulatory effect on B and T lymphocytes.[47] Venom-specific IgG4 antibodies are also implicated in the marked suppression of IgE and clinical reaction in beekeepers who get very large numbers of stings.[19] One study found immunological changes, associated with immune tolerance after 12 hours of rush VIT, which were maintained months later.[48,49]

Summary

VIT is unique in many ways, and yet in most ways it is a model for AIT. Selection of patients for VIT requires stratification of risk based on the natural history of the disease and known risk factors. There is a high frequency of mast cell disorders in patients with insect sting anaphylaxis. Baseline serum tryptase should be measured in all patients who are candidates for VIT and when considering the discontinuation of VIT. VIT is as safe as any AIT and remarkably safe even with 2–3 day rush regimens. VIT can be built up to maintenance dose with equal safety using 16 week, 8 week, or 2–3 day regimens. Cardiovascular medications (beta-blockers and ACE inhibitors) may increase the risk of severe reaction to stings, but may be continued when medically necessary. VIT is up to 98% effective in preventing anaphylaxis and induces sustained unresponsiveness in almost 70% of patients who are treated for 5 years or more. Decades of observation and investigation have identified the high-risk factors for severe sting anaphylaxis, and those that indicate a likely lack of sustained unresponsiveness in about 30% of those treated (despite 98% efficacy). Although not as well characterized as the Hymenoptera venoms, immunotherapy with whole body extracts of imported fire ants is used with essentially the same methods and similar outcomes.[50]

References

1. Golden DB. Insect sting allergy and venom immunotherapy: a model and a mystery. *J Allergy Clin Immunol*. 2005;115:439−447.
2. Golden DBK, Demain J, Freeman T, et al. Stinging insect hypersensitivity: a practice parameter update 2016. *Ann Allergy Asthma Immunol*. 2017;118:28−54.
3. Golden DBK, Marsh DG, Freidhoff LR, et al. Natural history of Hymenoptera venom sensitivity in adults. *J Allergy Clin Immunol*. 1997;100:760−766.
4. Sturm GJ, Kranzelbinder B, Schuster C, et al. Sensitization to Hymenoptera venoms is common, but systemic sting reactions are rare. *J Allergy Clin Immunol*. 2014;133: 1635−1643.
5. Golden DBK, Marsh DG, Kagey-Sobotka A, et al. Epidemiology of insect venom sensitivity. *JAMA*. 1989;262:240−244.
6. Bilo BM, Bonifazi F. Epidemiology of insect-venom anaphylaxis. *Curr Opin Allergy Clin Immunol*. 2008;8:330−337.
7. Reisman RE. Natural history of insect sting allergy: relationship of severity of symptoms of initial sting anaphylaxis to re-sting reactions. *J Allergy Clin Immunol*. 1992;90: 335−339.
8. Golden DBK, Kagey-Sobotka A, Lichtenstein LM. Survey of patients after discontinuing venom immunotherapy. *J Allergy Clin Immunol*. 2000;105:385−390.
9. Muller UR, Ring J. When can immunotherapy for insect allergy be stopped? *J Allergy Clin Immunol Prac*. 2015;3:324−328.
10. Reisman RE. Duration of venom immunotherapy: relationship to the severity of symptoms of initial insect sting anaphylaxis. *J Allergy Clin Immunol*. 1993;92: 831−836.
11. Muller UR. Elevated baseline serum tryptase, mastocytosis and anaphylaxis. *Clin Exp Allergy*. 2009;39:620−622.
12. Rueff F, Przybilla B, Bilo MB, et al. Predictors of severe systemic anaphylactic reactions in patients with Hymenoptera venom allergy: importance of baseline serum tryptase − a study of the EAACI interest group on insect venom hypersensitivity. *J Allergy Clin Immunol*. 2009;124:1047−1054.
13. Bonadonna P, Perbellini O, Passalacqua G, et al. Clonal mast cell disorders in patients with systemic reactions to Hymenoptera stings and increased serum tryptase levels. *J Allergy Clin Immunol*. 2009;123:680−686.

14. Alvarez-Twose I, Gonzalez-de-Olano D, Sanchez-Munoz L, et al. Validation of the REMA score for predicting mast cell clonality and systemic mastocytosis in patients with systemic mast cell activation symptoms. *Int Arch Allergy Immunol.* 2012;157: 275−280.

15. Niedoszytko M, Bonadonna P, Oude-Elberink JNG, Golden DBK. Epidemiology, diagnosis, and treatment of Hymenoptera venom allergy in mastocytosis patients. Mastocytosis (Akin C, Alam R, eds.) *Immunol Allergy Clin N Am.* 2014;34:365−381.

16. Brockow K, Jofer C, Behrendt H, Ring J. Anaphylaxis in patients with mastocytosis: a study on history, clinical features and risk factors in 120 patients. *Allergy.* 2008;63: 226−232.

17. Vos BJPR, Anrooij B, Doormaal JJ, Dubois AEJ, Oude-Elberink JNG. Fatal anaphylaxis to yellow jacket stings in mastocytosis: options for identification and treatment of at risk patients. *J Allergy Clin Immunol: In Pract.* 2017;5:1264−1271.

18. Pravettoni V, Piantanida M, Primavesi L, Forti S, Pastorello EA. Basal platelet-activating factor acetylhydrolase: prognostic marker of severe Hymenoptera venom anaphylaxis. *J Allergy Clin Immunol.* 2014;133:1218−1220.

19. Varga EM, Kausar F, Aberer W, et al. Tolerant beekeepers display venom-specific functional IgG4 antibodies in the absence of specific IgE. *J Allergy Clin Immunol.* 2013;131: 1419−1421.

20. Stoevesandt J, Hain J, Kerstan A, Trautmann A. Over- and underestimated parameters in severe Hymenoptera venom-induced anaphylaxis: cardiovascular medication and absence of urticaria/angioedema. *J Allergy Clin Immunol.* 2012;130:698−704.

21. Muller U, Haeberli G. Use of beta-blockers during immunotherapy for Hymenoptera venom allergy. *J Allergy Clin Immunol.* 2005;115:606−610.

22. Plunkett G, Jacobson RS, Golden DBK. Hymenoptera venoms used to produce allergen extracts. *Ann Allergy Asthma Immunol.* 2017;118:649−654.

23. Golden DB, Bernstein DI, Freeman TM, Tracy JM, Lang DM, Nicklas RA. AAAAI/ACAAI joint venom extract shortage task force report. *J Allergy Clin Immunol Prac.* 2017;5:330−332.

24. Freeman TM, Hyghlander R, Ortiz A, Martin ME. Imported fire ant immunotherapy: effectiveness of whole body extracts. *J Allergy Clin Immunol.* 1992;90:210−215.

25. Konstantinou GN, Manoussakis E, Douladiris N, et al. A 5-year venom immunotherapy protocol with 50 mcg maintenance dose: safety and efficacy in school children. *Pediatr Allergy Immunol.* 2011;22:393−397.

26. Golden DBK. Rush venom immunotherapy: ready for prime time? *J Allergy Clin Immunol Prac.* 2017;5:804−805.

27. Hunt KJ, Valentine MD, Sobotka AK, Benton AW, Amodio FJ, Lichtenstein LM. A controlled trial of immunotherapy in insect hypersensitivity. *N Engl J Med.* 1978; 299:157−161.

28. Goldberg A, Confino-Cohen R. Bee venom immunotherapy − how early is it effective? *Allergy.* 2010;65:391−395.

29. Muller UR, Jutel M, Reimers A, et al. Clinical and immunologic effects of H1 antihistamine preventive medication during honeybee venom immunotherapy. *J Allergy Clin Immunol.* 2008;122:1001−1007.

30. Wohrl S, Gamper S, Hemmer W, Heinze G, Stingl G, Kinaciyan T. Premedication with montelukast reduces large local reactions of allergen immunotherapy. *Int Arch Allergy Immunol.* 2007;144:137−142.

31. Goldberg A, Confino-Cohen R. Rush venom immunotherapy in patients experiencing recurrent systemic reactions to conventional venom immunotherapy. *Ann Allergy.* 2003;91:405−410.

32. Galera C, Soohun N, Zankar N, Caimmi S, Gallen C, Demoly P. Severe anaphylaxis to bee venom immunotherapy: efficacy of pretreatment with omalizumab. *J Investig Allergol Clin Immunol.* 2009;19:225−229.

33. Kontou-Fili K. High omalizumab dose controls recurrent reactions to venom immunotherapy in indolent systemic mastocytosis. *Allergy.* 2008;63:376−378.

34. Rueff F, Wenderoth A, Przybilla B. Patients still reacting to a sting challenge while receiving conventional Hymenoptera venom immunotherapy are protected by increased venom doses. *J Allergy Clin Immunol.* 2001;108:1027−1032.

35. Golden DBK, Johnson K, Addison BI, Valentine MD, Kagey-Sobotka A, Lichtenstein LM. Clinical and immunologic observations in patients who stop venom immunotherapy. *J Allergy Clin Immunol.* 1986;77:435−442.

36. Goldberg A, Confino-Cohen R. Maintenance venom immunotherapy administered at 3-month intervals is both safe and efficacious. *J Allergy Clin Immunol.* 2001;107:902−906.

37. Goldberg A, Confino-Cohen R. Effectiveness of maintenance bee venom immunotherapy administered at 6 month intervals. *Ann Allergy Asthma Immunol.* 2007;99:352−357.

38. Golden DBK, Kwiterovich KA, Kagey-Sobotka A, Valentine MD, Lichtenstein LM. Discontinuing venom immunotherapy: outcome after five years. *J Allergy Clin Immunol.* 1996;97:579−587.

39. Golden DBK, Kwiterovich KA, Addison BA, Kagey-Sobotka A, Lichtenstein LM. Discontinuing venom immunotherapy: extended observations. *J Allergy Clin Immunol.* 1998;101:298−305.

40. Cox L. Advantages and disadvantages of accelerated immunotherapy schedules. *J Allergy Clin Immunol.* 2008;122:432−434.

41. Keating MU, Kagey-Sobotka A, Hamilton RG, Yuninger JW. Clinical and immunologic follow-up of patients who stop venom immunotherapy. *J Allergy Clin Immunol.* 1991;88:339−348.

42. Lerch E, Muller U. Long-term protection after stopping venom immunotherapy. *J Allergy Clin Immunol.* 1998;101:606−612.

43. Golden DBK. Long-term outcome after venom immunotherapy. *Curr Opin Allergy Clin Immunol.* 2010;10:337−341.

44. Golden DBK, Lawrence ID, Kagey-Sobotka A, Valentine MD, Lichtenstein LM. Clinical correlation of the venom-specific IgG antibody level during maintenance venom immunotherapy. *J Allergy Clin Immunol.* 1992;90:386−393.

45. Akdis CA, Blesken T, Akdis M, et al. Role of interleukin 10 in specific immunotherapy. *J Clin Investig.* 1998;102:98−106.

46. Jutel M, Akdis M, Blaser K, Akdis CA. Are regulatory T cells the target of venom immunotherapy? *Curr Opin Allergy Clin Immunol.* 2005;5:365−369.

47. Varga EM, Francis JN, Zach MS, Klunker S, Aberer W, Durham SR. Time course of serum inhibitory activity for facilitated allergen-IgE binding during bee venom immunotherapy in children. *Clin Exp Allergy.* 2009;39:1353−1357.

48. Michils A, Baldassarre S, Ledent C, Mairesse M, Gossart B, Duchateau J. Early effect of ultrarush venom immunotherapy on the IgG antibody response. *Allergy.* 2000;55:455−462.

49. Michils A, Ledent C, Mairesse M, Gossart B, Duchateau J. Wasp venom immunotherapy changes IgG antibody specificity. *Clin Exp Allergy.* 1997;27:1036–1042.

50. Steigelman DA, Freeman TM. Imported fire ant allergy: case presentation and review of incidence, prevalence, diagnosis and current treatment. *Ann Allergy Asthma Immunol.* 2013;111:242–245.

Mechanisms of allergen immunotherapy

Mechanisms of subcutaneous allergen immunotherapy against inhaled aeroallergens

7

Natasha C. Gunawardana, MRCP [1,2], **Stephen R. Durham, FRCP** [1,2]

[1]*Allergy and Clinical Immunology, Royal Brompton Hospital, London, United Kingdom;* [2]*Allergy and Clinical Immunology, National Heart and Lung Institute, Imperial College London, United Kingdom*

Introduction

Subcutaneous allergen immunotherapy (SCIT) involves giving injections of allergen extract in incremental doses generally weekly for 3—4 months followed by monthly maintenance injections for 3—4 years. SCIT is indicated in patients with allergic rhinoconjunctivitis with/without mild asthma in whom a dominant allergen is responsible for symptoms, with objective confirmation of IgE sensitivity. SCIT is a disease modifying treatment that has been in use clinically for over 100 years. The first trial was performed by Noon and Freeman in 1911 and involved a subcutaneous grass pollen extract.[1] Injections given 1—2 weekly resulted in a marked increase in tolerance to a conjunctival grass pollen challenge. They noted that if injections were too frequent or too excessive they led to systemic allergic reactions.

SCIT is effective in reducing symptom and medication scores[2] and is able to induce long-term tolerance, with persistence of clinical benefit on subsequent allergen exposure for years after the treatment has finished. SCIT appears at least as effective as antiallergic medications[3] that, in contrast to SCIT, have to be taken continually to be effective. In addition, SCIT has been shown to reduce asthma symptoms and medication scores, and decrease specific bronchial hyperreactivity.[4] SCIT remains the most commonly used form of immunotherapy[5] although this may change, with the advent of alternative effective and safer methods of delivery such as sublingual immunotherapy (SLIT).

Allergic diseases are characterized by the induction and maintenance of type 2 T lymphocyte responses; cardinal features include Th2 memory T cells, the production of the key cytokines IL-4, IL-5, IL-9, and IL-13, the presence of allergen-specific IgE and blood and tissue eosinophilia. SCIT acts on both the cellular and humoral arms of the allergic response. A greater understanding of the mechanisms of SCIT has already had widespread implications in determining novel approaches for immunotherapy[6] and in discovering novel potential biomarkers for monitoring disease severity and the response to treatment.[7] The precise mechanisms for long-term tolerance after

Immunotherapies for Allergic Disease. https://doi.org/10.1016/B978-0-323-54427-6.00007-9

immunotherapy remain unclear. In this chapter, we review the known immunological effects of SCIT given for the treatment of patients with rhinoconjunctivitis with/without bronchial asthma and IgE sensitivity to common inhaled aeroallergens.

Mechanisms of SCIT Studies

There is a high level of heterogeneity in methodology used in studies of SCIT that has implications for translatability of both clinical and mechanistic findings.[8] An ARIA-GA[2]LEN position paper highlighted the need for careful selection of candidates with moderate—severe disease, a dominant allergen provoking symptoms and confirmation of IgE sensitivity.[9] Compared to trials of pharmacotherapy, immunotherapy trials are often long term and suffer from lower average symptom scores due to pollen-free days and seasonal variation year on year in pollen counts as well as high dropout rates.[9] There are the confounding effects of high placebo responses, placebo unmasking due to local side effects in participants within actively treated arms and access to rescue medication in both arms, all of which may confound the separation of responders from nonresponders to treatment. Mechanistic studies require samples to be taken at baseline and at intervals during treatment and after treatment withdrawal. The duration of SCIT and the relative timing of sequential samples are particularly relevant to understand the immunological mechanisms underlying the induction and maintenance of long-term tolerance.

For seasonal allergens, aeroallergen sampling is necessary in and out of the pollen season for comparison that can be logistically challenging. To mitigate the problem of variability of natural allergen exposures, clinical surrogates, including nasal allergen challenge, conjunctival allergen provocation, and the use of environmental allergen exposure chambers, have been used. These approaches enable reproducible allergen exposures that may be repeated before and at intervals during treatment.[10] This enables a more standardized comparison between groups and importantly the ability to assess each patient effectively as their own control by comparing their individual measurements pre—post treatment.

In human studies, peripheral blood and serum sampling have been the main stay in assessing immunological changes during SCIT. Local changes in the target organ have also been evaluated by sampling nasal mucosal lining fluid, taking brushings or curettage of the nasal epithelium and the performance of repeated nasal biopsies. These techniques are important to understand the local changes on allergen exposure (e.g., during the early- and late phases of the allergic response) and differences between local and peripheral immune responses.

The particular aeroallergen studied, the type of allergen extract used, and the immunotherapy regimen employed may result in markedly different immunological changes. For example, among the grasses, there is extensive cross-reactivity for the major pollen allergens.[11] The use of an immunotherapy preparation dominant for one grass pollen[12] has been shown to result in clinical benefits against all Northern temperate grasses. Approximately 60% of patient with aeroallergen allergy and likely to be sensitized to minor pollen pan allergens such as profilin and polcalcin that may or may not be clinically relevant.[13,14] Other idiosyncrasies of allergens include the known protease activity of house dust mite (HDM) that activates innate immune responses by mimicking pattern-associated molecular patterns[15,16] and may play a role in the response to immunotherapy.[17] The advent of molecular allergology has resulted in the cloning of most major allergens.[18] This has enabled the production of hypoallergenic mutants that retain immunogenicity but do not cross-link IgE thereby reducing the risk of anaphylaxis. Novel adjuvants have been developed that enable delayed allergen absorption and modify the immune response to injected allergens. Immunotherapy mechanisms are therefore likely to vary, depending on the type of allergen, the route of administration, different delivery systems, and the presence/absence of adjuvants or coinjected immune modifiers.[19]

New techniques for monitoring immune cell responses such as HLA tetramer analysis of antigen-specific T-cell populations are dependent on the specificity of the allergen peptides recognized by an individual's immune phenotype.

Desensitization and reduction of local mast cells, basophils, and eosinophils

Mast cells and basophils are granulated cells that have the high affinity IgE receptor (FcεRI) expressed on their surface. Mast cells are resident locally in tissues.[20] On antigen presentation cross-linking of specific IgE (sIgE) bound to high affinity FcεRI receptor on the mast cell surface causes degranulation and release of preformed histamine and other vasoactive amines, the release of type 2 cytokines including IL-4 and IL-13, and newly derived proinflammatory lipids from arachidonic acid that include leukotrienes C4, D4, and E4 and prostaglandin D2. Basophils are found in the circulation and are recruited into tissues during the late phase of allergic inflammation. Basophil-derived IL-4 and 13 induce IgE class switch recombination of B cells, activate innate lymphoid cells (ILC) in response to allergen,[21] and may possibly have a role in increasing antigen presentation to Th2 cells.[22] The number of eosinophils in the blood and local tissues increases on exposure to allergen. Eosinophils release granular proteins such as major basic protein and eosinophil peroxidase that are toxic to respiratory epithelium. Eosinophils promote peripheral B-cell numbers, enhance plasma cell survival, and produce chemoattractants that recruit dendritic cells (DCs) and T effector cells.[23]

Aeroallergen and venom SCIT[24] cause an early desensitization of mast cells. Ragweed SCIT over 8 months reduced local mast cell and basophil mediators histamine, tosyl L arginine methyl ester-esterase, and tryptase in response to nasal challenge early in treatment.[25] c kit (CD117) expression is necessary for migration and survival of mast cell progenitors and activation of mast cells. There are reductions in seasonal increases in c kit + mast cells and basophils in nasal biopsy samples after 2 years of treatment with grass pollen SCIT[26] (Fig. 7.1[27]). Mast cell numbers in the skin are decreased following successful grass pollen SCIT.[28]

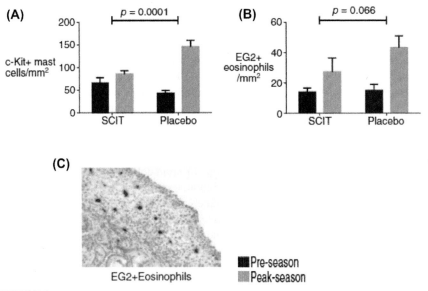

FIGURE 7.1

Effects of 2 years grass pollen SCIT on seasonal (A) c-Kit + mast cells (B) EG2+ eosinophils in the nasal mucosa. (C) Staining for activation marker EG2+ on eosinophils. Abbreviations: *SCIT*, subcutaneous immunotherapy.

From Matsuoka T, Shamji MH, Durham SR. Allergen immunotherapy and tolerance Allergol Int. 2013;62(4): 403-413. https://doi.org/10.2332/allergolint.13-RAI-0650; with permission.

The mechanisms of mast cell desensitization are not fully known. Blocking antibodies generated by immunotherapy (see later) may competitively bind allergen-preventing activation via the FcεRI.[29] There is also the potential that binding of these IgG antibodies to the low affinity IgG receptor FcγRIIb that may inhibit FcεRI signaling.[30] Histamine itself has regulatory functions, down regulating both Th1 and Th2 cell activation via the histamine receptor 2.[31] Following venom immunotherapy, there is upregulation of histamine receptor 2[24] that could also be a potential mechanism of suppression.

Seasonal eosinophil infiltration in the nasal mucosa is reduced following grass pollen SCIT as determined by immunochemical staining of eosinophils using antibodies against the eosinophil markers MBP and EG2 on nasal biopsy[32,33] (Fig. 7.1, Ref. 27). This decrease is associated with a reduction in IL-5 expression and correlates with the clinical response to immunotherapy.[32] The number of nasal epithelial basophils, as well as eosinophils, is decreased following grass pollen SCIT.[34]

Eosinophil recruitment into tissues is dependent on specific endothelial adhesion molecules including intercellular adhesion molecule 1 (ICAM-1) and vascular adhesion molecule 1 (VCAM-1) and these are increased in allergic rhinitis.[35] There are decreases in ICAM locally in the conjunctiva following allergoid SLIT[36] and nasal mucosa following local nasal immunotherapy.[37] There are systemic decreases in soluble ICAM-1 and soluble VCAM-1 following HDM SCIT.[38] Following SCIT, there are reduced levels of the eosinophil chemokine eotaxin.[39]

Reduction of type 2 innate lymphoid cells

ILC have morphological characteristics similar to lymphocytes but lack T- or B-cell antigen receptors delineating antigen specificity and other lineage markers. ILCs represent important alternative sources of cytokines and are able to amplify T-cell-driven immune responses to allergens. They are classified into subgroups according to their ability to produce cytokines associated with particular T helper cell lineages. Type 2 innate lymphoid cells (ILC2) secrete large amounts of IL-5, IL-9 and IL-13 in response to epithelial derived IL-33, IL-25, thymic stromal lymphopoietin (TSLP) and leukotriene D4.[40]

In allergic rhinitis, on nasal allergen challenge there is a rapid recruitment of ILC2 to the nasal mucosa[41] and peripheral blood.[42] On seasonal exposure, there are 50% increases of ILC2 in peripheral blood.[43-45] There were no functional differences in cytokine production from ILC2 in allergic patients compared to nonallergic controls, however on transcriptomic analysis, allergic patients have an upregulation of proinflammatory activator protein 1 and nonallergic patients have increased transcription of genes NKG7, SOCS1, and TBX21 that downregulate inflammatory responses, specifically Th2 responses.[44]

SCIT for both grass[43] and HDM[46] reduces the proportion of c kit/CD117 + ILC2 cells in peripheral blood in patients with allergic rhinitis to similar levels seen in nonallergic control patients. Responders to HDM SCIT had lower levels of ILC2 cells postimmunotherapy compared to HDM SCIT nonresponders with decreased activation on ex vivo HDM stimulation.[46]

Human ILC2 cells express the prostaglandin D2 (PGD2) receptor chemoattractant receptor homologous molecule expressed on Th2 lymphocytes (CRTH2). PGD2 in vitro induces ILC2 chemotaxis.[47] There was less CRTH2 expression from ILC2 in responders to HDM SCIT with levels similar to healthy controls.[46] IL-35 from regulatory T cells (Treg) has an important role in inducing allergen tolerance with immunotherapy (see later). They are able to suppress ILC2 IL-5 and IL-13 production in vitro.[45] In a murine model of birch pollen SCIT, there were no changes in IL-33, IL-25, and TSLP production in the lung following SCIT.[48] However, the number of ILC2 recruited into lung tissue was markedly decreased along with the number of Th2 cells but there was no change in the functional ability of the ILC2 present in these mice to produce IL-5.

Loss of type 2 dendritic cell responses and increased DC tolerogenic responses

DCs are professional antigen presenting cells that have a key role in determining the direction of adaptive immune responses toward inflammatory and tolerogenic phenotypes.[49] DCs are divided into two major subsets: plasmacytoid DC (pDC) and myeloid/conventional DCs, which are further subdivided into two main groups. In view of the extremely low numbers of circulating DCs, laboratory studies of DC function in man have often involved the use of peripheral monocyte-derived DCs (moDC) as surrogates. Depending on antigenic, cellular, and molecular stimuli, immature DCs polarize their response to drive the differentiation of naïve T cells to distinct effector T-cell phenotypes.[50] DCs display a range of innate pattern recognition receptors including toll-like receptors (TLRs) and c-type lectin receptors (CLRs) that are likely to have roles in allergen recognition, processing, and the subsequent immune responses.[51,52]

DCs in allergy have a proallergenic phenotype. IL-33,[53] TSLP,[54] and IL-25[55] released from the epithelium in response to allergen prime DCs toward a "type 2" phenotype (termed DC2) that can be differentiated from other types of DCs by their cell surface markers and transcriptional profile. DC1 and DC17, respectively, produce IFNγ and IL 17 that are necessary for Th1 and Th17 priming the key cytokines required for the respective differentiation of these T helper cells. In contrast, DC2 cells in humans have not conclusively been shown to produce IL-4,[56] the main cytokine required for Th2 differentiation. In murine models, DC may produce IL-4 that acts in an autocrine fashion directly acting on the DC themselves.[57] Default immature tolergenic IL-10 producing DCreg have the capacity to induce allergen-specific regulatory T cells (Treg) that suppress immune responses to these allergens.[58,59]

In response to allergen, the epithelium produces CCL2 and CCL20, which recruit DCs into local tissue.[60] Compared to nonatopic controls, allergic individuals had increased numbers of mDC and pDCs in the nasal mucosa after nasal grass pollen allergen challenge and in the skin after injection of intradermal allergen[61] with no difference in the numbers of circulating DCs. In the same study, the investigators found a deficiency in DCreg IL-10 production and DC1 IL-12 and IFNα production in allergic individuals compared to controls. Subsequent T-cell-mDC cocultures from allergic patients supported Th2 and Th17 differentiation.

DCs express the high affinity IgE receptor FceRI in a trimeric form as opposed to the tetrameric form found on mast cells and basophils. The role of the DC FceRI is controversial. Allergen-IgE complexes bound to these receptors increase allergen uptake and antigen presentation to memory T cells. However, this may have a more important in the development of tolerogenic responses rather than potentiating Th2 deviation demonstrated in humanized murine models.[62,63]

pDC have been shown to demonstrate tolerogenic responses though this may be location specific.[64] Tonsillar (lymphoid) pDCs are able to induce FOX P3+ Treg from naïve T cells. These cells colocalize in tonsillar tissue. A study characterized pDC and mDC subgroups, antibody receptors, and CLR expression in a small number of patients after 1 year of multiple aeroallergen SCIT. The proportion of pDC increased with expression of FcεRI after 1 year of SCIT that may be in keeping with the tolerogenic role of these cells and the role of FcεRI expression on DCs.[65]

In addition, the activation of TLR9 on pDCs by its agonist CpG reduces the expression and function of FcεRI on pDCs and the activation of the IgE receptor conversely affects expression of TLR 9 on DCs.[66] Allergic subjects have increased expression of the IgE receptor and their ability to produce IFNα on CpG stimulation was impaired, implying a reciprocal antagonism between FcεRI and the expression of type 1 interferons by DCs,[67] which is believed to explain how anti-IgE treatment may augment DC interferon α production and inhibit seasonal viral induced asthma exacerbations in children.[68] Whether SCIT might prevent virus induced asthma exacerbations by a similar mechanism is supported by a recent study of HDM SCIT that restored this innate immune response in peripheral pDCs by a 3—5-fold increase in IFNα production in response to CpG.[66]

SCIT may also have an impact on CLR receptor expression patterns in different populations of mDCs to match those observed in healthy controls. This implies an underlying change in how allergen may be recognized by these cells.[65] This may be of particular interest in house dust mite immunotherapy, where binding of HDM to the CLR DC SIGN, has been shown to downregulate its expression and skew immune responses to a Th2 type.[52]

A recent series of studies characterized moDC responses after grass pollen SLIT by transcriptomic analysis.[69,70] After SLIT moDC showed a reduction in the DC2 markers CD141, GATA3, OX40 ligand, and receptor-interacting serine/threonine-protein kinase 4 (RIPK4) with an upregulation of DCreg associated markers that correlated with clinical outcomes. Furthermore, these changes were replicated using a simple RT-PCR test on peripheral blood and correlated with the response to SLIT implying potential use as a biomarker of response. This requires further investigation in a larger population. Whether a similar DC signature occurs after SCIT is yet to be determined.

Decreases in Th2 lymphocyte responses

SCIT has long been known to alter CD4+ T helper cell responses and subset proportions, with several nonexclusive potential mechanisms described: a decrease in Th2 cells through either anergy or deletion, an increase in Treg and immune deviation in favor of Th1 responses. In addition, there are effects on newly describe subsets of T cells such as T follicular helper cells and T follicular regulatory cells.[71]

In the nasal mucosa, suppression of allergen induced late responses is accompanied by a decrease in CD4+ T cells and an increase in interferon gamma (IFNγ)-expressing cells and decrease in Th2 cells positive for IL-4 mRNA.[33,72] This is supported by the loss of Th2 cytokines in the nasal mucosa after allergen challenge.[73,74] On intradermal grass pollen challenge following successful SCIT there is a similar reduction in IL-4 mRNA positive lymphocytes in late-phase skin responses.[75,76]

In peripheral blood, it is difficult to identify rare allergen-specific T helper cells among the whole population of T cells. Tetramer analysis uses four bioengineered MHC class II molecules specific for major antigen epitopes that are used to bind antigen-specific T cells ex vivo restricted to specific HLA DR phenotypes.[77] Through tetramer analysis, certain allergen epitopes have been found responsible for eliciting the allergic Th2 cell responses that dominate the T-cell repertoire.[78] Immunotherapy treated and nonallergic individuals, had low frequencies of allergen Th2 cells, with Th1 and type 1 regulatory T cell (Tr1) immunotypes instead being the dominant CD4+ cell immunotypes toward these epitopes. In allergic individuals, allergic epitopes can also generate Tr1 and Th1 responses; however, these are at a lower frequency than pathogenic Th2 responses.[78] Allergen-specific Th2 cells have been shown to be short lived, terminally differentiated and exhibit less of the apoptosis inhibitor Bcl 2.[78]

By identifying and studying these antigen-specific T cells, it has recently been possible to describe a Th2 cell subset that is present in both aeroallergen and food allergy, distinguishing them from other Th2 cells necessary for normal immune function. This subset of Th2 cells are characterized by expression of the chemoattractant receptor CRTH2, the natural killer cell marker CD161, and the homing receptor CD49d in human terminally differentiated (CD27- CCR7- and CD 7-) CD4+ T cells. They have been termed Th2A cells[79] and may be a future biomarker of both the allergy and immunotherapy responses.

Following SCIT, there was a selective depletion of this cell population shown in both alder pollen allergy[77] and grass pollen allergy[74] and OIT for peanut.[79] Two years after continuous grass pollen SCIT, there are reduced frequencies of MHC-restricted allergen-specific CCR4+ CRTH2+ CD161+ T cells and increased frequencies of CD27+ cells consistent with a loss of allergen-specific Th2 cells (Fig. 7.2[74]). One year off therapy, this phenotypic profile reverted with increased frequencies of CRTH2+ and CD161+ cells and reduced frequencies of CD27+ cells mirroring a loss of symptomatic tolerance. There is sharper drop in these Th2 cells with SCIT than SLIT that reaches significance by year 2.[74]

Th1 immunodeviation and changes in Th2/Th1 ratios

There have been several reports that aeroallergen SCIT may increase Th1 cells or increase the proportion of Th1 cells relative to Th2 cells. There are more cells expressing IFNγ mRNA in the nasal mucosa[33,72,80] in skin biopsies following intradermal allergen.[75] There is a more controversial increase in peripheral blood Th1 cells after SCIT demonstrated by ex vivo cell cultures[73,81−84] and determined by IFNγ in cell culture supernatants. However, this may be due to a reduction in Th2 cells and a change in the ratio to Th1 cells. The changes in levels of nasal IFNγ following nasal allergen challenge correlated inversely with seasonal symptoms after immunotherapy.[33,85]

The recent work using tetramer analysis[77,78] showed no alteration in allergen-specific Th1 cells following immunotherapy and again that deletion of epitope-specific Th2 cells may possibly be responsible for the observed change in Th2/Th1 ratios.[78]

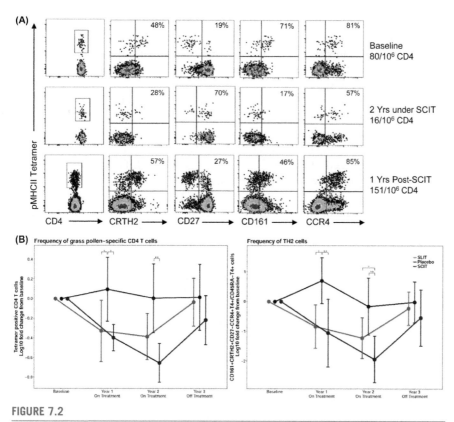

FIGURE 7.2

(A) Changes to allergen-specific T cells after 2 years grass pollen SCIT and after 1 year off treatment. (B) Changes in allergen-specific T cells and Th2 cells and relationship to clinical parameters after 2 years grass pollen SCIT and after 1 year off treatment.

From Renand A, Shamji MH, Harris KM et al. Synchronous immune alterations mirror clinical response during allergen immunotherapy. J Allergy Clin Immunol. 2018;141(5):1750–1760. https://doi.org/10.1016/j.jaci. 2017.09.041; with permission.

Increase in T regulatory cells and IL-10 mediated effects

Treg are a heterogenous group of T cells with a suppressive capacity relevant in all forms of immune tolerance toward environmental proteins, cancer cells, and transplanted organs and control the development of autoimmunity and allergic disease.[86] There is controversy in the classification of Treg subtypes. Treg can be classified into thymus derived and peripherally derived groups. Peripheral Treg are composed of mainly IL-10 producing Tr1 cells and FOXP3+ Treg. Peripheral FOXP3+ cells can be hard to distinguish from thymic T reg cells, although novel markers such as Helios[87] and neuropilin-1 may be used to differentiate them.[88] Treg inhibit allergic inflammation by producing suppressive cytokines including IL-10, TGF-β, and IL-35, causing apoptosis of effector T cells via granzymes and perforins and suppressing DC activation. This leads to the suppression of effector cells (mast cells and basophils), eosinophils, Th2 cells, B cells, DCs, and inflamed tissue cells.[89] In vitro, IL-10 can inhibit IgE production, increase blocking IgG4 production, and inhibit proliferative T-cell responses.[90,91]

Treg are important in the maintenance of tolerance in healthy individuals and in high allergen exposure populations such as beekeepers.[92] Venom SCIT induces peripheral and local epithelial Treg and is accompanied by an increase in IL-10 production.[90] For aeroallergen SCIT, there is an increase in local and peripheral IL-10 + cells and TGF-β+ cells[93,94] (Fig. 7.3[27]) and both FOXP3+[95,96] and Tr1 cells have been linked with clinical efficacy.[97] SCIT induces FOXP3+ peripheral Treg in nasal mucosa[95] with no effect on thymic Treg in tonsillar tissue (lymphoid tissue) based on immunohistochemistry. A detailed study of T-cell subset changes during birch pollen SCIT documented an increase in antigen-specific Tr1 cells by the end of the induction phase that resulted in a decreased ratio of allergen-specific IL-5+ Th2/Tr1 cells.[81] In contrast, CD4+CD25 + CD127low Treg cell numbers did not change. Although untreated and SCIT-treated subjects developed enhanced Th2 cell responses during the birch pollen season, only SCIT-treated patients experienced elevated numbers of allergen-specific Tr1 cells, which were associated with diminished clinical symptoms. In coculture assays, allergen-specific Tr1 cells showed an IL-10- and dose-dependent inhibition of CD4+CD25+ T effector cells. In a study of peripheral blood T-cell cultures after HDM SCIT, IL-10, and TGFβ suppressed antigen-specific responses in these patients that were restored following blockade of the effects of these two cytokines.[91] However, 1 year after grass pollen SCIT, in antigen stimulated peripheral blood cultures there were increased IL10 + CD4 + CD25 + T cells compared to placebo the amounts of IL 10 produced by these cells was not high enough to inhibit Th2 cytokine production.[98]

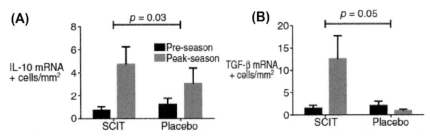

FIGURE 7.3

Effects of 2 years grass pollen SCIT on IL-10 and TGF-β mRNA + cells in the nasal mucosa. Abbreviations: *IL-10*, interleukin 10; *SCIT*, subcutaneous immunotherapy; *TGF-β*, transforming growth factor beta.

From Matsuoka T, Shamji MH, Durham SR. Allergen immunotherapy and tolerance Allergol Int. 2013;62(4): 403–413. https://doi.org/10.2332/allergolint.13-RAI-0650; with permission.

A recent study in birch pollen allergic individuals shows that antigen-specific Th2 responses develop despite a quantitative and qualitative normal Treg compartment.[99] In keeping with this the number of HLA restricted allergen-specific Tr1 cells following grass pollen SCIT did not change toward specific epitopes and the main mechanism of immunotherapy may be the loss of Th2 cells.[78]

Reduced T follicular helper cells and increased T follicular regulatory cells

T follicular helper cells (Tfh) reside in the marginal zones of B-cell germinal follicles within lymph nodes.[100] They are essential for B cells to make antibody through affinity maturation and isotype switching producing B-cell survival and selection signals. FoxP3+ thymus-derived Treg can express Bcl-6 and express the homing molecule CXCR5 and migrate into germinal centers.[101] Following interactions with SLAM associated protein, CD28, and B cell, these develop into a distinct population of T follicular regulatory cells (Tfr) that share characteristics with both follicular cells and T regs suppressing Tfh cell responses and B cells.[102] Following SCIT in peripheral blood, there is a reduction in Tfh cells and an increase in Tfr potentially under the influence of IL-2.[103] In a recent study, there were less Tfr cells in tonsillar (secondary lymphoid tissue) in patients with allergic rhinitis than healthy controls, which correlates to findings in peripheral blood, despite total Treg numbers and CXCR5- cells being unchanged.[71] In addition, when cocultured with Tfh cells and B cells, Tfr cells from AR patients were defective in suppression of IgE production but not IgM, IgG, or IgA. The ratio of Tfr/Tfh cells significantly correlated with the clinical response to HDM SCIT.

Increase in B regulatory cells

B-cell immune responses are mediated by antigen presentation to T cells, secretion of cytokines and differentiation to plasma cells, and subsequent secretion of antibodies.[104] In lymphoid tissue, B cells interact with T cells leading to B-cell proliferation and the formation of germinal centers. B cells undergo class switching, recombination, and somatic hypermutation. Affinity maturation leads to selection of the cells that have the highest affinity for the antigen. Fully differentiated plasma cells produce one isotype of antibody. Long lasting memory B cells and plasma cells persist and are considerably easier to activate than naïve B cells. They continue to produce affinity matured antibodies. In murine models, IgE responses are usually short lived and usually directed toward plasma cell responses, as opposed to memory B-cell responses or potentiating further interactions with T cells. B cells express the low affinity IgE receptor CD23 and have an important role in allergen presentation.[105,106]

Similar to Treg, there are a group of immunosuppressive B cells termed B regulatory cells (Breg) that release immune-regulatory cytokines IL-10, TGFβ, and IL-35 to support the differentiation of Treg and suppresses inflammation in autoimmune disease, infection, and allergy.[107] In patients with high allergen exposure such as beekeepers and patients before after bee pollen immunotherapy, IL-10 producing Breg (BR1) suppress whole peripheral blood mononuclear cell (PMBC) proliferation responses.[108] IgG4 was produced 10 times higher in the IL-10 positive B cells on stimulation with TLR9 ligand. Recently, similar changes in population of B cells were demonstrated after HDM SCIT with increased fractions of Breg after HDM SCIT.[109] IgG4 and IgA HDM antigen-specific Der p1 B cells increased after immunotherapy to a greater extent in responders to immunotherapy than nonresponders. Similar increases in Breg cells have been shown following grass pollen SCIT, which also correlates to clinical outcomes.[110]

Initial increase followed by persistent decrease in IgE

Following SCIT, there are transient increases in serum IgE that also occurs for all routes of immunotherapy and all types of allergen. For seasonal aeroallergens, there is then a blunting of seasonal increases over subsequent seasons. The transient increase is not accompanied by increased side effects. Prolonged SCIT over several years can lead to a decrease in allergen-specific IgE that may be a contributing factor in long-term tolerance.[74,111] Despite the importance of IgE in generating responses, there is a paucity of IgE positive B cells in vivo. Tonsillar germinal center IgG-expressing B cells cultured with IL-4 and anti-CD40L underwent sequential class switching to generate IgE secreting plasma cells, which implies that IgE memory may reside within the IgG memory B-cell population.[112]

Generation of blocking IgG and IgA antibodies

The generation of a serum-blocking factor was initially shown by Cooke in 1935, with the passive transfer of inhibitory activity by injecting serum of patients having undergone ragweed SCIT under the skin of allergic patients.[113] This blocking activity is thought to reside in IgG and IgA compartments.

Following SCIT, in the serum, there are 10−100-fold increases in IgG, IgG4 having the greatest proportionate increase within 6−12 weeks of starting immunotherapy.[113] IgG can compete with IgE for binding of allergen and prevent FcεRI cross-linking and downstream effects, and inhibit basophil reactivity in vitro.[114−116] It can also block binding to low affinity FcεRII on B cells inhibiting IgE-facilitated antigen presentation to T cells.[105,117] The IgG4 to IgG1 ratio correlated with clinical symptoms scores.[118]

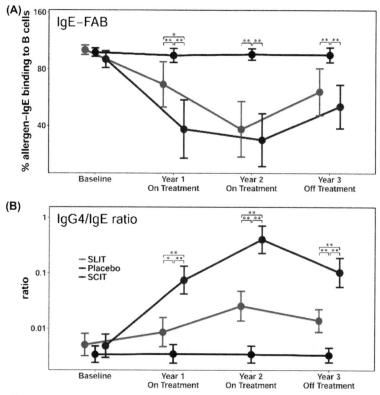

FIGURE 7.4

Effects of 2 years grass pollen SCIT, SLIT, and placebo on (A) IgE functional antibody binding (IgE-FAB) and (B) IgG4/IgE ratio after 2 years on treatment and 1 year off treatment.

From Renand A, Shamji MH, Harris KM et al. Synchronous immune alterations mirror clinical response during allergen immunotherapy. J Allergy Clin Immunol. *2018;141(5):1750–1760. https://doi.org/10.1016/j.jaci.2017.09.041; with permission.*

The IgE functional antibody binding (FAB) assay detects the effect of these antibodies on CD23-mediated B-cell antigen presentation (Fig. 7.4[74]). It correlates modestly with clinical outcomes and has been used as a surrogate measure of the blocking capacity of immunotherapy-generated antibodies.[106,119] This blocking ability is antigen specific.[120] After 2 years of immunotherapy and then discontinuation, IgG and IgG4 levels decrease to near preimmunotherapy levels but, despite this, residual blocking activity is maintained.[121] Similar changes have been shown for other aeroallergens.[122]

Increased nasal-specific IgG and IgA has been demonstrated following SCIT.[123] This did not correlate to serum antibody levels for IgG. SCIT with genetically modified derivatives of birch pollen increased IgG1, IgG2, and IgG4 and IgA in nasal fluid, which was associated with reduced nasal allergen challenge symptoms.[124] Nasal fluid is more effective at blocking IgE FAB than sera. Following grass pollen SCIT nasal IgG4 was induced with increased inhibitory activity in the nasal fluid than serum that was blocked by depletion of IgG.[125] The nasal fluid inhibitory activity is correlated better with clinical outcomes than immunoreactive IgG levels. There is nasal mucosal IgE antibody production in allergic rhinitis, with increased concentrations of B cells and plasma cells compared to peripheral blood and local class switch recombination to IgE synthesis[126] The more effective IgE FAB in nasal fluid may be as increased effective blocking IgG4 antibodies are also formed locally on allergen exposure. However, as IgE genes are downstream of IgG4, it is not possible that the same B cells class switch from IgE to produce IgG4.[127]

Recently, a trial involving the direct administration of allergen-specific IgG4 antibody to the major cat allergen Fel-D1 was able to prevent allergen challenge-induced symptoms.[128] As this does not require the administration of allergen to change the underlying immune response, this is termed passive immunotherapy.

How novel mechanisms can improve aeroallergen SCIT

Increasing knowledge of the mechanism of allergen immunotherapy aims to improve future strategies for aeroallergen immunotherapy. The aims are to make immunotherapy faster with fewer injections, with greater efficacy and more convenient treatment regimens for patients. Table 7.1[128–145] summarizes some of the novel approaches that have been used to modify aeroallergen SCIT based on knowledge of the mechanisms of SCIT, enhancing tolerogenic responses and reducing allergenicity. To date these approaches have shown varying degrees of efficacy, whereas none have shown significant benefits over conventional aeroallergen SCIT in the context of head-to-head controlled trials that are urgently needed.

Summary

Aeroallergen SCIT is the archetypal model of allergen immunotherapy. Knowledge gained from study of the mechanisms has had implications for improving allergen immunotherapy and in recognizing potential biomarkers of clinical response. Furthermore, understanding the mechanisms of allergen-specific tolerance during allergen immunotherapy may have implications for treatment and tolerance induction in the context of organ-specific autoimmune disease and protection against rejection following organ transplantation.

Key mechanisms of aeroallergen SCIT are the suppression of effector cells; mast cells, eosinophils, and basophils; changes to how an allergen is recognized by DCs toward tolerant immune responses; loss of allergen-specific Th2 responses;

Table 7.1 Modifications to SCIT, mechanisms of action, and example studies.

		Mechanistic concept	Example studies
Allergen derivatives	Allergoids	Physically or chemically modified whole allergen to reduce IgE binding while preserving immunogenicity	(Corrigan, 2005) Grass
	Recombinant allergens	Manufactured directly from cDNA, allows identification of relevant, hypoallergenic allergens in immunotherapy	(Jutel, 2005) Grass (Pauli, 2008) Birch
	T-cell peptides	Non-IgE-reactive amino acid sequences recognized by T cells	(Circassia, unpublished) HDM (Couroux, 2015) Cat (Circassia, unpublished) Fel d 1
	Contiguous overlapping peptides	All possible T-cell epitopes with disrupted IgE epitopes	(Spertini 2016) Birch
	B-cell peptides	Non-IgE-reactive peptides bound to carrier protein	(Niederberger 2018) Grass
	Hydrolyzed peptides	Hydrolysis whole allergen, epitopes for T and B cells, reduced IgE-binding	(Mosges 2018)
	Passive immunotherapy	Antiallergen IgG antibodies	(Orengo 2018) Cat
Adjuvants	Depots	Adsorbs allergen, triggers innate and Th1 responses.	(Leynadier, 2018) Calcium phosphate plus 5 grass pollen extract Pollinex combined with L-tyrosine (see later)
	TLR agonists	TLR 4 and TLR 9 agonists increase Th1 immune responses and/or induce treg responses	(Drachenberg, 2001) Grass + MPL + L-tyrosine SCIT (Creticos, 2006) A. artemisiifolia and CpG motif. Ragweed + CpG: Failed phase 3 (DuBuske 2011) Modified allergens from 13 grasses tyrosine adsorbed with adjuvant MPL
	Nanoparticles	Particles that encapsulate allergen, enhance delivery, prevent IgE binding	(Basomba 2002) Liposomes + HDM SC

Continued

Table 7.1 Modifications to SCIT, mechanisms of action, and example studies.—*cont'd*

	Mechanistic concept	Example studies
Virus-like particles	Derived from viral capsids, stimulate innate mechanisms	(Senti 2009) HDM combined with QbG10 VLP given SC
		(Klimek 2011) TLR 9 CpG inside VLP, no allergen, given SC.
Allergen + Anti-IgE (omalizumab)	Binds free IgE, reduces allergic side effects, and increases tolerability	(Kuehr 2002) Birch and grass pollen SCIT + anti-IgE
		(Kopp 2009) Depigmented glutaraldehyde polymerized grass pollen allergoid + anti-IgE SCIT
Allergen + anti-IL-4		(Chaker 2016) Grass pollen SCIT + anti-IL-4, RDBPCT. No difference in late-phase skin response

increased T reg responses with or without an increase in Th1 responses; the generation of B reg responses; and production of effective blocking antibodies.

Currently, there are still no effective methods of identifying which patients are likely to respond to immunotherapy, to know when patients have achieved sustained tolerance and predictive markers for significant allergic side effects. The aim is to make immunotherapy safer, less expensive, and more convenient for patients. Through the study of SCIT mechanisms, we may eventually be able to understand the underlying process of sensitization and how this leads to clinical disease.

References

1. Noon L. Prophylactic inoculation against hay fever. *Lancet*. 1911;177(4580): 1572–1573. https://doi.org/10.1016/S0140-6736(00)78276-6.
2. Calderon MA, Alves B, Jacobson M, Hurwitz B, Sheikh A, Durham S. Allergen injection immunotherapy for seasonal allergic rhinitis. *Cochrane Database Syst Rev*. 2007; (1):CD001936. https://doi.org/10.1002/14651858.cd001936.pub2.
3. Matricardi P, Kuna P, Panetta V, Wahn U, Narkus A. Subcutaneous immunotherapy and pharmacotherapy in seasonal allergic rhinitis: a comparison based on meta-analyses. *J Allergy Clin Immunol*. 2011;128(4):791–799.e6. https://doi.org/10.1016/j.jaci.2011.03.049.

4. Abramson MJ, Puy RM, Weiner JM. Injection allergen immunotherapy for asthma. *Cochrane Database Syst Rev.* 2010;8:CD001186. https://doi.org/10.1002/14651858.cd001186.pub2.

5. Kora J, Tankersley MS, ACAAI Immunotherapy, Diagnostics Committee. Perception and practice of sublingual immunotherapy among practicing allergists in the United States: a follow-up survey. *Ann Allergy Asthma Immunol.* 2013;110(3):194−197.e4. https://doi.org/10.1016/j.anai.2012.12.014.

6. Klimek L, Pfaar O, Bousquet J, Senti G, Kündig T. Allergen immunotherapy in allergic rhinitis: current use and future trends. *Expert Rev Clin Immunol.* 2017;13(9):897−906. https://doi.org/10.1080/1744666x.2017.1333423.

7. Shamji M, Kappen J, Akdis M, et al. Biomarkers for monitoring clinical efficacy of allergen immunotherapy for allergic rhinoconjunctivitis and allergic asthma: an EAACI Position Paper. *Allergy.* 2017;72(8):1156−1173. https://doi.org/10.1111/all.13138.

8. Pfaar O, Alvaro M, Cardona V, Hamelmann E, Mösges R, Kleine-Tebbe J. Clinical trials in allergen immunotherapy: current concepts and future needs. *Allergy.* 2018;73(9):1775−1783. https://doi.org/10.1111/all.13429.

9. Bousquet J, Schünemann H, Bousquet P, et al. How to design and evaluate randomized controlled trials in immunotherapy for allergic rhinitis: an ARIA-GA2LEN statement. *Allergy.* 2011;66(6):765−774. https://doi.org/10.1111/j.1398-9995.2011.02590.x.

10. Pepper AN, Ledford DK. Nasal and ocular challenges. *J Allergy Clin Immunol.* 2018;141(5):1570−1577. https://doi.org/10.1016/j.jaci.2017.11.066.

11. Laffer S, Vrtala S, Duchêne M, et al. IgE-binding capacity of recombinant timothy grass (Phleum pratense) pollen allergens. *J Allergy Clin Immunol.* 1994;94(1):88−94. https://doi.org/10.1016/0091-6749(94)90075-2.

12. Durham SR, Emminger W, Kapp A, et al. SQ-standardized sublingual grass immunotherapy: confirmation of disease modification 2 years after 3 years of treatment in a randomized trial. *J Allergy Clin Immunol.* 2012;129(3):717−725.e5. https://doi.org/10.1016/j.jaci.2011.12.973.

13. Asero R, Mistrello G, Amato S. Detection of pan-allergens in commercial pollen extracts for allergen immunotherapy. *Ann Allergy Asthma Immunol.* 2016;117(2):180−185. https://doi.org/10.1016/j.anai.2016.05.010.

14. Ruiz-García M, del Potro M, Fernández-Nieto M, Barber D, Jimeno-Nogales L, Sastre J. Profilin: a relevant aeroallergen? *J Allergy Clin Immunol.* 2011;128(2):416−418. https://doi.org/10.1016/j.jaci.2011.03.008.

15. Hammad H, Plantinga M, Deswarte K, et al. Inflammatory dendritic cells—not basophils—are necessary and sufficient for induction of Th2 immunity to inhaled house dust mite allergen. *J Exp Med.* 2010;207(10):2097−2111. https://doi.org/10.1084/jem.20101563.

16. Trompette A, Divanovic S, Visintin A, et al. Allergenicity resulting from functional mimicry of a Toll-like receptor complex protein. *Nature.* 2009;457(7229):585. https://doi.org/10.1038/nature07548.

17. Calderón MA, Linneberg A, Kleine-Tebbe J, et al. Respiratory allergy caused by house dust mites: what do we really know? *J Allergy Clin Immunol.* 2015;136(1):38−48. https://doi.org/10.1016/j.jaci.2014.10.012.

18. Valenta R, Karaulov A, Niederberger V, et al. Molecular aspects of allergens and allergy. *Adv Immunol.* 2018;138:195−256. https://doi.org/10.1016/bs.ai.2018.03.002.

19. Gunawardana NC, Durham SR. New approaches to allergen immunotherapy. *Ann Allergy Asthma Immunol.* 2018;121(3):293–305. https://doi.org/10.1016/j.anai.2018.07.014.

20. Kabashima K, Nakashima C, Nonomura Y, et al. Biomarkers for evaluation of mast cell and basophil activation. *Immunol Rev.* 2018;282(1):114–120. https://doi.org/10.1111/imr.12639.

21. Motomura Y, Morita H, Moro K, et al. Basophil-derived interleukin-4 controls the function of natural helper cells, a member of ILC2s, in lung inflammation. *Immunity.* 2014;40(5):758–771. https://doi.org/10.1016/j.immuni.2014.04.013.

22. Siracusa MC, Kim BS, Spergel J, Artis D. Basophils and allergic inflammation. *J Allergy Clin Immunol.* 2013;132(4):789–801. https://doi.org/10.1016/j.jaci.2013.07.046.

23. Spencer LA, Weller PF. Functions of tissue-resident eosinophils. *Nat Rev Immunol.* 2017;17(12):746. https://doi.org/10.1038/nri.2017.95.

24. Novak N, Mete N, Bussmann C, et al. Early suppression of basophil activation during allergen-specific immunotherapy by histamine receptor 2. *J Allergy Clin Immunol.* 2012;130(5):1153–1158.e2. https://doi.org/10.1016/j.jaci.2012.04.039.

25. Iliopoulos O, Proud D, Adkinson NF, et al. Effects of immunotherapy on the early, late, and rechallenge nasal reaction to provocation with allergen: changes in inflammatory mediators and cells. *J Allergy Clin Immunol.* 1991;87(4):855–866. https://doi.org/10.1016/0091-6749(91)90134-a.

26. Nouri-Aria KT, Pilette C, Jacobson MR, Watanabe H, Durham SR. IL-9 and c-Kit+ mast cells in allergic rhinitis during seasonal allergen exposure: effect of immunotherapy. *J Allergy Clin Immunol.* 2005;116(1):73–79. https://doi.org/10.1016/j.jaci.2005.03.011.

27. Matsuoka T, Shamji MH, Durham SR. Allergen immunotherapy and tolerance. *Allergol Int.* 2013;62(4):403–413. https://doi.org/10.2332/allergolint.13-RAI-0650.

28. Durham, Varney, Gaga, et al. Grass pollen immunotherapy decreases the number of mast cells in the skin. *Clin Exp Allergy.* 1999;29(11):1490–1496. https://doi.org/10.1046/j.1365-2222.1999.00678.x.

29. Lichtenstein LM, Norman PS, Winkenwerder WL. Clinical and in vitro studies on the role of immunotherapy in ragweed hay fever. *Am J Med.* 1968;44(4):514–524. https://doi.org/10.1016/0002-9343(68)90052-1.

30. MacGlashan D, Moore G, Muchhal U. Regulation of IgE-mediated signalling in human basophils by CD32b and its role in Syk down-regulation. *Clin Exp Allergy.* 2014;44(5):713–723. https://doi.org/10.1111/cea.12155.

31. Jutel M, Watanabe T, Klunker S, et al. Histamine regulates T-cell and antibody responses by differential expression of H1 and H2 receptors. *Nature.* 2001;413(6854):420. https://doi.org/10.1038/35096564.

32. Wilson DR, Nouri-Aria KT, Walker SM, et al. Grass pollen immunotherapy: symptomatic improvement correlates with reductions in eosinophils and IL-5 mRNA expression in the nasal mucosa during the pollen season. *J Allergy Clin Immunol.* 2001;107(6):971–976. https://doi.org/10.1067/mai.2001.115483.

33. Durham SR, Ying S, Varney VA, et al. Grass pollen immunotherapy inhibits allergen-induced infiltration of CD4+ T lymphocytes and eosinophils in the nasal mucosa and increases the number of cells expressing messenger RNA for interferon-γ. *J Allergy Clin Immunol.* 1996;97(6):1356–1365. https://doi.org/10.1016/s0091-6749(96)70205-1.

34. Wilson D, Irani A-MA, Walker S, et al. Grass pollen immunotherapy inhibits seasonal increases in basophils and eosinophils in the nasal epithelium. *Clin Exp Allergy*. 2001; 31(11):1705−1713. https://doi.org/10.1046/j.1365-2222.2001.01231.x.

35. Montefort S, Feather I, Wilson S, et al. The expression of leukocyte-endothelial adhesion molecules is increased in perennial allergic rhinitis. *Am J Respir Cell Mol Biol*. 1992;7(4):393−398. https://doi.org/10.1165/ajrcmb/7.4.393.

36. Passalacqua G, Albano M, Fregonese L, et al. Randomised controlled trial of local allergoid immunotherapy on allergic inflammation in mite-induced rhinoconjunctivitis. *Lancet*. 1998;351(9103). https://doi.org/10.1016/S0140-6736(97)07055-4.

37. Passalacqua G, Albano M, Ruffoni S, et al. Nasal immunotherapy to Parietaria: evidence of reduction of local allergic inflammation. *Am J Resp Crit Care*. 1995;152(2): 461−466. https://doi.org/10.1164/ajrccm.152.2.7633693.

38. Ohashi Y, Nakai Y, Tanaka A, et al. Clinical role of soluble adhesion molecules during immunotherapy for perennial allergic rhinitis. *Arch Otolaryngol Head Neck Surg*. 1998; 124(1):41−45. https://doi.org/10.1001/archotol.124.1.41.

39. Scadding G, Eifan A, Lao-Araya M, et al. Effect of grass pollen immunotherapy on clinical and local immune response to nasal allergen challenge. *Allergy*. 2015;70(6): 689−696. https://doi.org/10.1111/all.12608.

40. Neill DR, Wong S, Bellosi A, et al. Nuocytes represent a new innate effector leukocyte that mediates type-2 immunity. *Nature*. 2010;464(7293):1367. https://doi.org/10.1038/nature08900.

41. Dhariwal J, Cameron A, Trujillo-Torralbo M-B, et al. Mucosal type 2 innate lymphoid cells are a key component of the allergic response to aeroallergens. *Am J Resp Crit Care*. 2017;195(12):1586−1596. https://doi.org/10.1164/rccm.201609-1846oc, 15.

42. Doherty TA, Scott D, Walford HH, et al. Allergen challenge in allergic rhinitis rapidly induces increased peripheral blood type 2 innate lymphoid cells that express CD84. *J Allergy Clin Immunol*. 2014;133(4):1203−1205.e7. https://doi.org/10.1016/j.jaci.2013.12.1086.

43. Simhadri VR, Mariano JL, Zenarruzabeitia O, et al. Seasonal increases in peripheral innate lymphoid type 2 cells are inhibited by subcutaneous grass pollen immunotherapy. *J Allergy Clin Immunol*. 2014;134(5):1193−1195.e4. https://doi.org/10.1016/j.jaci.2014.07.029.

44. Lombardi V, Beuraud C, Neukirch C, et al. Circulating innate lymphoid cells are differentially regulated in allergic and nonallergic subjects. *J Allergy Clin Immunol*. 2016; 138(1):305−308. https://doi.org/10.1016/j.jaci.2015.12.1325.

45. Shamji MH, Layhadi JA, Achkova D, et al. Role of Interleukin-35 in sublingual allergen immunotherapy. *J Allergy Clin Immunol*. 2019;143(3):1131−1142. https://doi.org/10.1016/j.jaci.2018.06.041.

46. Mitthamsiri W, Pradubpongsa P, Sangasapaviliya A, Boonpiyathad T. Decreased CRTH2 expression and response to allergen Re-stimulation on innate lymphoid cells in patients with allergen-specific immunotherapy. *Allergy Asthma Immunol Res*. 2018;10(6):662−674. https://doi.org/10.4168/aair.2018.10.6.662.

47. Simon KL, Anderson SM, Garabedian EK, Moratto D, Sokolic RA, Candotti F. Prostaglandin D2 regulates human type 2 innate lymphoid cell chemotaxis. *J Allergy Clin Immunol*. 2014;133(3):899−901.e3. https://doi.org/10.1016/j.jaci.2013.09.020.

48. Rijt LS, Logiantara A, Canbaz D, Ree R. Birch pollen-specific subcutaneous immunotherapy reduces ILC2 frequency but does not suppress IL-33 in mice. *Clin Exp Allergy*. 2018;48(11):1402−1411. https://doi.org/10.1111/cea.13254.

49. Collin M, Bigley V. Human dendritic cell subsets: an update. *Immunology*. 2018;154(1): 3–20. https://doi.org/10.1111/imm.12888.

50. Pulendran B, Tang H, Manicassamy S. Programming dendritic cells to induce TH2 and tolerogenic responses. *Nat Immunol*. 2010;11(8):647. https://doi.org/10.1038/ni.1894.

51. Schülke S, Vieths S. Dendritic cell targeting with C-type lectins for improvement of allergen immunotherapy. *J Allergy Clin Immunol*. 2016;138(2):568–570. https://doi.org/10.1016/j.jaci.2016.06.006.

52. Huang H-J, Lin Y-L, Liu C-F, Kao H-F, Wang J-Y. Mite allergen decreases DC-SIGN expression and modulates human dendritic cell differentiation and function in allergic asthma. *Mucosal Immunol*. 2011;4(5):519. https://doi.org/10.1038/mi.2011.17.

53. Rank MA, Kobayashi T, Kozaki H, Bartemes KR, Squillace DL, Kita H. IL-33–activated dendritic cells induce an atypical TH2-type response. *J Allergy Clin Immunol*. 2009;123(5):1047–1054. https://doi.org/10.1016/j.jaci.2009.02.026.

54. Soumelis V, Reche PA, Kanzler H, et al. Human epithelial cells trigger dendritic cell–mediated allergic inflammation by producing TSLP. *Nat Immunol*. 2002;3(7):673–680. https://doi.org/10.1038/ni805.

55. Wang Y-H, Angkasekwinai P, Lu N, et al. IL-25 augments type 2 immune responses by enhancing the expansion and functions of TSLP-DC–activated Th2 memory cells. *J Exp Med*. 2007;204(8):1837–1847. https://doi.org/10.1084/jem.20070406.

56. MacDonald AS, Maizels RM. Alarming dendritic cells for Th2 induction. *J Exp Med*. 2008;205(1):13–17. https://doi.org/10.1084/jem.20072665.

57. Maroof A, Penny M, Kingston R, et al. Interleukin-4 can induce interleukin-4 production in dendritic cells. *Immunology*. 2006;117(2):271–279. https://doi.org/10.1111/j.1365-2567.2005.02305.x.

58. Schülke S. Induction of interleukin-10 producing dendritic cells as a tool to suppress allergen-specific T helper 2 responses. *Front Immunol*. 2018;9:455. https://doi.org/10.3389/fimmu.2018.00455.

59. Steinbrink K, Wölfl M, Jonuleit H, Knop J, Enk A. Induction of tolerance by IL-10-treated dendritic cells. *J Immunol*. 1997;159(10):4772–4780.

60. Pichavant M, Charbonnier A-S, Taront S, et al. Asthmatic bronchial epithelium activated by the proteolytic allergen Der p 1 increases selective dendritic cell recruitment. *J Allergy Clin Immunol*. 2005;115(4):771–778. https://doi.org/10.1016/j.jaci.2004.11.043.

61. Pilette C, Jacobson M, Ratajczak C, et al. Aberrant dendritic cell function conditions Th2-cell polarization in allergic rhinitis. *Allergy*. 2013;68(3):312–321. https://doi.org/10.1111/all.12090.

62. Sallmann E, Reininger B, Brandt S, et al. High-affinity IgE receptors on dendritic cells exacerbate Th2-dependent inflammation. *J Immunol*. 2011;187(1):164–171. https://doi.org/10.4049/jimmunol.1003392.

63. Platzer B, Baker K, Vera M, et al. Dendritic cell-bound IgE functions to restrain allergic inflammation at mucosal sites. *Mucosal Immunol*. 2014;8(3):516. https://doi.org/10.1038/mi.2014.85.

64. Palomares O, Rückert B, Jartti T, et al. Induction and maintenance of allergen-specific FOXP3+ Treg cells in human tonsils as potential first-line organs of oral tolerance. *J Allergy Clin Immunol*. 2012;129(2):510–520.e9. https://doi.org/10.1016/j.jaci.2011.09.031.

65. Lundberg K, Rydnert F, Broos S, Andersson M, Greiff L, Lindstedt M. Allergen-specific immunotherapy alters the frequency, as well as the FcR and CLR expression

profiles of human dendritic cell subsets. *PLoS One*. 2016;11(2):e0148838. https://doi.org/10.1371/journal.pone.0148838.

66. Tversky J, Bieneman A, Chichester K, Hamilton R, Schroeder J. Subcutaneous allergen immunotherapy restores human dendritic cell innate immune function. *Clin Exp Allergy*. 2010;40(1):94−102. https://doi.org/10.1111/j.1365-2222.2009.03388.x.

67. Gill MA, Liu AH, Calatroni A, et al. Enhanced plasmacytoid dendritic cell antiviral responses after omalizumab. *J Allergy Clin Immunol*. 2018;141(5):1735−1743.e9. https://doi.org/10.1016/j.jaci.2017.07.035.

68. Teach SJ, Gill MA, Togias A, et al. Preseasonal treatment with either omalizumab or an inhaled corticosteroid boost to prevent fall asthma exacerbations. *J Allergy Clin Immunol*. 2015;136(6):1476−1485. https://doi.org/10.1016/j.jaci.2015.09.008.

69. Gueguen C, Bouley J, Moussu H, et al. Changes in markers associated with dendritic cells driving the differentiation of either TH2 cells or regulatory T cells correlate with clinical benefit during allergen immunotherapy. *J Allergy Clin Immunol*. 2016;137(2):545−558. https://doi.org/10.1016/j.jaci.2015.09.015.

70. Zimmer A, Bouley J, Mignon M, et al. A regulatory dendritic cell signature correlates with the clinical efficacy of allergen-specific sublingual immunotherapy. *J Allergy Clin Immunol*. 2012;129(4):1020−1030. https://doi.org/10.1016/j.jaci.2012.02.014.

71. Yao Y, Wang Z-C, Wang N, et al. Allergen immunotherapy improves defective follicular regulatory T cells in patients with allergic rhinitis. *J Allergy Clin Immunol*. 2019;144(1):118−128. https://doi.org/10.1016/j.jaci.2019.02.008.

72. Tulic MK, Fiset P-O, Christodoulopoulos P, et al. Amb a 1−immunostimulatory oligodeoxynucleotide conjugate immunotherapy decreases the nasal inflammatory response. *J Allergy Clin Immunol*. 2004;113(2):235−241. https://doi.org/10.1016/j.jaci.2003.11.001.

73. Klimek D, Jarman C, Riechelmann R-K. Short-term preseasonal birch pollen allergoid immunotherapy influences symptoms, specific nasal provocation and cytokine levels in nasal secretions, but not peripheral T-cell responses, in patients with allergic rhinitis. *Clin Exp Allergy*. 1999;29(10):1326−1335. https://doi.org/10.1046/j.1365-2222.1999.00651.x.

74. Renand A, Shamji MH, Harris KM, et al. Synchronous immune alterations mirror clinical response during allergen immunotherapy. *J Allergy Clin Immunol*. 2018;141(5):1750−1760. https://doi.org/10.1016/j.jaci.2017.09.041.

75. Varney V, Hamid Q, Gaga M, et al. Influence of grass pollen immunotherapy on cellular infiltration and cytokine mRNA expression during allergen-induced late-phase cutaneous responses. *J Clin Invest*. 1993;92(2):644−651. https://doi.org/10.1172/jci116633.

76. Durham SR, Walker SM, Varga E-M, et al. Long-term clinical efficacy of grass-pollen immunotherapy. *N Engl J Med*. 1999;341(7):468−475. https://doi.org/10.1056/nejm199908123410702.

77. Wambre E, DeLong JH, James EA, LaFond RE, Robinson D, Kwok WW. Differentiation stage determines pathologic and protective allergen-specific CD4+ T-cell outcomes during specific immunotherapy. *J Allergy Clin Immunol*. 2012;129(2):544−551.e7. https://doi.org/10.1016/j.jaci.2011.08.034.

78. Wambre E, DeLong JH, James EA, et al. Specific immunotherapy modifies allergen-specific CD4+ T-cell responses in an epitope-dependent manner. *J Allergy Clin Immunol*. 2014;133(3):872−879.e7. https://doi.org/10.1016/j.jaci.2013.10.054.

79. Wambre E, Bajzik V, DeLong JH, et al. A phenotypically and functionally distinct human T$_H$2 cell subpopulation is associated with allergic disorders. *Sci Transl Med.* 2017; 9:401. https://doi.org/10.1126/scitranslmed.aam9171.

80. Wachholz PA, Nouri-Aria KT, Wilson DR, et al. Grass pollen immunotherapy for hayfever is associated with increases in local nasal but not peripheral Th1 : Th2 cytokine ratios. *Immunology.* 2002;105(1):56–62. https://doi.org/10.1046/j.1365-2567.2002.01338.x.

81. Möbs C, Slotosch C, Löffler H, Jakob T, Hertl M, Pfützner W. Birch pollen immunotherapy leads to differential induction of regulatory T cells and delayed helper T cell immune deviation. *J Immunol.* 2010;184(4):2194–2203. https://doi.org/10.4049/jimmunol.0901379.

82. Eer C, Siemann U, Bohle B, et al. Immunological changes during specific immunotherapy of grass pollen allergy: reduced lymphoproliferative responses to allergen and shift from TH2 to TH1 in T-cell clones specific for Phl p 1, a major grass pollen allergen. *Clin Exp Allergy.* 1997;27(9):1007–1015. https://doi.org/10.1111/j.1365-2222.1997.tb01252.x.

83. Till S, Walker S, Dickason R, et al. IL-5 production by allergen-stimulated T cells following grass pollen immunotherapy for seasonal allergic rhinitis. *Clin Exp Immunol.* 1997;110(1):114–121. https://doi.org/10.1111/j.1365-2249.1997.494-ce1392.x.

84. Guerra F, Carracedo J, Solana-Lara R, Sánchez-Guijo P, Ramírez R. TH2 lymphocytes from atopic patients treated with immunotherapy undergo rapid apoptosis after culture with specific allergens. *J Allergy Clin Immunol.* 2001;107(4):647–653. https://doi.org/10.1067/mai.2001.112263.

85. Benjaponpitak S, Oro A, Maguire P, Marinkovich V, DeKruyff RH, Umetsu DT. The kinetics of change in cytokine production by CD4+ T cells during conventional allergen immunotherapy. *J Allergy Clin Immunol.* 1999;103(3):468–475. https://doi.org/10.1016/s0091-6749(99)70473-2.

86. Palomares O, Akdis M, Martín-Fontecha M, Akdis CA. Mechanisms of immune regulation in allergic diseases: the role of regulatory T and B cells. *Immunol Rev.* 2017; 278(1):219–236. https://doi.org/10.1111/imr.12555.

87. Gottschalk RA, Corse E, Allison JP. Expression of Helios in peripherally induced Foxp3+ regulatory T cells. *J Immunol.* 2012;188(3):976–980. https://doi.org/10.4049/jimmunol.1102964.

88. Yadav M, Louvet C, Davini D, et al. Neuropilin-1 distinguishes natural and inducible regulatory T cells among regulatory T cell subsets in vivo. *J Exp Med.* 2012;209(10): 1713–1722. https://doi.org/10.1084/jem.20120822.

89. Akdis CA, Akdis M. Mechanisms of immune tolerance to allergens: role of IL-10 and Tregs. *J Clin Invest.* 2014;124(11):4678–4680. https://doi.org/10.1172/jci78891.

90. Akdis C, Blesken T, Akdis M, Wüthrich B, Blaser K. Role of interleukin 10 in specific immunotherapy. *J Clin Invest.* 1998;102(1):98–106. https://doi.org/10.1172/jci2250.

91. Jutel M, Akdis M, Budak F, et al. IL-10 and TGF-β cooperate in the regulatory T cell response to mucosal allergens in normal immunity and specific immunotherapy. *Eur J Immunol.* 2003;33(5):1205–1214. https://doi.org/10.1002/eji.200322919.

92. Meiler F, Zumkehr J, Klunker S, Rückert B, Akdis CA, Akdis M. In vivo switch to IL-10–secreting T regulatory cells in high dose allergen exposure. *J Exp Med.* 2008; 205(12):2887–2898. https://doi.org/10.1084/jem.20080193.

93. Pilette C, Nouri-Aria KT, Jacobson MR, et al. Grass pollen immunotherapy induces an allergen-specific IgA2 antibody response associated with mucosal TGF-β expression. *J Immunol.* 2007;178(7):4658–4666. https://doi.org/10.4049/jimmunol.178.7.4658.

94. Nouri-Aria KT, Wachholz PA, Francis JN, et al. Grass pollen immunotherapy induces mucosal and peripheral IL-10 responses and blocking IgG activity. *J Immunol.* 2004; 172(5):3252–3259. https://doi.org/10.4049/jimmunol.172.5.3252.

95. Radulovic S, Jacobson MR, Durham SR, Nouri-Aria KT. Grass pollen immunotherapy induces Foxp3-expressing CD4+ CD25+ cells in the nasal mucosa. *J Allergy Clin Immunol.* 2008;121(6):1467–1472. https://doi.org/10.1016/j.jaci.2008.03.013, 1472.e1.

96. Ling EM, Smith T, Nguyen DX, et al. Relation of CD4+CD25+ regulatory T-cell suppression of allergen-driven T-cell activation to atopic status and expression of allergic disease. *Lancet.* 2004;363(9409):608–615. https://doi.org/10.1016/s0140-6736(04) 15592-x.

97. Möbs C, Ipsen H, Mayer L, et al. Birch pollen immunotherapy results in long-term loss of Bet v 1–specific TH2 responses, transient TR1 activation, and synthesis of IgE-blocking antibodies. *J Allergy Clin Immunol.* 2012;130(5):1108–1116.e6. https:// doi.org/10.1016/j.jaci.2012.07.056.

98. Francis JN, Till SJ, Durham SR. Induction of IL-10+CD4+CD25+ T cells by grass pollen immunotherapy. *J Allergy Clin Immunol.* 2003;111(6):1255–1261. https:// doi.org/10.1067/mai.2003.1570.

99. Bacher P, Heinrich F, Stervbo U, et al. Regulatory T cell specificity directs tolerance versus allergy against aeroantigens in humans. *Cell.* 2016;167(4):1067–1078.e16. https://doi.org/10.1016/j.cell.2016.09.050.

100. Kemeny D. The role of the T follicular helper cells in allergic disease. *Cell Mol Immunol.* 2012;9(5):386–389. https://doi.org/10.1038/cmi.2012.31.

101. Linterman MA, Pierson W, Lee SK, et al. Foxp3+ follicular regulatory T cells control the germinal center response. *Nat Med.* 2011;17(8):975. https://doi.org/10.1038/ nm.2425.

102. Chung Y, Tanaka S, Chu F, et al. Follicular regulatory T cells expressing Foxp3 and Bcl-6 suppress germinal center reactions. *Nat Med.* 2011;17(8):983. https://doi.org/ 10.1038/nm.2426.

103. Schulten V, Tripple V, Seumois G, et al. Allergen-specific immunotherapy modulates the balance of circulating Tfh and Tfr cells. *J Allergy Clin Immunol.* 2018;141(2): 775–777.e6. https://doi.org/10.1016/j.jaci.2017.04.032.

104. Wong R, Bhattacharya D. Basics of memory B-cell responses: lessons from and for the real world. *Immunology.* 2019;156(2):120–129. https://doi.org/10.1111/imm.13019.

105. van Neerven R, Wikborg T, Lund G, et al. Blocking antibodies induced by specific allergy vaccination prevent the activation of CD4+ T cells by inhibiting serum-IgE-facilitated allergen presentation. *J Immunol.* 1999;163(5):2944–2952.

106. Wachholz PA, Soni N, Till SJ, Durham SR. Inhibition of allergen-IgE binding to B cells by IgG antibodies after grass pollen immunotherapy. *J Allergy Clin Immunol.* 2003; 112(5):915–922. https://doi.org/10.1016/s0091-6749(03)02022-0.

107. van de Veen W. The role of regulatory B cells in allergen immunotherapy. *Curr Opin Allergy Clin Immunol.* 2017;17(6):447. https://doi.org/10.1097/aci.0000000000000400.

108. van de Veen W, Stanic B, Yaman G, et al. IgG4 production is confined to human IL-10–producing regulatory B cells that suppress antigen-specific immune responses. *J Allergy Clin Immunol.* 2013;131(4):1204–1212. https://doi.org/10.1016/j.jaci.2013.01.014.

109. Boonpiyathad T, Sokolowska M, Morita H, et al. Der p 1-specific regulatory T-cell response during house dust mite allergen immunotherapy. *Allergy.* 2019;74(5):976—985. https://doi.org/10.1111/all.13684, 2019.

110. Zissler UM, Jakwerth CA, Guerth FM, et al. Early IL-10 producing B-cells and coinciding Th/Tr17 shifts during three year grass-pollen AIT. *Ebiomedicine.* 2018;36. https://doi.org/10.1016/j.ebiom.2018.09.016.

111. Gleich GJ, Zimmermann EM, Henderson LL, Yunginger JW. Effect of immunotherapy on immunoglobulin E and immunoglobulin G antibodies to ragweed antigens: a six-year prospective study. *J Allergy Clin Immunol.* 1982;70(4):261—271. https://doi.org/10.1016/0091-6749(82)90062-8.

112. Ramadani F, Bowen H, Upton N, et al. Ontogeny of human IgE-expressing B cells and plasma cells. *Allergy.* 2017;72(1):66—76. https://doi.org/10.1111/all.12911.

113. Cooke RA, Barnard JH, Hebald S, Stull A. Serological evidence of immunity with coexisting sensitization in a type of human allergy (hay fever). *J Exp Med.* 1935;62(6):733—750. https://doi.org/10.1084/jem.62.6.733.

114. Ejrnaes A, Svenson M, Lund G, Larsen J, Jacobi H. Inhibition of rBet v 1-induced basophil histamine release with specific immunotherapy -induced serum immunoglobulin G: no evidence that FcγRIIB signalling is important. *Clin Exp Allergy.* 2006;36(3):273—282. https://doi.org/10.1111/j.1365-2222.2006.02442.x.

115. Lambin P, Bouzoumou A, Murrieta M, et al. Purification of human IgG4 subclass with allergen-specific blocking activity. *J Immunol Methods.* 1993;165(1):99—111. https://doi.org/10.1016/0022-1759(93)90111-j.

116. Leynadier F, Abuaf N, Halpern G, Murrieta M, Garcia-Duarte C, Dry J. Blocking IgG antibodies after rush immunotherapy with mites. *Ann Allergy.* 1986;57(5):325—329.

117. Würtzen P, Lund G, Lund K, Arvidsson M, Rak S, Ipsen H. A double-blind placebo-controlled birch allergy vaccination study II: correlation between inhibition of IgE binding, histamine release and facilitated allergen presentation. *Clin Exp Allergy.* 2008;38(8):1290—1301. https://doi.org/10.1111/j.1365-2222.2008.03020.x.

118. GEHLHAR SCHLAAK, BECKER BUFE. Monitoring allergen immunotherapy of pollen-allergic patients: the ratio of allergen-specific IgG4 to IgG1 correlates with clinical outcome. *Clin Exp Allergy.* 1999;29(4):497—506. https://doi.org/10.1046/j.1365-2222.1999.00525.x.

119. Shamji MH, Wilcock LK, Wachholz PA, et al. The IgE-facilitated allergen binding (FAB) assay: validation of a novel flow-cytometric based method for the detection of inhibitory antibody responses. *J Immunol Methods.* 2006;317(1—2):71—79. https://doi.org/10.1016/j.jim.2006.09.004.

120. Dodev T, Bowen H, Shamji M, et al. Inhibition of allergen-dependent IgE activity by antibodies of the same specificity but different class. *Allergy.* 2015;70(6):720—724. https://doi.org/10.1111/all.12607.

121. James LK, Shamji MH, Walker SM, et al. Long-term tolerance after allergen immunotherapy is accompanied by selective persistence of blocking antibodies. *J Allergy Clin Immunol.* 2011;127(2):509—516.e5. https://doi.org/10.1016/j.jaci.2010.12.1080.

122. McHugh SM, Lavelle B, Kemeny DM, Patel S, Ewan PW. A placebo-controlled trial of immunotherapy with two extracts of Dermatophagoides pteronyssinus in allergic rhinitis, comparing clinical outcome with changes in antigen-specific IgE, IgG, and IgG subclasses. *J Allergy Clin Immunol.* 1990;86(4):521—531. https://doi.org/10.1016/s0091-6749(05)80208-8.

123. Platts-Mills T, von Maur R, Ishizaka K, Norman P, Lichtenstein L. IgA and IgG anti-ragweed antibodies in nasal secretions. Quantitative measurements of antibodies and correlation with inhibition of histamine release. *J Clin Invest*. 1976;57(4): 1041−1050. https://doi.org/10.1172/jci108346.

124. Reisinger J, Horak F, Pauli G, et al. Allergen-specific nasal IgG antibodies induced by vaccination with genetically modified allergens are associated with reduced nasal allergen sensitivity. *J Allergy Clin Immunol*. 2005;116(2):347−354. https://doi.org/10.1016/j.jaci.2005.04.003.

125. Shamji MH, Kappen J, Abubakar-Waziri H, et al. Nasal allergen neutralising IgG4 antibodies block IgE-mediated responses: novel biomarker of subcutaneous grass pollen immunotherapy. *J Allergy Clin Immunol*. 2018;143(3):1067−1076. https://doi.org/10.1016/j.jaci.2018.09.039.

126. Takhar P, Smurthwaite L, Coker HA, et al. Allergen drives class switching to IgE in the nasal mucosa in allergic rhinitis. *J Immunol*. 2005;174(8):5024−5032. https://doi.org/10.4049/jimmunol.174.8.5024.

127. Aalberse R. The role of IgG antibodies in allergy and immunotherapy. *Allergy*. 2011; 66(s95):28−30. https://doi.org/10.1111/j.1398-9995.2011.02628.x.

128. Orengo J, Radin A, Kamat V, et al. Treating cat allergy with monoclonal IgG antibodies that bind allergen and prevent IgE engagement. *Nat Commun*. 2018;9(1):1421. https://doi.org/10.1038/s41467-018-03636-8.

129. Corrigan C, Kettner J, Doemer C, Cromwell O, Narkus A, Group S. Efficacy and safety of preseasonal-specific immunotherapy with an aluminium-adsorbed six-grass pollen allergoid. *Allergy*. 2005;60(6):801−807. https://doi.org/10.1111/j.1398-9995.2005.00790.x.

130. Jutel M, Jaeger L, Suck R, Meyer H, Fiebig H, Cromwell O. Allergen-specific immunotherapy with recombinant grass pollen allergens. *J Allergy Clin Immunol*. 2005; 116(3):608−613. https://doi.org/10.1016/j.jaci.2005.06.004.

131. Pauli G, Larsen TH, Rak S, et al. Efficacy of recombinant birch pollen vaccine for the treatment of birch-allergic rhinoconjunctivitis. *J Allergy Clin Immunol*. 2008;122(5): 951−960. https://doi.org/10.1016/j.jaci.2008.09.017.

132. Couroux P, Patel D, Armstrong K, Larché M, Hafner R. Fel d 1-derived synthetic peptide immuno-regulatory epitopes show a long-term treatment effect in cat allergic subjects. *Clin Exp Allergy*. 2015;45(5):974−981. https://doi.org/10.1111/cea.12488.

133. Spertini F, DellaCorte G, Kettner A, et al. Efficacy of 2 months of allergen-specific immunotherapy with Bet v 1−derived contiguous overlapping peptides in patients with allergic rhinoconjunctivitis: results of a phase IIb study. *J Allergy Clin Immunol*. 2016;138(1):162−168. https://doi.org/10.1016/j.jaci.2016.02.044.

134. Niederberger V, Neubauer A, Gevaert P, et al. Safety and efficacy of immunotherapy with the recombinant B-cell epitope−based grass pollen vaccine BM32. *J Allergy Clin Immunol*. 2018;142(2):497−509.e9. https://doi.org/10.1016/j.jaci.2017.09.052.

135. Mösges R, Kasche E, Raskopf E, et al. A randomized, double-blind, placebo-controlled, dose-finding trial with Lolium perenne peptide immunotherapy. *Allergy*. 2018;73(4): 896−904. https://doi.org/10.1111/all.13358.

136. Leynadier F, Banoun L, Dollois B, et al. Immunotherapy with a calcium phosphate-adsorbed five-grass-pollen extract in seasonal rhinoconjunctivitis: a double-blind, placebo-controlled study. *Clin Exp Allergy*. 2001;31(7):988−996. https://doi.org/10.1046/j.1365-2222.2001.01145.x.

137. Drachenberg K, Wheeler A, Stuebner P, Horak F. A well-tolerated grass pollen-specific allergy vaccine containing
a novel adjuvant, monophosphoryl lipid A, reduces allergic symptoms after only four preseasonal injections. *Allergy.* 2001;56(6):498–505. https://doi.org/10.1034/j.1398-9995.2001.056006498.x.

138. Creticos PS, Schroeder JT, Hamilton RG, et al. Immunotherapy with a ragweed–toll-like receptor 9 agonist vaccine for allergic rhinitis. *N Eng J Med.* 2006;355(14): 1445–1455. https://doi.org/10.1056/nejmoa052916.

139. Buske L, Frew AJ, Horak F, et al. Ultrashort-specific immunotherapy successfully treats seasonal allergic rhinoconjunctivitis to grass pollen. *Allergy Asthma Proc.* 2011;32(3): 239–247. https://doi.org/10.2500/aap.2011.32.3453 (9).

140. Basomba A, Tabar AI, de Rojas DF, et al. Allergen vaccination with a liposome-encapsulated extract of Dermatophagoides pteronyssinus : a randomized, double-blind, placebo-controlled trial in asthmatic patients. *J Allergy Clin Immunol.* 2002; 109(6):943–948. https://doi.org/10.1067/mai.2002.124465.

141. Senti G, Johansen P, Haug S, et al. Use of A-type CpG oligodeoxynucleotides as an adjuvant in allergen-specific immunotherapy in humans: a phase I/IIa clinical trial. *Clin Exp Allergy.* 2009;39(4):562–570. https://doi.org/10.1111/j.1365-2222.2008.03191.x.

142. Klimek L, Willers J, Hammann-Haenni A, et al. Assessment of clinical efficacy of CYT003-QbG10 in patients with allergic rhinoconjunctivitis: a phase IIb study. *Clin Exp Allergy.* 2011;41(9):1305–1312. https://doi.org/10.1111/j.1365-2222.2011.03783.x.

143. Kuehr J, Brauburger J, Zielen S, et al. Efficacy of combination treatment with anti-IgE plus specific immunotherapy in polysensitized children and adolescents with seasonal allergic rhinitis. *J Allergy Clin Immunol.* 2002;109(2):274–280.

144. Kopp M, Hamelmann E, Zielen S, et al. Combination of omalizumab and specific immunotherapy is superior to immunotherapy in patients with seasonal allergic rhino-conjunctivitis and co-morbid seasonal allergic asthma. *Clin Exp Allergy.* 2009;39(2): 271–279. https://doi.org/10.1111/j.1365-2222.2008.03121.x.

145. Chaker AM, Shamji MH, Dumitru FA, et al. Short-term subcutaneous grass pollen immunotherapy under the umbrella of anti–IL-4: a randomized controlled trial. *J Allergy Clin Immunol.* 2016;137(2):452–461.e9. https://doi.org/10.1016/j.jaci.2015.08.046.

Sublingual immunotherapy: aeroallergen and venom*

8

Christopher A. Coop, MD[1]**, Theodore M. Freeman, MD**[2]

[1]*Department of Allergy and Immunology, Allergist, Allergy and Immunology Clinic, Wilford Hall Ambulatory Surgical Center, San Antonio, TX, United States;* [2]*San Antonio Asthma and Allergy Clinic, Owner, Allergy Immunology, San Antonio, TX, United States*

ABBREVIATIONS

Amb a 1	Ambrosia artemisiifolia major allergen 1
DF	*Dermatophagoides farina*
DP	*Dermatophagoides pteronyssinus*
FDA	US Federal Drug Administration
HDM	house dust mite
Ig	immunoglobulin
IL	interleukin
SCIT	subcutaneous Immunotherapy
SLIT	sublingual immunotherapy
TGF-β	transforming growth factor-beta
Th1	T helper cells type 1
Th2	T helper cells type 2
USD	Unites States Dollars

Introduction

Sublingual immunotherapy (SLIT) has been used for many years in Europe, and its acceptance is gaining traction in the United States, especially with the US Federal Drug Administration (FDA) approval of SLIT tablets for grasses, ragweed, and dust mites. Specific immunotherapy is proven to desensitize the immune system from airborne allergens. SLIT is felt to be a safer alternative to subcutaneous immunotherapy (SCIT) with a decreased risk of systemic anaphylactic reactions and no know fatalities to date.

Successful SLIT trials have been conducted for allergic rhinoconjunctivitis, asthma, atopic dermatitis, and even the prevention of asthma and atopy. In general,

---

* The opinions or assertions herein are the private views of the authors and are not to be construed as reflecting the views of the Department of the Air Force or the Department of Defense.

Immunotherapies for Allergic Disease. https://doi.org/10.1016/B978-0-323-54427-6.00008-0

aeroallergen SCIT seems to be more effective than SLIT. However, there are more safety concerns with SCIT, and SCIT is generally given in a medical setting, whereas SLIT can be given at home. For venom allergy, SCIT is proven to be effective. In contrast, there is little evidence that venom SLIT is effective.

Aeroallergen SLIT studies have been published for house dust mite (HDM), cat epithelia, trees, grasses, and weeds. SLIT is administered as liquid drops or dissolvable tablets to the oral mucosa. Typically, the drops or tablets are held under the tongue for up to 2 min for epithelial absorption. The optimal time for the allergen to be under the tongue is based on pharmokinetic studies, in which the allergen was tagged with a radioisotope and then followed over 48 h.[1] SLIT for aeroallergens is considered to be cost effective for allergic rhinoconjunctivitis and asthma.

Early studies of sublingual immunotherapy

One of the earliest SLIT studies involved 41 patients with cat allergy-induced rhino-conjunctivitis.[1] The patients were randomized to receive a standardized cat extract (~40 mcg Fel d 1) or placebo for 105 days. The treatment efficacy was measured by changes in symptoms during 90 min of exposure in an apartment containing cat dander. There were not significant changes in symptoms between the active SLIT group and the placebo group. In addition, no significant changes were found between the two groups in the cat-specific immunoglobulin (Ig)G and IgE levels and the prick skin tests. The short amount of time of the SLIT treatment in this trial may have affected the outcomes.

Another SLIT trial was conducted in 58 patients with seasonal rhinoconjunctivitis caused by grass pollens.[2] Subjects were randomized to receive a standardized SLIT allergen preparation (Stallergènes; Anthony, France) or a matched placebo for 17 weeks. The actively treated patients had significantly decreased rhinitis and conjunctivitis symptoms during the grass pollen season when compared to placebo. Furthermore, SLIT patients used significantly less allergy medications. There were minimal side effects in the SLIT group. The authors concluded that grass pollen SLIT is effective, easy to self-administer, inexpensive, and safe.

A Canadian study analyzed ragweed SLIT drops.[3] A standardized extract of ragweed allergen or placebo was administered daily to 83 patients before and during the ragweed pollen season (July–October 2001). The patients in the ragweed SLIT group had significantly less sneezing and nasal pruritus and their ragweed-specific IgE and IgG4 levels significantly increased during the trial period.

Tonnel et al. evaluated HDM SLIT in a placebo-controlled trial of 32 patients for 2 years.[4] Seventeen patients received a placebo extract and 15 subjects received a *Dermatophagoides pteronyssinus* and *Dermatophagoides farinae* 50/50 allergen extract. The dust mite SLIT group had significantly decreased total rhinitis, blocked nose, and nasal itching scores in the first and second years. Skin reactivity to house dust mites was significantly decreased in the active group who received HDM extract.

Sublingual immunotherapy tablets

There are several SLIT tablets that have been approved by the FDA for the treatment of allergic rhinitis and/or allergic rhinoconjunctivitis. Oralair is a grass pollen allergy tablet that contains five types of northern grass pollen (Sweet Vernal, Orchard, Perennial Rye, Timothy, and Kentucky Blue Grass) and is approved for patients aged 10–65 years old.[5] Oralair SLIT tablets are initiated 4 months before the expected onset of grass pollen season and then continued throughout the grass pollen season. Grastek is another SLIT grass tablet that has Timothy grass pollen. It is approved for ages 5–65.[6] Grastek SLIT tablets are typically prescribed 12 weeks before the expected onset of each grass pollen season, and then the patient will continue treatment throughout the grass pollen season.

Ragwitek is an SLIT tablet that incorporates short ragweed pollen for patients aged 18–65 years old.[7] It is recommended that patients take Ragwitek 12 weeks before the expected onset of ragweed pollen season and then continue treatment throughout the ragweed season. Recently, Odactra was approved by the FDA.[8] It is an HDM (*Dermatophagoides farinae* and *Dermatophagoides pteronyssinus*) allergen extract indicated for allergic rhinoconjunctivitis in patients 18 through 65 years old. Because house dust mite is a perennial allergen, Odactra is recommended to be used every day of the year. Table 8.1 has details regarding the SLIT tablets.

The SLIT tablets are prescribed as one tablet daily placed under the tongue where the tablet will dissolve within 10 s.[5–8] The tablets should not be swallowed. The first dose of the sublingual tablets should be administered under the supervision of a physician, and the patient should be observed for 30 min following the initial dose. The most common adverse reactions of SLIT tablets are throat irritation,

Table 8.1 U.S. Federal drug administration (FDA) approved sublingual immunotherapy tablets.

SLIT tablet	Aeroallergen(s)	Ages of approval	Dosing
Oralair	Sweet Vernal, Orchard, Perennial Rye, Timothy and Kentucky Blue grass	10–65 years old	100/300 IR tablets, start 4 months prior and continue through grass season
Grastek	Timothy grass	5–65 years old	2800 BAU tablet, start 12 weeks prior and continue through grass season
Ragwitek	Short ragweed	18–65 years old	12 Amb a 1-unit tablet, start 12 weeks prior and continue through ragweed season
Odactra	Dermatophagoides farinae and Dermatophagoides pteronyssinus	18–65 years old	12 SQ-house dust mite tablet, everyday use

*BAU, bioequivalent allergy units; *IR, index of reactivity; *SQ, standardized quality.

mouth pruritus/pain, swelling of the lips and tongue, nausea, stomach pain, and taste alteration. Contraindications for the use of the SLIT tablets include asthma that is severe or uncontrolled, a history of a systemic or local allergic reaction to sublingual immunotherapy and a history of eosinophilic esophagitis.[2] Additionally, patients should not use the tablets if they have a hypersensitivity to any of the inactive ingredients contained in the tablets.

There is a black box warning for the SLIT tablets in the United States.[5–8] The black box states that the tablets can cause life-threatening allergic reactions including anaphylaxis and severe laryngopharyngeal restriction. It also mentions that the tablets should not be given to patient with unstable asthma. It instructs physicians to give the first dose of the tablet in the medical office and observe patients for 30 min following the initial dose. Patients should also be prescribed an epinephrine autoinjector, and they should be instructed on the appropriate use of the epinephrine autoinjector. Patients should seek immediate medical care if the epinephrine autoinjector is used. Finally, the SLIT tablets should not be prescribed to patients who are unresponsive to epinephrine and inhaled bronchodilators such as those patients taking β-blockers or patients with medical conditions who may not survive a serious allergic reaction.

The wholesale price of both Grastek and Ragwitek was ∼10 per pill, or $247.50 for a 30-day supply, when they were initially approved—according to information from Merck. The wholesale price of Oralair is $12 per pill, or $300 for a 30-day supply according to Greer Laboratories, which is marketing the drug in the United States.[9] Odactra is expected to be at a similar cost per pill when compared to the other SLIT tablets. The costs of the SLIT tablets can be offset by insurance coverage and other programs sponsored by the pharmaceutical companies.

Mechanisms of sublingual immunotherapy

There are several proposed immunologic mechanisms of SLIT. The oral mucosa provides an environment to promote tolerance to allergens. When the allergens of SLIT are taken up by the oral mucosa, tolerogenic dendritic cells support the differentiation of T helper cells type 1 (Th1).[10] This represents a shift from the allergic disease promoting T helper cells type 2 (Th2) responses to a Th1 inflammatory response.

SLIT promotes the induction of interleukin (IL)-10 producing regulatory T cells and the production of transforming growth factor-beta (TGF-β). IL-10 and TGF-β suppress allergen-specific T-cell responses.[11] Sublingual grass pollen immunotherapy is also associated with increases in sublingual Foxp3-expressing cells and elevated allergen-specific IgG and IgA antibodies.[12,13] These antibodies block allergen IgE complex formation and contribute to an antiinflammatory environment.

Scadding et al. analyzed biopsies from the sublingual mucosa of 14 grass pollen SLIT treated-atopic patients, 9 placebo-treated atopic patients, and 8 normal controls.[12] Foxp3+ cells were significantly increased in the oral epithelium of

Table 8.2 Immunologic changes from sublingual immunotherapy.

1 Shift to T helper cells type 1 (Th1) from Th2 cells
2 Induction of IL-10
3 Increased regulatory T cells
4 Production of transforming growth factor beta (TGF-β)
5 Increased sublingual Foxp3-expressing cells
6 Elevated specific IgG1/IgG4 and IgA
7 Decreased levels of CD80, CD86
8 Decreased IL-4 and IL-5 production

SLIT-treated patients when compared to the placebo-treated patients. Additionally, the IgG1 and IgG4 levels were significantly increased in the biopsies of those patients who had received SLIT. During the peak season, the IgA1 and IgA2 levels were increased in the patients receiving SLIT.

SLIT-treated patients were compared to patients being treated with symptomatic therapy alone in a 3-year trial.[14] The clinical benefits as measured by symptoms scores and medication use were significantly better in the patients undergoing prolonged SLIT. Immunologically, SLIT resulted in increased IL-10 production, increased programmed cell death ligand 1 expression and increased allergen-specific IgG4 levels. There were also decreased levels of CD80, CD86 expression and IL-4 production in the SLIT patients.

O'Hehir et al. conducted a randomized double-blind placebo-controlled study of HDM SLIT for 12 months in 30 patients to evaluate immunologic markers.[15] Compared to placebo, the SLIT group had significantly decreased serum IL-5 production at 6 and 12 months of therapy. Additionally, the active SLIT group had increased serum levels of IL-10 and TGF-β. The SLIT group had increased regulatory T cells and serum Der p 2 specific IgG4 levels. The authors concluded that TGF-β mediates the immunological suppression seen in HDM SLIT. The immunologic changes of SLIT are shown in Table 8.2.

Efficacy and safety of sublingual immunotherapy
Allergic rhinoconjunctivitis

SLIT for allergic rhinoconjunctivitis has been evaluated in double-blind placebo-controlled trials. In general, higher doses of SLIT are more effective than lower doses. Grazax (Timothy grass tablet) was evaluated in a 5-year double-blind, placebo-controlled trial.[16] The trial included 2 years of blinded follow-up after completion of a 3-year period of treatment. Participants were adults with a history of moderate-to-severe grass pollen-induced allergic rhinoconjunctivitis with symptoms inadequately controlled by medications. The patients could have asthma. The investigational treatment was initiated 4—8 months before the anticipated start of the grass pollen season.

A total of 238 participants completed the trial. The mean rhinoconjunctivitis daily symptom score was reduced by 25% ($P \leq .004$) in the grass allergy SLIT tablet group compared with the placebo group over the five grass pollen seasons. There was a significant difference in the percentage of days with severe symptoms during the peak grass pollen exposure when compared with placebo (49%−63%, $P \leq .0001$). Efficacy of the grass tablet was supported by significant effects on the allergen-specific antibody response (IgG4 levels and IgE-blocking factor). There were no major safety issues.

Another double-blind placebo-controlled study of Grazax focused on efficacy and quality-of-life measures in 855 patients with seasonal allergic rhinoconjunctivitis.[17,18] These patients were randomized to receive Grazax once a day versus placebo and they started therapy 8 weeks before the start of the grass pollen season and continued throughout the pollen season. If patients had allergic symptoms, they received loratadine or placebo as rescue medication. Assessments were made by a quality-of-life questionnaire. The findings of this trial showed that the grass allergen SLIT tablets improved allergic rhinoconjunctivitis quality-of-life scores. The Grazax tablets also reduced symptoms greater than the rescue antihistamine alone.

Oralair, the five grass pollen SLIT tablet, has also been evaluated for clinical efficacy in double-blind placebo-controlled studies. Didier et al. conducted a trial of 633 patients who were treated for either 2 or 4 months before the grass pollen season and during the grass pollen season with active SLIT tablets or placebo.[19] These patients were treated for three consecutive seasons. The primary outcome was the average adjusted symptom score (symptom score adjusted for rescue medication use). Other outcomes were symptoms, rescue medication use, quality of life, and safety assessments. The mean average adjusted symptom score was reduced by 36.0% and 34.5% at season 3 in both active treatment groups (2- and 4-month preseason/coseason SLIT tablet) when compared with placebo ($P < .0001$ for both groups). Improvements were also seen in symptoms scores, medication scores, and quality-of-life assessments. Adverse events were mainly local reactions that improved in subsequent seasons.

Oralair was found to be efficacious in another randomized placebo-controlled trial.[20] A total of 473 adults with grass pollen allergic rhinoconjunctivitis were randomized to receive Oralair or placebo for 4 months before grass season and then throughout the grass pollen season. A combined symptom and medication rescue score was used to evaluate the patients. The mean daily combined score was significantly lower in the active SLIT tablet treatment group when compared to the placebo group during the pollen season. The most frequent reported adverse events were oral pruritus, throat irritation, and nasopharyngitis. No reports of anaphylaxis were observed and epinephrine was not used by any patient. There is additional objective data showing that Oralair is safe and effective for up to 5 years of treatment and some of these trials included patients with asthma.[21−23]

There have been several studies evaluating the effectiveness and safety of Ragwitek, the ragweed SLIT tablet. Creticos et al. conducted a randomized double-blind placebo-controlled trial of 784 adult patients with allergic rhinoconjunctivitis.[24]

Patients self-administered 1.5, 6, or 12 units of Ambrosia artemisiifolia major allergen 1 (Amb a 1) SLIT tablets for 52 weeks or they took a placebo. The combined medication and symptom scores of the patients receiving the 12 unit Amb a one ragweed SLIT tablets were significantly improved during the peak and the entire ragweed season when compared with placebo. The SLIT tablets were well tolerated and there were no reported systemic allergic reactions.

An additional trial of 565 patients was conducted with the ragweed SLIT tablets.[25] Patients were randomized to receive either the daily ragweed tablet of 6 or 12 Amb a 1 units for 52 weeks. During peak ragweed season, the patients who took the 6 and 12 Amb a 1 unit ragweed tablets showed 21% and 27% improvement in total combined score (symptoms and medication use) versus placebo ($P < .05$). Most of the adverse events were mild, oral reactions; however, one patient in the 6-Amb a 1 unit group received epinephrine for localized pharyngeal edema at an emergency facility.

HDM SLIT tablets have been evaluated in several clinical trials. One study evaluated 427 adults with HDM-induced allergic rhinitis.[26] Patients were randomized in a double-blind, placebo-controlled study to receive HDM SLIT tablets [500 index of reactivity (IR) tablets or 300IR tablets] or placebo. The patients received the treatment once daily for 1 year and then were followed for the subsequent year. Both HDM SLIT tablets significantly reduced the mean average adjusted symptom scores when compared with placebo. The efficacy of the SLIT tablets was maintained during the treatment free follow-up phase of 1 year. The onset of action of the SLIT tablets was 4 months. The only adverse events were localized reactions. There were no reports of anaphylaxis in this study.

Another HDM SLIT tablet study was conducted by Demoly et al. of 992 adult patients.[27] Patients with moderate-to-severe allergic rhinitis from HDM were randomized in a double-blind, placebo-controlled trial. Subjects received either 6 standardized quality (SQ)-HDM, 12 SQ-HDM or placebo tablets daily for 1 year. The results of the trial showed that patients receiving the 12 SQ-HDM SLIT tablets had significant improvement in their rhinitis symptoms, medication, and quality-of-life scores starting at 14 weeks and continuing throughout the trial. The active treatment was well tolerated with minimal adverse events.

Asthma

SLIT appears to be safe and effective in asthmatic patients. An early study by Bousquet et al. found HDM SLIT to be effective in asthmatic patients.[28] In this trial, 85 patients with HDM-induced asthma received either placebo or SLIT with a standardized *Dermatophagoides pteronyssinus* (DP)-*D. farinae* (DF) 50/50 extract for 24 months. The SLIT group had a significant decrease in their asthma medication use and a significant improvement in their quality-of-life scores. They also had significant improvements in their lung function and decreased bronchial hyperreactivity compared to placebo. The SLIT group showed a significant increase in specific IgE DP, IgE DF, IgG4 DP, and IgG4 DF levels after SLIT.

Wang et al. conducted a randomized double-blind placebo-controlled trial of dust mite allergic asthmatic patients.[29] Patients received an aqueous, standardized, 300 index of reactivity mixture of DP and DF extracts or a placebo daily for 12 months. Subjects in the actively treated group with moderate, persistent asthma were better able to achieve control of their asthma by the asthma control questionnaire. They also had a greater mean reduction in their inhaled corticosteroid use when compared to the placebo group. The moderate persistent asthma group was defined as patients taking 401–800 μg of budesonide per day.

Another study of 604 subjects demonstrated that HDM SLIT tablets helped mild-to-moderate asthma patients to reduce their inhaled corticosteroid dose.[30] Patients received SLIT tablets for 1 year, and the mean difference between the active and placebo group was a reduction in daily ICS dose of 81 μg.

Nolte et al. reported on four separate trials of a total of 2467 patients who were randomized to placebo or 1.5, 6, or 12 Amb a 1 units.[31] These studies included patients with asthma and allergic rhinoconjunctivitis and lasted 28–52 weeks. The focus of this analysis was safety and tolerability of the ragweed SLIT tablet. In general, more adverse events were reported in the 6 and 12 Amb a 1 unit groups when compared to placebo. Most of these adverse events were local application site reactions occurring in the first few days of treatment. The asthmatic patients did not report worsening of their symptoms. There was no angioedema that led to airway obstruction or respiratory compromise, and patients did not have anaphylactic shock or life-threatening reactions.

A systematic review of 63 studies with 5131 patients analyzed SLIT for the treatment of allergic rhinoconjunctivitis and asthma.[32] The review concluded that there is strong evidence showing that SLIT improves asthma symptoms. Eight of 13 studies reported a greater than 40% improvement in asthma symptoms. For allergic rhinoconjunctivitis, 9 of 36 studies demonstrated a greater than 40% improvement in symptoms for patients using SLIT. Additionally, 16 of 41 studies reported that medication use for asthma and allergies decreased by more than 40% for the SLIT patients.

A Cochrane Database review evaluated 52 studies with 5077 patients who had received SLIT for asthma.[33] Most of the studies were double-blind placebo controlled, and most of the participants had mild or intermittent asthma. In general, SLIT immunotherapy was beneficial when compared to placebo for patients with asthma. However, the authors had difficulty analyzing most of the studies due to lack of data for outcomes such as asthma exacerbations, quality-of-life measures, and the use of different symptom and medication scores. There were very few serious adverse events in the trials, and most of the adverse events were local reactions.

Odactra (ALK, Hosham Deenmark) has been approved with the indication for asthma in Europe.

Prevention of asthma and atopy

There is evidence that SLIT can prevent the development of asthma. Valovirta et al. conducted a double-blind placebo-controlled trial of 812 children with grass pollen allergic rhinoconjunctivitis but no medical history or signs of asthma.[34] The subjects received the standard quality (SQ) grass SLIT tablet (GRAZAX 75,000 SQ-T/2800 BAU) or placebo for 3 years of treatment and then were followed for an additional 2 years. Those patients who received the SQ timothy grass SLIT tablet had a significantly reduced risk of experiencing asthma symptoms or using asthma medications at the end of the trial (odds ratio $= 0.66$, $P < .036$) and during the 2-year posttreatment follow-up period. Additionally, the total IgE, timothy grass pollen-specific IgE, and skin prick test reactivity to grass pollen were all reduced in the active group when compared to placebo.

Regarding the prevention of atopy, Zolkipli evaluated 111 infants less than age 1 in a prospective, randomized, double-blind, placebo-controlled trial.[35] The infants had a high risk of atopy defined as having 2 or greater first degree relatives with allergic disease. The subjects had negative skin prick test responses to common allergens (HDM, grass pollen, cat, peanut, milk, and egg) at randomization. High dose HDM immunotherapy extract versus placebo solution was administered orally twice daily for 12 months. The children were assessed every 3 months. There was a significant reduction in sensitization to any of the common allergens in the active SLIT group compared to the placebo group. The adverse events were mild and comparable in each group.

A retrospective study of 302 patients investigated the long term and preventive effects of grass HDM or parietaria SLIT.[36] In this trial, only 1% of patients without asthma who received SLIT reported an onset of respiratory symptoms and only 9.6% of patients undergoing new skin tests showed new sensitizations. The clinical benefits of SLIT were strongly linked to the length of treatment. The patients with long-lasting benefits of SLIT were treated for a mean length of time of 29.1 months, while patients showing a return to pre-SLIT conditions only received SLIT for a mean of 13.3 months.

Atopic dermatitis

There are a few clinical trials supporting the use of SLIT for the treatment of atopic dermatitis. Pajno et al. conducted a randomized double-blind placebo-controlled trial of HDM SLIT in 56 children with atopic dermatitis.[37] These children were sensitized to dust mites alone and did not have food allergy or chronic asthma. SLIT or placebo was given for 18 months in addition to standard therapy. The children receiving dust mite SLIT had a significant improvement in their SCORAD score (scoring atopic dermatitis) and had a significant reduction in their medication use. These significant differences were seen in the patients with mild-to-moderate atopic dermatitis only. Two patients had to stop SLIT because of an exacerbation of their dermatitis.

Another open study of SLIT was published in dust mite sensitized children with atopic dermatitis.[38] A total of 57 children received dust mite SLIT or placebo for 72 weeks. The active SLIT group had a significantly reduced SCORAD score when compare with the standard treatment. SLIT was well tolerated. Adverse events consisted only of immediate and transient local events.

SLIT with DF drops was evaluated in 107 patients with atopic dermatitis.[39] After 12 months, the active SLIT treatment group had significantly reduced average daily drug scores and visual analogue scores. The treatment group also had a higher level of serum-specific IgG4 than the control group at 6 and 12 months of therapy.

Finally, Gendelman and Lang completed a systematic review of SLIT for the treatment of atopic dermatitis.[40] They found that many studies reported clinical improvement in atopic dermatitis symptoms with SLIT; however, there were methodological shortcomings in many of these studies. These flaws included lack of a control group, lack of randomization, allocation concealment, and the fact that many of the enrolled subjects did not complete the entire protocol.

A review of the safety and efficacy of SLIT for atopic dermatitis was conducted by Cox and Calderon.[3]

Pediatric studies

SLIT has been found to be safe and effective in the pediatric population. Bufe et al. evaluated 253 children ages 5–16 years in a randomized placebo-controlled European trial.[41] The children had grass pollen-induced rhinoconjunctivitis with or without asthma. The patients received the Grazax timothy grass pollen SLIT tablet or placebo starting 8–23 weeks before the grass pollen season in 2007. They continued treatment throughout the entire grass season. The median rhinoconjunctivitis symptom, medication, and asthma symptom scores were all statistically significantly improved in the active treatment group compared to placebo. Oral pruritus was the most common adverse event occurring in 40 subjects. There were no serious treatment-related adverse events.

Di Rienzo et al. demonstrated that HDM SLIT was effective and safe in asthmatic children.[42] Sixty children with allergic asthma and rhinitis due to mites were divided into two matched groups (35 children received SLIT for 4–5 years and 25 received standard drug therapy). The SLIT group had better asthma control, and the mean peak expiratory flow results were significantly higher in the active SLIT group than in the control group after 10 years. There were no serious adverse events.

A North American study of 345 children (5–17 years old) was conducted evaluating timothy grass SLIT tablets (15 μg of Phl p 5) versus placebo.[43] Treatment was started 16 weeks before grass season and continued throughout grass season. Significant improvements were seen in symptom scores, medication scores, and rhinoconjunctivitis quality-of-life scores. Phl p 5 specific IgG4 and IgE-blocking factor levels were significantly higher at the peak and end of the grass pollen season ($P < .001$). In this study, adverse events were mild and transient; however, 1 grass SLIT tablet patient experienced lip angioedema, dysphagia, and cough.

A safety study of 195 children who received HDM SLIT tablets was published in 2016.[44] Dust mite allergic children received an HDM SLIT tablet [6 standardized quality (SQ) or 12 SQ)] or placebo once daily for 28 days. Generally, the two HDM SLIT tablet doses were well tolerated. There were no serious adverse events, anaphylactic reactions, or localized swellings in the mouth or throat. Approximately 6% of the patients in the active group discontinued the SLIT tablets because of adverse events.

There is evidence that SLIT may be ineffective in children. In one trial, 168 children aged 6–18 years with allergic rhinitis were randomly assigned to receive placebo or mixed grass pollen SLIT for 2 years.[45] The mean daily total symptom score did not differ between the children in the active SLIT group compared to placebo. Additionally, there were no differences between the groups in rescue medication free days and quality-of-life measures.

Another study of HDM SLIT was conducted in 251 children with allergic rhinitis.[46] The participants received either SLIT or placebo for 2 years. There was no difference in the symptom or medication scores between the two groups after the treatment period.

Sublingual versus subcutaneous immunotherapy

In general, SCIT appears to be more effective than SLIT, and SLIT is safer than SCIT; however, direct comparison studies are lacking. One early trial evaluated dust mite SLIT drops, SCIT, and sublingual placebo drops in 36 patients with rhinitis and asthma for 1 year.[47] The patients treated with dust mite SLIT had significantly decreased rhinitis symptoms but their asthma scores were unchanged. The medication scores decreased significantly for both active groups when compared to their baseline scores. Additionally, dust mite IgG4 concentrations were significantly higher in both the SLIT and SCIT groups after 1 year.

Another trial of 71 individuals with birch pollen-induced rhinoconjunctivitis were studied in a 3-year placebo-controlled randomized trial of SLIT versus SCIT.[48] For the active groups (SLIT and SCIT), symptom and medication scores were significantly improved compared to placebo. The clinical efficacy of SLIT was not statistically different from SCIT. SLIT appeared safer overall with only local mild side effects. The SCIT group had a few serious systemic side effects.

Di Bona et al. published an indirect meta-analysis-based comparison between SCIT and SLIT in the treatment of seasonal allergic rhinitis from grass allergens.[49] The analysis included 36 double-blind randomized controlled trials (3013 patients and 2768 controls). The treatment efficacy was determined as the standardized mean difference in symptom and medication scores of SCIT or SLIT compared to placebo. The SCIT symptom and medication scores were significantly higher than the SLIT (drops and tablets) scores, and the authors concluded that SCIT was more effective for seasonal allergic rhinitis due to grass pollen.

Chelladurai et al. accomplished a systematic review of eight trials comparing the effectiveness of SCIT versus SLIT for the treatment of allergic rhinoconjunctivitis and asthma.[50] There was low-grade evidence supporting the effectiveness of SCIT over SLIT for asthma symptom reduction and medication use. There was moderate grade evidence for SCIT over SLIT for nasal and eye symptom reduction. SLIT was found to be safer overall, and there was one report of anaphylaxis in a child treated with SCIT.

Allergists use of sublingual immunotherapy

Two surveys had been published regarding the use of SLIT among practicing allergists in the United States. The first survey was published in 2008 and reported that only 5.9% of allergists in the Unites States were using SLIT.[51] The majority of the allergists (61.7%) were not using SLIT because it was not approved by the FDA. Those allergists using SLIT had it reimbursed by patients paying out of their pocket. Most of the allergists perceived SLIT to be as effective as SCIT. The majority of the allergists (81.8%) gave the first dose of SLIT in their office, and only 41.5% of practicing allergists gave epinephrine injectors to their SLIT patients. Some practitioners required their patients to administer all of the SLIT doses in their office.

A second follow-up survey of practicing allergists and SLIT was published in 2013.[52] In this survey, 11.4% of allergists reported using SLIT. In addition, the lack of FDA approval of SLIT was a deterrent for its use among practitioners. The majority of the respondents believed that SLIT was safer than SCIT. In this survey, only 43% of the practicing allergists felt that SLIT had equal efficacy when compared to SCIT. Most of the allergists gave at least the first dose of SLIT in their office under medical supervision, and most allergists prescribed an epinephrine injector for their SLIT patients. In general, more allergists in the United States are prescribing SLIT, and this number should continue to increase with the FDA approval of the various SLIT tablets.

Cost effectiveness of sublingual immunotherapy

There have been a few studies analyzing the cost effectiveness of sublingual immunotherapy. Berto et al. evaluated the cost effectiveness of sublingual immunotherapy in 135 children with allergic rhinitis and asthma in Italy.[53] The children included in the analysis had 1 year of data before receiving SLIT and then 3 years of data while receiving SLIT. The outcome measures included number of exacerbations, doctor visits, and absence from school. The direct costs were money spent on medications, specialist visits, and SLIT. The indirect costs were parental work loss. The authors found a substantial reduction in all of the outcome measures during the SLIT period when compared to the period before the patients received SLIT. The average annual cost per patient was 2672 Euros/$3143 USD before the initiation of SLIT and 629 Euros/$740 UDS per year while the patients were receiving SLIT.

An open-label randomized clinical trial compared the costs of SLIT versus SCIT.[54] There were 19 patients receiving SLIT, 23 patients on SCIT, and a control group of 22 patients. The outcome measures were Rhinoconjunctivitis Quality-of-Life Questionnaire score, visual analog scale score, symptomatic medication reduction, and direct and indirect costs. The SLIT and SCIT patients had similar clinical outcomes. Over 3 years of treatment, SLIT was found to be more cost effective (3-year expenditures per patient on SLIT were 684 Euros/$798 USD and 1004 Euros/$1171 USD for patients on SCIT).

Ariano et al. conducted an economic evaluation of SLIT versus symptomatic treatment in 70 patients with allergic asthma due to HDM.[55] Fifty of the patients received HDM SLIT, and 20 patients were treated with symptomatic drugs for 3 years. The trial continued for an additional 2 years after stopping SLIT for a total of 5 years. For the first year only, the patients who received SLIT had a higher mean annual cost but this mean annual cost became significantly lower after the first year and continued for the full 5 years of the trial.

Finally, the grass allergen tablet (Grazax) was compared with symptomatic medication in seven Northern European countries in a prospective pharmacoeconomic analysis over a 9-year time period.[56] The grass allergen tablet was clinically superior to symptomatic treatment showing a significant increase in the number of quality of life years gained. Furthermore, for the grass tablet SLIT group, there was significantly less use of rescue medications (loratadine and budesonide) and less hours missed from work. The authors concluded that the grass allergen tablet is a cost effective intervention for the prevention of grass pollen-induced rhinoconjunctivitis for a tablet price below 6 Euro ($7 USD).

A comprehensive systematic review of AIT found it to be cost effective at about 6 years after initiation.[4]

Sublingual immunotherapy for venom allergy
Venom immunotherapy for systemic reactions

Currently, SLIT is not recommended for venom allergy because of lack of large clinical studies showing efficacy.[57] There has been one study showing that SLIT for venom allergy may be an effective treatment. A small study of 21 patients with systemic reactions to wasp venom was published in 2009.[58,59] The patients were treated with a sublingual Vespula venom extract until a maintenance dose of 100,000 standardized quality units of venom extract weekly was reached. The maintenance dose was 10 drops of pure venom extract 3 times a week (corresponding to 100 μg of venom extract). Four of the patients underwent sting challenges and only one patient experienced throat constriction. Regarding adverse events, two patients had mild reactions (dysphagia and itching) during the induction phase of the trial, and no adverse events were reported during the maintenance phase. The authors concluded that large multicenter studies are needed to further investigate the safety and efficacy of SLIT in patient with Hymenoptera venom allergy.

Venom immunotherapy for large local reactions

There is limited data regarding SLIT venom immunotherapy for large local reactions to hymenoptera. A randomized, double-blind, placebo-controlled study was conducted involving patients with large local reactions (LLRs) who were monosensitized to honeybee.[60] After a baseline sting challenge, the patients were randomized to either SLIT or placebo for 6 months. Patients underwent a 6-week build-up period followed by maintenance with 525 μg of venom monthly. A sting challenge was repeated after 6 months.

A total of 26 patients completed the study. In the active group, the median of the peak maximal diameter of the LLRs decreased from 20.5 to 8.5 cm ($P = .014$). There was no change in the placebo group. The diameter of the LLRs was reduced by more than 50% in 57% of patients. There was one case of generalized urticaria that occurred in a placebo-treated patient at the 6-month sting challenge. There were no adverse events in the SLIT group. The authors concluded that honeybee SLIT significantly reduced the size of LLRs, and there were no adverse events. They recommended further large trials to investigate the effectiveness of this treatment.

Conclusion

SLIT has been used in Europe for many years, and its use is increasing in the United States. SLIT has been shown to be effective for allergic rhinoconjunctivitis, asthma, and atopic dermatitis; however, it may not be as effective as SCIT. SLIT offers the advantage of being safer and more convenient. It can be self-administered at home by patients, and there is a decreased risk of systemic reactions with SLIT. SLIT appears to be cost effective.

The mechanisms of SLIT are similar to SCIT. These mechanisms are a shift from Th2 to Th1 cells, induction of IL-10 and production of TGF-β. Regulatory T cells and specific IgG1/IgG4 and IgA may also be involved in the immunologic response of SLIT.

One disadvantage to SLIT is patients with multiple aeroallergen sensitivities who require many allergens for immunotherapy. It is preferable for these patients to receive SCIT as the dosing is less onerous. Another limitation of SLIT in the United States is the lack of FDA approval for many aeroallergens. Currently, SLIT is only approved by the FDA for grasses, ragweed, and HDM.

SLIT as a treatment for systemic reactions from venom allergy is not recommended currently because of the lack of large studies showing efficacy. There is one small study showing benefit of SLIT for large local reactions from bee venom, and this may be a consideration for some patients. Definitely more research is needed regarding SLIT for venom allergy.

References

1. Nelson HS, Oppenheimer J, Vatsia GA, et al. A double-blind, placebo-controlled evaluation of sublingual immunotherapy with standardized cat extract. *J Allergy Clin Immunol*. 1993;92(2):229–236.

2. Sabbah A, Hassoun S, Le Sellin J, et al. A double-blind, placebo-controlled trial by the sublingual route of immunotherapy with a standardized grass pollen extract. *Allergy.* 1994;49(5):309–313.

3. Bowen T, Greenbaum J, Charbonneau Y, et al. Canadian trial of sublingual swallow immunotherapy for ragweed rhinoconjunctivitis. *Ann Allergy Asthma Immunol.* 2004; 93(5):425–430.

4. Tonnel AB, Scherpereel A, Douay B, et al. Allergic rhinitis due to house dust mites: evaluation of the efficacy of specific sublingual immunotherapy. *Allergy.* 2004;59(5): 491–497.

5. Oralair® (Sweet Vernal, Orchard, Perennial Rye, Timothy, and Kentucky Blue Grass Mixed Pollens Allergen Extract- https://www.fda.gov/downloads/biologicsbloodvaccines/allergenics/ucm391580.pdf.

6. Grastek® (Timothy Grass Pollen Allergen Extract) Tablet- https://www.fda.gov/downloads/BiologicsBloodVaccines/Allergenics/UCM393184.pdf.

7. Ragwitek® (Short Ragweed Pollen Allergen Extract) Tablet-https://www.fda.gov/downloads/biologicsbloodvaccines/allergenics/ucm393600.pdf.

8. Odactra® House Dust Mite (Dermatophagoides farinae and Dermatophagoides pteronyssinus) Allergen Extract Tablet- https://www.fda.gov/downloads/biologicsbloodvaccines/allergenics/ucm544382.pdf.

9. https://www.rxlist.com/script/main/art.asp?articlekey=178133.

10. Jay DC, Nadeau KC. Immune mechanisms of sublingual immunotherapy. *Curr Allergy Asthma Rep.* 2014;14(11):473.

11. Allam J-P, Würtzen PA, Reinartz M, et al. Phl p 5 resorption in human oral mucosa leads to dose-dependent and time-dependent allergen binding by oral mucosal Langerhans cells, attenuates their maturation, and enhances their migratory and TGF-β1 and IL-10-producing properties. *J Allergy Clin Immunol.* 2010;126:638–645.

12. Scadding GW, Shamji MH, Jacobson MR, et al. Sublingual grass pollen immunotherapy is associated with increases in sublingual Foxp3-expressing cells and elevated allergen-specific immunoglobulin G4, immunoglobulin A and serum inhibitory activity for immunoglobulin E-facilitated allergen binding to B cells. *Clin Exp Allergy.* 2010;40(4): 598–606.

13. James LK, Shamji MH, Walker SM, et al. Long-term tolerance after allergen immunotherapy is accompanied by selective persistence of blocking antibodies. *J Allergy Clin Immunol.* 2011;127:509–516.

14. Piconi S, Trabattoni D, Rainone V, et al. Immunological effects of sublingual immunotherapy: clinical efficacy is associated with modulation of programmed cell death ligand 1, IL-10, and IgG4. *J Immunol.* 2010;185(12):7723–7730.

15. O'Hehir RE, Gardner LM, de Leon MP, et al. House dust mite sublingual immunotherapy: the role for transforming growth factor-beta and functional regulatory T cells. *Am J Respir Crit Care Med.* 2009;180(10):936–947.

16. Durham SR, Emminger W, Kapp A, et al. SQ-standardized sublingual grass immunotherapy: confirmation of disease modification 2 years after 3 years of treatment in a randomized trial. *J Allergy Clin Immunol.* 2012;129(3):717–725.

17. Durham SR, Yang WH, Pedersen MR, et al. Sublingual immunotherapy with once-daily grass allergen tablets: a randomized controlled trial in seasonal allergic rhinoconjunctivitis. *J Allergy Clin Immunol.* 2006;117(4):802–809.

18. Rak S, Yang WH, Pedersen MR, et al. Once-daily sublingual allergen-specific immuno-therapy improves quality of life in patients with grass pollen-induced allergic rhinocon-junctivitis: a double-blind, randomized study. *Qual Life Res.* 2007;16(2):191—201.

19. Didier A, Worm M, Horak F, et al. Sustained 3-year efficacy of pre- and coseasonal 5-grass-pollen sublingual immunotherapy tablets in patients with grass pollen-induced rhinoconjunctivitis. *J Allergy Clin Immunol.* 2011;128(3):559—566.

20. Cox LS, Casale TB, Nayak AS, et al. Clinical efficacy of 300IR 5-grass pollen sublingual tablet in a US study: the importance of allergen-specific serum IgE. *J Allergy Clin Immunol.* 2012;130(6):1327—1334.

21. Didier A, Wahn U, Horak F, et al. Five-grass-pollen sublingual immunotherapy tablet for the treatment of grass-pollen-induced allergic rhinoconjunctivitis: 5 years of experience. *Expert Rev Clin Immunol.* 2014;10(10):1309—1324.

22. Didier A, Malling HJ, Worm M, et al. Post-treatment efficacy of discontinuous treatment with 300IR 5-grass pollen sublingual tablet in adults with grass pollen-induced allergic rhinoconjunctivitis. *Clin Exp Allergy.* 2013;43(5):568—577.

23. Malling HJ, Montagut A, Melac M, et al. Efficacy and safety of 5-grass pollen sublingual immunotherapy tablets in patients with different clinical profiles of allergic rhinoconjunctivitis. *Clin Exp Allergy.* 2009;39(3):387—393.

24. Creticos PS, Maloney J, Bernstein DI, et al. Randomized controlled trial of a ragweed allergy immunotherapy tablet in North American and European adults. *J Allergy Clin Immunol.* 2013;131(5):1342—1349.

25. Nolte H, Hébert J, Berman G, et al. Randomized controlled trial of ragweed allergy immunotherapy tablet efficacy and safety in North American adults. *Ann Allergy Asthma Immunol.* 2013;110(6):450—456.

26. Bergmann KC, Demoly P, Worm M, et al. Efficacy and safety of sublingual tablets of house dust mite allergen extracts in adults with allergic rhinitis. *J Allergy Clin Immunol.* 2014;133(6):1608—1614.

27. Demoly P, Emminger W, Rehm D, et al. Effective treatment of house dust mite-induced allergic rhinitis with 2 doses of the SQ HDM SLIT-tablet: results from a randomized, double-blind, placebo-controlled phase III trial. *J Allergy Clin Immunol.* 2016;137(2): 444—451.

28. Bousquet J, Scheinmann P, Guinnepain MT, et al. Sublingual-swallow immunotherapy (SLIT) in patients with asthma due to house-dust mites: a double-blind, placebo-controlled study. *Allergy.* 1999;54(3):249—260.

29. Wang L, Yin J, Fadel R, et al. House dust mite sublingual immunotherapy is safe and appears to be effective in moderate, persistent asthma. *Allergy.* 2014;69(9):1181—1188.

30. Mosbech H, Deckelmann R, de Blay F, et al. Standardized quality (SQ) house dust mite sublingual immunotherapy tablet (ALK) reduces inhaled corticosteroid use while main-taining asthma control: a randomized, double-blind, placebo-controlled trial. *J Allergy Clin Immunol.* 2014;134(3):568—575.

31. Nolte H, Amar N, Bernstein DI, et al. Safety and tolerability of a short ragweed sublin-gual immunotherapy tablet. *Ann Allergy Asthma Immunol.* 2014;113(1):93—100.

32. Lin SY, Erekosima N, Kim JM, et al. Sublingual immunotherapy for the treatment of allergic rhinoconjunctivitis and asthma: a systematic review. *J Am Med Assoc.* 2013; 309(12):1278—1288.

33. Normansell R, Kew KM, Bridgman AL. Sublingual immunotherapy for asthma. *Cochrane Database Syst Rev.* 2015;(8):CD011293.

34. Valovirta E, Petersen TH, Piotrowska T, et al. Results from the 5-year SQ grass sublingual immunotherapy tablet asthma prevention (GAP) trial in children with grass pollen allergy. *J Allergy Clin Immunol*. 2017. pii: S0091-6749(17)31088-6.

35. Zolkipli Z, Roberts G, Cornelius V, et al. Randomized controlled trial of primary prevention of atopy using house dust mite allergen oral immunotherapy in early childhood. *J Allergy Clin Immunol*. 2015;136(6):1541−1547.

36. Madonini E, Agostinis F, Barra R, et al. Long-term and preventive effects of sublingual allergen-specific immunotherapy: a retrospective, multicentric study. *Int J Immunopathol Pharmacol*. 2003;16(1):73−79.

37. Pajno GB, Caminiti L, Vita D, et al. Sublingual immunotherapy in mite-sensitized children with atopic dermatitis: a randomized, double-blind, placebo-controlled study. *J Allergy Clin Immunol*. 2007;120(1):164−170.

38. Di Rienzo V, Cadario G, Grieco T, et al. Sublingual immunotherapy in mite-sensitized children with atopic dermatitis: a randomized, open, parallel-group study. *Ann Allergy Asthma Immunol*. 2014;113(6):671−673.

39. Qin YE, Mao JR, Sang YC, et al. Clinical efficacy and compliance of sublingual immunotherapy with Dermatophagoides farinae drops in patients with atopic dermatitis. *Int J Dermatol*. 2014;53(5):650−655.

40. Gendelman SR, Lang DM. Sublingual immunotherapy in the treatment of atopic dermatitis: a systematic review using the GRADE system. *Curr Allergy Asthma Rep*. 2015; 15(2):498.

41. Bufe A, Eberle P, Franke-Beckmann E, et al. Safety and efficacy in children of an SQ-standardized grass allergen tablet for sublingual immunotherapy. *J Allergy Clin Immunol*. 2009;123(1):167−173.

42. Di Rienzo V, Marcucci F, Puccinelli P, et al. Long-lasting effect of sublingual immunotherapy in children with asthma due to house dust mite: a 10-year prospective study. *Clin Exp Allergy*. 2003;33(2):206−210.

43. Blaiss M, Maloney J, Nolte H, et al. Efficacy and safety of timothy grass allergy immunotherapy tablets in North American children and adolescents. *J Allergy Clin Immunol*. 2011;127(1):64−71.

44. Maloney J, Prenner BM, Bernstein DI, et al. Safety of house dust mite sublingual immunotherapy standardized quality tablet in children allergic to house dust mites. *Ann Allergy Asthma Immunol*. 2016;116(1):59−65.

45. Röder E, Berger MY, Hop WC, et al. Sublingual immunotherapy with grass pollen is not effective in symptomatic youngsters in primary care. *J Allergy Clin Immunol*. 2007; 119(4):892−898.

46. de Bot CM, Moed H, Berger MY, et al. Sublingual immunotherapy not effective in house dust mite-allergic children in primary care. *Pediatr Allergy Immunol*. 2012;23(2): 150−158.

47. Mungan D, Misirligil Z, Gürbüz L. Comparison of the efficacy of subcutaneous and sublingual immunotherapy in mite-sensitive patients with rhinitis and asthma–a placebo controlled study. *Ann Allergy Asthma Immunol*. 1999;82(5):485−490.

48. Khinchi MS, Poulsen LK, Carat F, et al. Clinical efficacy of sublingual and subcutaneous birch pollen allergen-specific immunotherapy: a randomized, placebo-controlled, double-blind, double-dummy study. *Allergy*. 2004;59(1):45−53.

49. Di Bona D, Plaia A, Leto-Barone MS, et al. Efficacy of subcutaneous and sublingual immunotherapy with grass allergens for seasonal allergic rhinitis: a meta-analysis-based comparison. *J Allergy Clin Immunol*. 2012;130(5):1097−1107.

50. Chelladurai Y, Suarez-Cuervo C, Erekosima N, et al. Effectiveness of subcutaneous versus sublingual immunotherapy for the treatment of allergic rhinoconjunctivitis and asthma: a systematic review. *J Allergy Clin Immunol Pract.* 2013;1(4):361−369.
51. Tucker MH, Tankersley MS. ACAAI Immunotherapy and Diagnostics Committee. Perception and practice of sublingual immunotherapy among practicing allergists. *Ann Allergy Asthma Immunol.* 2008;101(4):419−425.
52. Sikora JM, Tankersley MS. ACAAI Immunotherapy and Diagnostics Committee. Perception and practice of sublingual immunotherapy among practicing allergists in the United States: a follow-up survey. *Ann Allergy Asthma Immunol.* 2013;110(3): 194−197.
53. Berto P, Bassi M, Incorvaia C, et al. Cost effectiveness of sublingual immunotherapy in children with allergic rhinitis and asthma. *Eur Ann Allergy Clin Immunol.* 2005;37(8): 303−308.
54. Pokladnikova J, Krcmova I, Vlcek J. Economic evaluation of sublingual vs subcutaneous allergen immunotherapy. *Ann Allergy Asthma Immunol.* 2008;100(5):482−489.
55. Ariano R, Berto P, Incorvaia C, et al. Economic evaluation of sublingual immunotherapy vs. symptomatic treatment in allergic asthma. *Ann Allergy Asthma Immunol.* 2009; 103(3):254−259.
56. Bachert C, Vestenbaek U, Christensen J, et al. Cost-effectiveness of grass allergen tablet (GRAZAX) for the prevention of seasonal grass pollen induced rhinoconjunctivitis - a Northern European perspective. *Clin Exp Allergy.* 2007;37(5):772−779.
57. Ruëff F, Bilò MB, Jutel M, et al. Sublingual immunotherapy with venom is not recommended for patients with Hymenoptera venom allergy. *J Allergy Clin Immunol.* 2009; 123(1):272−273.
58. Patriarca G, Nucera E, Roncallo C, et al. Sublingual desensitization in patients with wasp venom allergy: preliminary results. *Int J Immunopathol Pharmacol.* 2008;21(3): 669−677.
59. Patriarca G, Nucera E, Roncallo C, et al. Sublingual immunotherapy with venom for patients with Hymenoptera venom allergy. *J Allergy Clin Immunol.* 2009;124(2):385.
60. Severino MG, Cortellini G, Bonadonna P, et al. Sublingual immunotherapy for large local reactions caused by honeybee sting: a double-blind, placebo-controlled trial. *J Allergy Clin Immunol.* 2008;122(1):44−48.

Further reading

1. Passalacqua G, Altrinetti V, Mariani G, et al. Pharmacokinetics of radiolabelled Par j 1 administered intranasally to allergic and healthy subjects. *Clin Exp Allergy.* 2005;35: 880−883.
2. Antico A, Fante R. Esophageal hypereosinophilia induced by grass sublingual immunotherapy. *J Allergy Clin Immunol.* 2014.
3. Cox L, Calderon MA. Allergen immunotherapy for atopic dermatitis: is there room for debate? *J Allergy Clin Immunol Pract.* 2016;4:435−444.
4. Meadows A, Kaambwa B, Novielli N, et al. A systematic review and economic evaluation of subcutaneous and sublingual allergen immunotherapy in adults and children with seasonal allergic rhinitis. *Health Technology Assessment.* 2013;17. vi, xi-xiv, 1-322.

Food tolerance, allergy, and allergen unresponsiveness

Hsi-en Ho, MD [1]**, Cecilia Berin, PhD** [1,2]

[1]*Division of Pediatric Allergy and Immunology, Icahn School of Medicine at Mount Sinai, New York, NY, United States;* [2]*Pediatrics, Mount Sinai School of Medicine, New York, NY, United States*

Food antigen-specific immune responses in health

A key feature of a healthy immune system is the ability to distinguish pathogenic antigens from innocuous ones. Accordingly, oral tolerance is the default immune response to food antigens in a healthy individual. Food tolerance is an active immune process. It begins with the digestion and uptake of food antigens in the small intestine, followed by the initiation of immune response at the gut-associated lymphoid tissues and regional lymph nodes. This multistep process involves the following:

(1) the transmission of food antigens from the gut lumen to the lamina propria,
(2) the capturing and processing of antigens by resident antigen-presenting cells,
(3) the transfer of antigen to regional lymphoid tissues,
(4) antigen presentation and initiation of T-cell response in the lymphoid tissues, and finally
(5) the migration of effector immune cells back to the gut.

In a healthy individual, the T-cell response is thought to be characterized by the formation of regulatory T (Treg) cells, which are capable of actively suppressing food-specific IgE production, Th2 lineage generation, and mast cell activation, resulting in a state of oral tolerance.

The first step in the development of food-antigen-specific immune response is the digestion and acquisition of food peptides. After ingestion, food proteins are broken down into smaller peptides and amino acids by gastric acid and digestive enzymes in the stomach, duodenum, and jejunum. A small portion of intact food antigens do escape digestion and can be found at the gut mucosa. In this form, they can be presented by antigen-presenting cells, and they are therefore immunologically active. A healthy gut mucosa is an effective barrier, which is upheld by tight junctions between enterocytes. However, there are multiple mechanisms in which food antigens can be transmitted from the gut lumen to the lamina propria. First, food antigens can be taken up by microfold cells, or M cells. The M cells are flattened gut epithelial cells that overlie Peyer's patches and are specialized in the uptake of particulate antigens, such as bacterial and viral particles. Peyer's patches have been shown to be the site of uptake of extensively heated milk[2] and egg antigens[3] as well as peanut antigens.[4] Soluble antigens can be absorbed via fluid phase endocytosis by enterocytes.[5] In this manner, soluble antigens can bypass the tight junctions between enterocytes. Third, small intestine goblet cells can form the goblet cell-associated antigen passage, which is a steady-state pathway that can be rapidly filled with luminal antigens and deliver them to the lamina propria.[6] Lastly, some intestinal mononuclear phagocytes, including dendritic cells, can extend dendrites between enterocytes without disrupting the tight junctions.[7] In this manner, they can reach into the intestinal lumen and acquire food peptides.[8]

Once food peptides have moved across the mucosal barrier, they can be captured by antigen-presenting cells. Dendritic cells process food antigens and carry them to T-cell areas of organized lymphoid structures for the initiation of adaptive immune response.[9] Relevant gastrointestinal lymphoid structures include the mesenteric lymph nodes (MLNs) and Peyer's patches. Mesenteric lymph nodes are the regional nodes that drain the gut through the lymphatic systems. Peyer's patches, on the other hand, are isolated lymphoid follicles found below mucosal epithelium in the small intestine. Through studies deploying immunological ablation of lymphoid structures or surgical removal of regional lymph nodes, MLNs have been shown to be necessary for the induction of food tolerance, whereas Peyer's patches can be dispensable.[9–11]

Dendritic cells are the key antigen-presenting cells that interact with naïve T cells in the MLNs, and they present food antigens on MHC class II molecules. In a healthy state, dendritic cells are central to the generation of Treg cells, which are essential for maintenance of oral tolerance. Murine studies have shown that the expansion of dendritic cells with their growth factors (such as Flt3L) can lead to enhanced oral tolerance.[12]

The activation of different DC subsets and differential expression of costimulatory molecules help to determine the ensuing immune response. Two subsets of dendritic cells are known to be involved in the induction of oral tolerance:

(1) CD11b+ CX3CR1+ cells, and
(2) CD103+ CX3CR1− CD11b+/− cells.

CD11b+CX3CR1+ cells are derived from monocytes. Based on transcription analysis, they are actually more akin to macrophages than dendritic cells. These cells can extend dendrites between intestinal epithelial cells to capture luminal antigens and transfer them to CD103+ dendritic cells.[8] CD11b+ CX3CR1+ cells do not themselves travel to the MLNs under steady state. However, under the influence of microbiota, these cells express high levels of IL-10, resulting in the local expansion of newly generated Treg cells.[13]

In contrast, CD103+ CX3CR1− CD11b+/− cells are derived from dendritic cell progenitors. These cells travel to MLNs and presents food antigens to naïve T cells under steady state.[14,15] Both murine and human CD103+ CX3CR1- dendritic cells express high levels of TGF-β and retinoid acid-synthesizing enzymes

(RALDH),[16,17] which produces retinoid acid from vitamin A. In addition, these cells also express the enzyme indoleamine-pyrrole 2,3-dioxygenase (IDO).[18] TGF-β, RALDH, and IDO are all key factors that promote the development of Treg cells in the MLNs. Furthermore, MLN CD103+ dendritic cells induce the upregulation of α4β7 integrin and CCR9 chemokine receptors in responding T cells in a retinoid acid-dependent manner.[19,20] Therefore, newly generated Treg cells preferentially migrate back to intestinal lamina propria to exert their regulatory functions at the site of antigen encounter.

The regulatory phenotype of CD103+ dendritic cells is enhanced by the unique mucosal milieu of the gut through two main mechanisms. First, under the influence of local goblet cell-derived mucin molecule, Muc2, CD103+ dendritic cells increase their expression of TGF-β and RALDH.[21] In fact, oral tolerance is impaired in the absence of Muc2 in murine models. Conversely, exogenous mucin can rescue the loss of food tolerance in Muc2 knockout mice. Second, the regulatory phenotype of CD103+ DCs is also promoted by local production of GM-CSF.[22] The source of GM-CSF has been shown to be intestinal innate lymphoid cells, which are in turn stimulated by IL-1β from macrophages under the influence of local bacterial flora. In the absence of both GM-CSF and IL-1β, the generation of inducible Treg cells has been shown to be impaired.[22]

The role of regulatory T cells in food tolerance

Regulatory T cells are the key suppressor cells that actively maintain oral tolerance to food antigens. Their tolerance-inducing role was first discovered through adoptive transfer murine models, in which the transfer of T lymphocytes confers oral tolerance to antigen-naïve recipients. It has subsequently been shown that intestinal tolerance in mice requires gut homing and expansion of Treg cells in the lamina propia.[13,23]

Treg cells comprise different subsets with suppressive capacity. Two broad subsets of Treg cells have been described:

(1) natural Treg (nTreg) cells, which are thymus-derived natural occurring CD4+CD25+ forkhead box protein 3 (FOXP3)+ Treg cells, and
(2) inducible Treg (iTreg) cells

which are generated in the periphery after antigenic stimulation, and include FOXP3+Treg cells, CD4+FOXP3− IL-10-producing Tr1 cells, and TGF-β-producing Th3 cells. Clinical observations have pointed toward the importance of FOXP3+ Treg cells in maintaining oral tolerance. Mutations in FOXP3 result in IPEX (Immune dysregulation, polyendocrinopathy, enteropathy) syndrome, which is marked by a loss of immune tolerance, severe autoimmunity, and food allergy.[24] The deletion of the forkhead domain of FOXP3 in the scurfy mice similarly results in elevated IgE, eosinophilia, dysregulated Th1 and Th2 cytokine production, and multiorgan inflammation.[25] It has been demonstrated in murine models that iTreg cells are essential for oral tolerance, whereas nTreg cells are not directly involved in oral tolerance induction.[13,26]

Treg cells exert their immune effects through a wide variety of mechanisms—many of which have been dissected in mice. First, Treg cells can directly inhibit DC maturation by utilizing surface inhibitory molecules, such as cytotoxic T-lymphocyte antigen-4 (CTLA-4).[27] Second, Treg cells can affect effector cells through cytolysis (with the secretion of granzyme B),[28] or metabolic disruption.[29] Third, Treg cells produce suppressor cytokines, such as IL-10 and TGF-β.[30] IL-10 inhibits the production of proinflammatory cytokines, chemokine, and chemokine receptors. In addition, it inhibits the expression of MHC-II and costimulatory molecules CD80/CD86 on dendritic cells, monocytes, and macrophages, resulting in indirect inhibition of effector T cell proliferation.[31,32] Furthermore, IL-10 directly inhibits T-cell function by suppressing CD28-dependent T-cell costimulation.[33] TGF-β is centrally involved in the generation of oral tolerance, and it has pleiotropic effects.[34,35] TGF-β inhibits lymphocyte proliferation, as well as Th1 and Th2 cell differentiation and survival.[36–38] Importantly, TGF-β induces the expression of FOXP3 in naïve CD4+ T cells, leading to generation and expansion of iTreg cells.[30] Through these various mechanisms, Treg cells directly or indirectly suppress almost all cell types contributing to allergic inflammation.[39] The cumulative immune effects of Treg cells in oral tolerance are broad, and they include the generation of tolerogenic DCs,[27] inhibition of allergen-specific IgE production,[40] inhibition of allergen-specific T cell response, inhibition of allergen-induced activation of mast cells and basophils,[41] and impairment of effector T cells infiltration into the inflamed tissue.[42]

Though not as extensively studied, a similar subset of B cells known as Regulatory B (Breg) cells may also minimize allergic inflammation and promote tolerance, mainly through the secretion of IL-10.[43] A recent study has shown that mesenteric IL-10-producing CD5+ Breg cells can suppress cow's milk casein-induced anaphylaxis in mice.[44]

It should be noted that there are still currently limited evaluations of Treg response to dietary antigens in human, especially at a young age when food-sensitization tends to occur. In general, it has been found that the frequency of allergen-specific T cells is very low in nonallergic individuals. However, it has been shown that the frequency of CD4+CD25+ Treg cells increase in children who outgrew milk allergy, suggesting that the development of oral tolerance in human does involve Treg cells, at least in the initial phase.[45] In another study, in vitro stimulation of peripheral blood Treg cells with milk protein results in decreased Treg cell counts and increased expression of Th2-deviation markers, GATA-3 and IRF-4, in samples from milk-allergic children as compared to those of control subjects.[46] An examination of antigen-specific Tregs found a very low frequency of Tregs specific for dietary antigens in healthy individuals, as compared to Tregs specific for aeroallergens,[47] calling into question the role of food antigen-specific Tregs in maintenance of oral tolerance to foods.

Role of immunoglobulins in oral tolerance

The contribution of antibodies in immune tolerance is not well understood. Experimental models of oral tolerance use suppression of immunization, including antibody responses, to measure tolerance. Antigen feeding promotes production of IgA antibodies that contribute to tolerance through immune exclusion at mucosal sites. Healthy human subjects can have detectable antigen-specific IgG to food allergens without clinical symptoms.[48] The LEAP study, in which early (<11 months old) introduction of peanut in children generated peanut tolerance, showed that tolerance was associated with an induction of peanut-specific IgG4.[49] This study indicated that IgGs could have an important role in development of oral tolerance. Mouse models have shown that passive transfer of mice with allergen-specific IgG can suppress the development of sensitization even in the presence of a strong mucosal adjuvant to break tolerance.[50] The mechanism by which IgG antibodies could prevent the development of sensitization is not well understood, but may relate to antibody-facilitated presentation of antigen. IgG-facilitated presentation of antigen via breast milk has been identified as promoting the development of Tregs and immune tolerance in mice through the neonatal Fc receptor.[51,52]

Development of food allergy

Food allergy is characterized by a deviation from the default state of oral tolerance as described so far in this chapter. This may be due to aberrant oral tolerance processes, or due to a lack of opportunity of oral tolerance combined with proallergic signals generated outside of the gastrointestinal tract. The latter refers to the dual allergen exposure hypothesis, which proposes that dietary avoidance of foods combined with exposure to foods through nonoral routes, such as eczematous skin, results in food allergy.[53] The weight of clinical and experimental evidence supports this hypothesis for peanut, but perhaps not for other foods. Although the precise mechanism has yet to be fully elucidated, food allergy is thought to arise from a lack of regulatory response combined with a Th2 response driving the pathophysiology of food allergy. Th2 lymphocytes and cells producing type 2 cytokines are known to induce antibody class-switch recombination toward IgE, support B-cell proliferation, and promote differentiation of naïve B cells into antibody-secreting plasma cells. IgE is the fundamental antibody that facilitates adverse reactions to food in allergic patients. Upon exposure to food allergens, food-specific IgE antibodies initiate the acute phase reaction by binding to high-affinity FcεR1 receptors on the surface of mast cells and basophils, resulting in cell degranulation of preformed molecules, including histamine, as well as rapidly synthesis of lipid mediators, cytokines, and chemokines. The development of food-specific IgE antibodies is a hallmark of allergen sensitization.

IL-4 is critical to the development of food allergy, and mice carrying a mutation in the IL-4 receptor that generates exaggerated signaling are susceptible to food allergy and can be sensitized by feeding antigen without exogenous adjuvant.[54] IL-4 is produced not only by conventional Th2 cells,[55] but also regulatory T cells,[46] innate lymphoid cells (type 2),[56] basophils,[57] and mast cells.[58] IL-13 that has overlapping functions with IL-4 is also produced by multiple cell types, including T lymphocytes,[59] ILC2s,[60] and mast cells.[61] IL-9 is a Th2-associated cytokine derived from T cells and a unique mucosal mast cell subset[62] that plays a key role in the development of food allergy through the expansion of mucosal mast cells.[62–64] Innate sources of Th2-associated cytokines can contribute to Th2 lymphocyte skewing during presentation of antigen to naïve T cells, and phenotypic modifications of DCs also contribute to Th2 skewing. In particular, OX40L expression is one molecule that has been shown to be involved in downstream Th2 skewing in food allergy.[55,65,66]

In murine models of food allergy, mucosal epithelial cells are implicated in the pathogenesis of food allergy as well. Mucosal epithelial cells have been shown to secrete Th2-promoting mediators, such as thymic stromal lymphopoietin (TSLP), IL-25,[67] and IL-33.[68] The blockage of IL-25, IL33, and TSLP receptors simultaneously with monoclonal antibodies is effective in suppressing food allergy development in mice, whereas blockage of individual receptors was found to be ineffective in suppressing established food allergy.[68] Others have shown that neutralization of IL-33 alone is effective in suppressing food allergic symptoms after sensitization has occurred.[69] IL-33 may also contribute to acute reactions to foods by enhancing IgE-mediated activation of mast cells.[70]

The role of microbiota in food tolerance versus allergy

A potential role of microbiota, or the community of microbes, in the development of oral tolerance versus food allergy remains poorly understood. In mice, an impaired gut microbiota may contribute to food allergy susceptibility.[71,72] Germ-free mice are more responsive than wild-type mice to oral sensitization, with exaggerated anaphylactic response upon challenge to food allergens.[71,73] Similarly, when wild-type mice are treated with antibiotics to alter their gut flora, they become more susceptible to the induction of food allergy. It should be noted that the interpretation of germ-free mice data can be difficult, as they are known to have an underdeveloped mucosal immune system; however, the comparable findings in antibiotic-treated mice support a general inhibitory effect of healthy gut flora in the development of IgE-mediated immune response. A food allergy susceptible phenotype in genetically predisposed (IL-4R gain of function) mice could be transmitted to germ-free mice by transferring the gut microbiota,[72] indicating that susceptibility resides within the microbiota, either through the presence of proallergic organisms or the absence of protective organisms. Studies in humans support the hypothesis that microbial composition can influence food allergy susceptibility. Early life differences in microbial composition have been identified in those who go on to develop sensitization to foods.[74,75] Longitudinal profiling has shown that microbial composition measured in stool of milk-allergic children in infancy was associated with milk allergy resolution by 8 years old.[76] As the molecular pathways in which the gut microbes influence food allergy susceptibilities are elucidated, such mechanistic insights may aid in the future design of allergen immunotherapy.

Oral tolerance, desensitization, and sustained unresponsiveness: mechanisms of therapeutically induced food tolerance

As described thus far in this chapter, the complex interactions between mucosal epithelium, various host immune cell subsets, microbiota, diet, and food allergens contribute to oral tolerance versus food allergy. However, there are still significant gaps in knowledge regarding the exact mechanism in which lifelong oral tolerance naturally develops. As such, current immunotherapies have yet to fully replicate this process, with a loss of clinical *unresponsiveness* in subjects once the exposure to the allergen has been discontinued for a period of time (i.e., 2–24 weeks).

To have a framework for evaluating the immune response to immunotherapy in food allergy, it is therefore essential to differentiate clinical desensitization and sustained unresponsiveness (SU) (or "remission") from oral tolerance. Oral tolerance describes a complete lack of clinical reactivity to an ingested food antigen, independent of continued antigen exposure. Oral tolerance is typically of natural occurrence. Desensitization describes an increase in clinical reactivity threshold to a food allergen while receiving ongoing therapy. Desensitization may translate to a lack of clinical reactivity after accidental food allergen exposure; it can commonly be achieved after months of immunotherapy, but crucially, this state is only maintained during active treatment. SU is a state of nonresponsiveness of unknown persistence. It describes a lack of clinical reactivity to a food allergen after active therapy has been discontinued for a period of time. It is typically achieved after several years of treatment and is observed in a subset of subjects. The state of SU is thought to require some level of ongoing allergen exposure to maintain this state, and some investigators have proposed to label it as a state of "remission" from food allergy. Importantly, it is not known if a food-allergic patient who has undergone immunotherapy will remain permanently unresponsive to the food allergen. SU is therefore regarded as a distinct immune state from the healthy, preallergic state of oral immune tolerance.

The immune basis of desensitization, SU/remission, and tolerance are still under active investigation. The LEAP study, in which early dietary peanut exposure led to a prevention of peanut allergy,[49] is an example of oral tolerance in humans. Even after a year of peanut avoidance, the tolerance induced by early dietary peanut exposure was maintained.[77] As discussed earlier, the generation of peanut-specific IgG4 was a striking finding of this study. Dietary peanut exposure also prevented the increase of peanut-IgE over time that was observed without exposure to dietary peanut. It is not known if early dietary peanut influenced the peanut-specific Th2 or Treg response in the LEAP cohort.

It is not known whether desensitization and SU following immunotherapy are mediated by distinct mechanisms, or whether these are arbitrary groupings. Although those who are categorized as desensitized do regain clinical reactivity, their threshold of reactivity is generally much higher than pretreatment, so there is a substantial and sustained impact of therapy in these individuals.[78] Immune parameters associated with SU include a lower level of specific IgE at baseline and after treatment.[78,79] Although one clinical trial found that IgG4 levels early in treatment were predictive of SU to egg[80] IgG4 levels have not been shown to discriminate between SU and desensitization in peanut allergy.[78,81] Demethylation of the Foxp3 promoter in T cells and an increase in frequency and function of Foxp3+ cells was identified as uniquely associated with SU in peanut allergy,[81] which suggested that SU, like oral tolerance, is Treg mediated.

There is more information on the impact of immunotherapy on the food-specific immune response without distinction of the outcome of desensitization versus SU. The most consistent finding across clinical trials is the induction of food-specific IgG4. Although IgG4 binds relatively weakly to activating Fc gamma receptors, it binds the inhibitory FcγRIIb receptor[82] and likely contributes to clinical tolerance through the suppression of IgE-mediated activation of mast cells and basophils.[50,83,84] Immunotherapy also has a significant impact on the food-specific T-cell response. Peanut-specific T-cell responses have been assayed with various methods, but a consistent finding of suppressed Th2 immunity is observed. Peanut allergy is associated with a heterogeneous Th2 response including highly differentiated Th2 cells expressing IL-4, IL-5, and IL-9 and other markers consistent with terminal differentiation.[85,86] Wambre and colleagues have called these cells Th2A cells, and found that the frequency of these cells is suppressed by allergen immunotherapy.[85] The suppression of Th2 responses, including multifunctional Th2 cells, was reported to be incomplete and Th2 responses rebounded after termination of oral immunotherapy treatment.[87,88] Study of peanut-specific T cells at the single cell level following immunotherapy has revealed a signature consistent with T-cell anergy,[89] which could provide an explanation for the transient suppression of Th2 immune responses. A deletion of Th2 cells or their allergen-specific precursors, which could then allow the loss of allergen-specific IgE, may be required for sustained effects of immunotherapy. However, the role of Th2 cells in the maintenance of long-lived IgE responses is poorly understood and it is unclear if deletion of these Th2 cells is necessary or sufficient to abolish the allergen-specific IgE response.

Summary

Oral tolerance prevents the development of food allergy in mouse models and infants at risk of peanut allergy. It is well established from mouse models that oral tolerance is mediated by peripheral Tregs that suppress the development of IgE and other effector responses. Recent work in human cohorts and mice has begun to highlight an important role for IgG responses in the development of primary immune tolerance. The ultimate goal of oral immunotherapy is to establish oral tolerance, a permanent state of immune tolerance. This may be an achievable goal in young children,[90] but in older children and adults immunotherapy results in clinical protection requiring sustained allergen exposure. Although there are common mechanisms shared between oral tolerance and oral immunotherapy, such as IgG4 and Tregs (See Fig. 9.1 for an overview of these mechanisms), the persistence of allergen-specific Th2 cells and their rebound after termination of therapy may explain the inability to induce permanent oral tolerance in individuals with an established food allergy. A greater understanding of the mechanisms involved in persistence of food-specific IgE and T cells with Th2 effector potential is needed to advance the field. Studying the immune basis of robust clinical responses to oral immunotherapy in very young children may provide an exciting opportunity to understand the immune basis of true tolerance to foods.

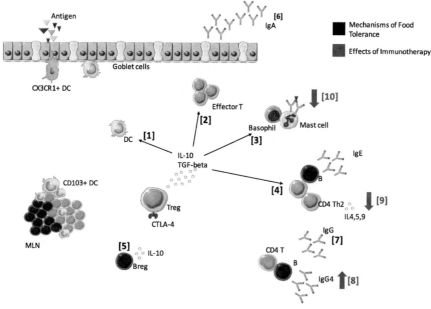

FIGURE 9.1

Overview of mechanisms of oral tolerance and response to immunotherapy. Antigen feeding elicits a number of immune pathways that contribute to oral tolerance. Antigen presentation by CD103+ DCs generates Tregs in the MLN, that through production of IL-10 and TGFb can suppress DCs (1), effector T cells (2), basophils (3), and the generation of allergen-specific IgE (4). In addition, these cytokines promote the generation of regulatory B cells producing IL-10 (5), IgA (6), and IgG4 (7) that also contribute to immune tolerance through immune exclusion and altered antigen presentation. Immune effects of oral immunotherapy share pathways of oral tolerance, including the generation of IgG4 (8), suppression of IgE (9), and suppression of mast cell and basophil activation.

References

1. Holt PG, Sly PD, Sampson HA, et al. Prophylactic use of sublingual allergen immuno-therapy in high-risk children: a pilot study. *J Allergy Clin Immunol.* 2013;132(4): 991−993. e991.
2. Roth-Walter F, Berin MC, Arnaboldi P, et al. Pasteurization of milk proteins promotes allergic sensitization by enhancing uptake through Peyer's patches. *Allergy.* 2008; 63(7):882−890.
3. Martos G, Lopez-Exposito I, Bencharitiwong R, Berin MC, Nowak-Wegrzyn A. Mech-anisms underlying differential food allergy response to heated egg. *J Allergy Clin Immu-nol.* 2011;127(4):990−997. e991-992.
4. Chambers SJ, Wickham MS, Regoli M, Bertelli E, Gunning PA, Nicoletti C. Rapid in vivo transport of proteins from digested allergen across pre-sensitized gut. *Biochem Biophys Res Commun.* 2004;325(4):1258−1263.
5. Berin MC, Kiliaan AJ, Yang PC, Groot JA, Taminiau JA, Perdue MH. Rapid transepithe-lial antigen transport in rat jejunum: impact of sensitization and the hypersensitivity reaction. *Gastroenterology.* 1997;113(3):856−864.
6. McDole JR, Wheeler LW, McDonald KG, et al. Goblet cells deliver luminal antigen to CD103+ dendritic cells in the small intestine. *Nature.* 2012;483(7389):345−349.
7. Rescigno M, Urbano M, Valzasina B, et al. Dendritic cells express tight junction proteins and penetrate gut epithelial monolayers to sample bacteria. *Nat Immunol.* 2001;2(4):361−367.
8. Mazzini E, Massimiliano L, Penna G, Rescigno M. Oral tolerance can be established via gap junction transfer of fed antigens from CX3CR1(+) macrophages to CD103(+) den-dritic cells. *Immunity.* 2014;40(2):248−261.
9. Worbs T, Bode U, Yan S, et al. Oral tolerance originates in the intestinal immune system and relies on antigen carriage by dendritic cells. *J Exp Med.* 2006;203(3):519−527.
10. Spahn TW, Fontana A, Faria AM, et al. Induction of oral tolerance to cellular immune responses in the absence of Peyer's patches. *Eur J Immunol.* 2001;31(4):1278−1287.
11. Spahn TW, Weiner HL, Rennert PD, et al. Mesenteric lymph nodes are critical for the induction of high-dose oral tolerance in the absence of Peyer's patches. *Eur J Immunol.* 2002;32(4):1109−1113.
12. Viney JL, Mowat AM, O'Malley JM, Williamson E, Fanger NA. Expanding dendritic cells in vivo enhances the induction of oral tolerance. *J Immunol.* 1998;160(12): 5815−5825.
13. Hadis U, Wahl B, Schulz O, et al. Intestinal tolerance requires gut homing and expansion of FoxP3+ regulatory T cells in the lamina propria. *Immunity.* 2011;34(2):237−246.
14. Bogunovic M, Ginhoux F, Helft J, et al. Origin of the lamina propria dendritic cell network. *Immunity.* 2009;31(3):513−525.
15. Schulz O, Jaensson E, Persson EK, et al. Intestinal CD103+, but not CX3CR1+, antigen sampling cells migrate in lymph and serve classical dendritic cell functions. *J Exp Med.* 2009;206(13):3101−3114.
16. Coombes JL, Siddiqui KR, Arancibia-Carcamo CV, et al. A functionally specialized pop-ulation of mucosal CD103+ DCs induces Foxp3+ regulatory T cells via a TGF-beta and retinoic acid-dependent mechanism. *J Exp Med.* 2007;204(8):1757−1764.
17. Jaensson E, Uronen-Hansson H, Pabst O, et al. Small intestinal CD103+ dendritic cells display unique functional properties that are conserved between mice and humans. *J Exp Med.* 2008;205(9):2139−2149.

18. Matteoli G, Mazzini E, Iliev ID, et al. Gut CD103+ dendritic cells express indoleamine 2,3-dioxygenase which influences T regulatory/T effector cell balance and oral tolerance induction. *Gut*. 2010;59(5):595–604.

19. Johansson-Lindbom B, Svensson M, Wurbel MA, Malissen B, Marquez G, Agace W. Selective generation of gut tropic T cells in gut-associated lymphoid tissue (GALT): requirement for GALT dendritic cells and adjuvant. *J Exp Med*. 2003;198(6):963–969.

20. Stenstad H, Ericsson A, Johansson-Lindbom B, et al. Gut-associated lymphoid tissue-primed CD4+ T cells display CCR9-dependent and -independent homing to the small intestine. *Blood*. 2006;107(9):3447–3454.

21. Shan M, Gentile M, Yeiser JR, et al. Mucus enhances gut homeostasis and oral tolerance by delivering immunoregulatory signals. *Science*. 2013;342(6157):447–453.

22. Mortha A, Chudnovskiy A, Hashimoto D, et al. Microbiota-dependent crosstalk between macrophages and ILC3 promotes intestinal homeostasis. *Science*. 2014;343(6178): 1249288.

23. Cassani B, Villablanca EJ, Quintana FJ, et al. Gut-Tropic T cells that express integrin alpha4beta7 and CCR9 are required for induction of oral immune tolerance in mice. *Gastroenterology*. 2011;141(6):2109–2118.

24. Torgerson TR, Linane A, Moes N, et al. Severe food allergy as a variant of IPEX syndrome caused by a deletion in a noncoding region of the FOXP3 gene. *Gastroenterology*. 2007;132(5):1705–1717.

25. Ramsdell F, Ziegler SF. FOXP3 and scurfy: how it all began. *Nat Rev Immunol*. 2014; 14(5):343–349.

26. Mucida D, Kutchukhidze N, Erazo A, Russo M, Lafaille JJ, Curotto de Lafaille MA. Oral tolerance in the absence of naturally occurring Tregs. *J Clin Investig*. 2005;115(7): 1923–1933.

27. Wing K, Onishi Y, Prieto-Martin P, et al. CTLA-4 control over Foxp3+ regulatory T cell function. *Science*. 2008;322(5899):271–275.

28. Cao X, Cai SF, Fehniger TA, et al. Granzyme B and perforin are important for regulatory T cell-mediated suppression of tumor clearance. *Immunity*. 2007;27(4):635–646.

29. Vignali DA, Collison LW, Workman CJ. How regulatory T cells work. *Nat Rev Immunol*. 2008;8(7):523–532.

30. Chen W, Jin W, Hardegen N, et al. Conversion of peripheral CD4+CD25- naive T cells to CD4+CD25+ regulatory T cells by TGF-beta induction of transcription factor Foxp3. *J Exp Med*. 2003;198(12):1875–1886.

31. de Waal Malefyt R, Abrams J, Bennett B, Figdor CG, de Vries JE. Interleukin 10(IL-10) inhibits cytokine synthesis by human monocytes: an autoregulatory role of IL-10 produced by monocytes. *J Exp Med*. 1991;174(5):1209–1220.

32. Timmann C, Fuchs S, Thoma C, et al. Promoter haplotypes of the interleukin-10 gene influence proliferation of peripheral blood cells in response to helminth antigen. *Genes Immun*. 2004;5(4):256–260.

33. Taylor A, Akdis M, Joss A, et al. IL-10 inhibits CD28 and ICOS costimulations of T cells via src homology 2 domain-containing protein tyrosine phosphatase 1. *J Allergy Clin Immunol*. 2007;120(1):76–83.

34. Kraus TA, Brimnes J, Muong C, et al. Induction of mucosal tolerance in Peyer's patch-deficient, ligated small bowel loops. *J Clin Investig*. 2005;115(8):2234–2243.

35. Miller A, Lider O, Roberts AB, Sporn MB, Weiner HL. Suppressor T cells generated by oral tolerization to myelin basic protein suppress both in vitro and in vivo immune

responses by the release of transforming growth factor beta after antigen-specific triggering. *Proc Natl Acad Sci U S A*. 1992;89(1):421—425.

36. Gorelik L, Constant S, Flavell RA. Mechanism of transforming growth factor beta-induced inhibition of T helper type 1 differentiation. *J Exp Med*. 2002;195(11): 1499—1505.

37. Gorelik L, Fields PE, Flavell RA. Cutting edge: TGF-beta inhibits Th type 2 development through inhibition of GATA-3 expression. *J Immunol*. 2000;165(9):4773—4777.

38. Heath VL, Kurata H, Lee HJ, Arai N, O'Garra A. Checkpoints in the regulation of T helper 1 responses. *Curr Top Microbiol Immunol*. 2002;266:23—39.

39. Palomares O, Yaman G, Azkur AK, Akkoc T, Akdis M, Akdis CA. Role of Treg in immune regulation of allergic diseases. *Eur J Immunol*. 2010;40(5):1232—1240.

40. Meiler F, Klunker S, Zimmermann M, Akdis CA, Akdis M. Distinct regulation of IgE, IgG4 and IgA by T regulatory cells and toll-like receptors. *Allergy*. 2008;63(11): 1455—1463.

41. Kashyap M, Thornton AM, Norton SK, et al. Cutting edge: CD4 T cell-mast cell interactions alter IgE receptor expression and signaling. *J Immunol*. 2008;180(4):2039—2043.

42. Ring S, Schafer SC, Mahnke K, Lehr HA, Enk AH. CD4+ CD25+ regulatory T cells suppress contact hypersensitivity reactions by blocking influx of effector T cells into inflamed tissue. *Eur J Immunol*. 2006;36(11):2981—2992.

43. van de Veen W, Stanic B, Wirz OF, Jansen K, Globinska A, Akdis M. Role of regulatory B cells in immune tolerance to allergens and beyond. *J Allergy Clin Immunol*. 2016; 138(3):654—665.

44. Kim AR, Kim HS, Kim DK, et al. Mesenteric IL-10-producing CD5+ regulatory B cells suppress cow's milk casein-induced allergic responses in mice. *Sci Rep*. 2016;6:19685.

45. Karlsson MR, Rugtveit J, Brandtzaeg P. Allergen-responsive CD4+CD25+ regulatory T cells in children who have outgrown cow's milk allergy. *J Exp Med*. 2004;199(12): 1679—1688.

46. Noval Rivas M, Burton OT, Wise P, et al. Regulatory T cell reprogramming toward a Th2-Cell-like lineage impairs oral tolerance and promotes food allergy. *Immunity*. 2015;42(3):512—523.

47. Bacher P, Heinrich F, Stervbo U, et al. Regulatory T cell specificity directs tolerance versus allergy against aeroantigens in humans. *Cell*. 2016;167(4):1067—1078. e1016.

48. Husby S, Oxelius VA, Teisner B, Jensenius JC, Svehag SE. Humoral immunity to dietary antigens in healthy adults. Occurrence, isotype and IgG subclass distribution of serum antibodies to protein antigens. *Int Arch Allergy Appl Immunol*. 1985;77(4):416—422.

49. Du Toit G, Roberts G, Sayre PH, et al. Randomized trial of peanut consumption in infants at risk for peanut allergy. *N Engl J Med*. 2015;372(9):803—813.

50. Burton OT, Tamayo JM, Stranks AJ, Koleoglou KJ, Oettgen HC. Allergen-specific IgG antibody signaling through FcgammaRIIb promotes food tolerance. *J Allergy Clin Immunol*. 2018;141(1):189—201. e183.

51. Mosconi E, Rekima A, Seitz-Polski B, et al. Breast milk immune complexes are potent inducers of oral tolerance in neonates and prevent asthma development. *Mucosal Immunology*. 2010;3(5):461—474.

52. Ohsaki A, Venturelli N, Buccigrosso TM, et al. Maternal IgG immune complexes induce food allergen-specific tolerance in offspring. *J Exp Med*. 2018;215(1):91—113.

53. Du Toit G, Sampson HA, Plaut M, Burks AW, Akdis CA, Lack G. Food allergy: update on prevention and tolerance. *J Allergy Clin Immunol*. 2018;141(1):30—40.

54. Mathias CB, Hobson SA, Garcia-Lloret M, et al. IgE-mediated systemic anaphylaxis and impaired tolerance to food antigens in mice with enhanced IL-4 receptor signaling. *J Allergy Clin Immunol.* 2011;127(3):795−805. e791-796.

55. Chu DK, Mohammed-Ali Z, Jimenez-Saiz R, et al. T helper cell IL-4 drives intestinal Th2 priming to oral peanut antigen, under the control of OX40L and independent of innate-like lymphocytes. *Mucosal Immunology.* 2014.

56. Noval Rivas M, Burton OT, Oettgen HC, Chatila T. IL-4 production by group 2 innate lymphoid cells promotes food allergy by blocking regulatory T-cell function. *J Allergy Clin Immunol.* 2016;138(3):801−811. e809.

57. Hussain M, Borcard L, Walsh KP, et al. Basophil-derived IL-4 promotes epicutaneous antigen sensitization concomitant with the development of food allergy. *J Allergy Clin Immunol.* 2018;141(1):223−234. e225.

58. Burton OT, Noval Rivas M, Zhou JS, et al. Immunoglobulin E signal inhibition during allergen ingestion leads to reversal of established food allergy and induction of regulatory T cells. *Immunity.* 2014;41(1):141−151.

59. Brandt EB, Munitz A, Orekov T, et al. Targeting IL-4/IL-13 signaling to alleviate oral allergen-induced diarrhea. *J Allergy Clin Immunol.* 2009;123(1):53−58.

60. Lee JB, Chen CY, Liu B, et al. IL-25 and CD4(+) TH2 cells enhance type 2 innate lymphoid cell-derived IL-13 production, which promotes IgE-mediated experimental food allergy. *J Allergy Clin Immunol.* 2016;137(4):1216−1225. e1211-1215.

61. Wang M, Takeda K, Shiraishi Y, et al. Peanut-induced intestinal allergy is mediated through a mast cell-IgE-FcepsilonRI-IL-13 pathway. *J Allergy Clin Immunol.* 2010; 126(2):306−316, 316 e301-312.

62. Chen CY, Lee JB, Liu B, et al. Induction of interleukin-9-producing mucosal mast cells promotes susceptibility to IgE-mediated experimental food allergy. *Immunity.* 2015; 43(4):788−802.

63. Forbes EE, Groschwitz K, Abonia JP, et al. IL-9- and mast cell-mediated intestinal permeability predisposes to oral antigen hypersensitivity. *J Exp Med.* 2008;205(4): 897−913.

64. Osterfeld H, Ahrens R, Strait R, Finkelman FD, Renauld JC, Hogan SP. Differential roles for the IL-9/IL-9 receptor alpha-chain pathway in systemic and oral antigen-induced anaphylaxis. *J Allergy Clin Immunol.* 2010;125(2):469−476. e462.

65. Blazquez AB, Berin MC. Gastrointestinal dendritic cells promote Th2 skewing via OX40L. *J Immunol.* 2008;180(7):4441−4450.

66. Chu DK, Llop-Guevara A, Walker TD, et al. IL-33, but not thymic stromal lymphopoietin or IL-25, is central to mite and peanut allergic sensitization. *J Allergy Clin Immunol.* 2013;131(1):187−200. e181-188.

67. Han H, Thelen TD, Comeau MR, Ziegler SF. Thymic stromal lymphopoietin-mediated epicutaneous inflammation promotes acute diarrhea and anaphylaxis. *J Clin Investig.* 2014;124(12):5442−5452.

68. Khodoun MV, Tomar S, Tocker JE, Wang YH, Finkelman FD. Prevention of food allergy development and suppression of established food allergy by neutralization of thymic stromal lymphopoietin, IL-25, and IL-33. *J Allergy Clin Immunol.* 2018;141(1): 171−179. e171.

69. Han H, Roan F, Johnston LK, Smith DE, Bryce PJ, Ziegler SF. IL-33 promotes gastrointestianl allergy in a TSLP-independent manner. *Mucosal Immunology.* 2017.

70. Galand C, Leyva-Castillo JM, Yoon J, et al. IL-33 promotes food anaphylaxis in epicutaneously sensitized mice by targeting mast cells. *J Allergy Clin Immunol.* 2016.

71. Stefka AT, Feehley T, Tripathi P, et al. Commensal bacteria protect against food allergen sensitization. *Proc Natl Acad Sci U S A*. 2014;111(36):13145−13150.

72. Noval Rivas M, Burton OT, Wise P, et al. A microbiota signature associated with experimental food allergy promotes allergic sensitization and anaphylaxis. *J Allergy Clin Immunol*. 2013;131(1):201−212.

73. Cahenzli J, Koller Y, Wyss M, Geuking MB, McCoy KD. Intestinal microbial diversity during early-life colonization shapes long-term IgE levels. *Cell Host & Microbe*. 2013; 14(5):559−570.

74. Azad MB, Konya T, Guttman DS, et al. Infant gut microbiota and food sensitization: associations in the first year of life. *Clin Exp Allergy*. 2015;45(3):632−643.

75. Savage JH, Lee-Sarwar KA, Sordillo J, et al. A prospective microbiome-wide association study of food sensitization and food allergy in early childhood. *Allergy*. 2018;73(1): 145−152.

76. Bunyavanich S, Shen N, Grishin A, et al. Early-life gut microbiome composition and milk allergy resolution. *J Allergy Clin Immunol*. 2016;138(4):1122−1130.

77. Du Toit G, Sayre PH, Roberts G, et al. Effect of avoidance on peanut allergy after early peanut consumption. *N Engl J Med*. 2016;374(15):1435−1443.

78. Vickery BP, Scurlock AM, Kulis M, et al. Sustained unresponsiveness to peanut in subjects who have completed peanut oral immunotherapy. *J Allergy Clin Immunol*. 2014; 133(2):468−475.

79. Wright BL, Kulis M, Orgel KA, et al. Component-resolved analysis of IgA, IgE, and IgG4 during egg OIT identifies markers associated with sustained unresponsiveness. *Allergy*. 2016;71(11):1552−1560.

80. Burks AW, Jones SM, Wood RA, et al. Oral immunotherapy for treatment of egg allergy in children. *N Engl J Med*. 2012;367(3):233−243.

81. Syed A, Garcia MA, Lyu SC, et al. Peanut oral immunotherapy results in increased antigen-induced regulatory T-cell function and hypomethylation of forkhead box protein 3 (FOXP3). *J Allergy Clin Immunol*. 2014;133(2):500−510. e511.

82. Bruhns P, Iannascoli B, England P, et al. Specificity and affinity of human Fcgamma receptors and their polymorphic variants for human IgG subclasses. *Blood*. 2009;113(16): 3716−3725.

83. Burton OT, Logsdon SL, Zhou JS, et al. Oral immunotherapy induces IgG antibodies that act through FcgammaRIIb to suppress IgE-mediated hypersensitivity. *J Allergy Clin Immunol*. 2014;134(6):1310−1317. e1316.

84. Santos AF, James LK, Bahnson HT, et al. IgG inhibits peanut-induced basophil and mast cell activation in peanut-tolerant children sensitized to peanut major allergens. *J Allergy Clin Immunol*. 2015.

85. Wambre E, Bajzik V, DeLong JH, et al. A phenotypically and functionally distinct human TH2 cell subpopulation is associated with allergic disorders. *Sci Transl Med*. 2017;9(401).

86. Chiang D, Chen X, Jones SM, et al. Single-cell profiling of peanut-responsive T cells in patients with peanut allergy reveals heterogeneous effector TH2 subsets. *J Allergy Clin Immunol*. 2018;141(6):2107−2120.

87. Wisniewski JA, Commins SP, Agrawal R, et al. Analysis of cytokine production by peanut-reactive T cells identifies residual Th2 effectors in highly allergic children who received peanut oral immunotherapy. *Clin Exp Allergy : Journal of the British Society for Allergy and Clinical Immunology*. 2015;45(7):1201−1213.

88. Gorelik M, Narisety SD, Guerrerio AL, et al. Suppression of the immunologic response to peanut during immunotherapy is often transient. *J Allergy Clin Immunol.* 2015;135(5): 1283−1292.

89. Ryan JF, Hovde R, Glanville J, et al. Successful immunotherapy induces previously unidentified allergen-specific CD4+ T-cell subsets. *Proc Natl Acad Sci U S A.* 2016;113(9): E1286−E1295.

90. Vickery BP, Berglund JP, Burk CM, et al. Early oral immunotherapy in peanut-allergic preschool children is safe and highly effective. *J Allergy Clin Immunol.* 2017;139(1): 173−181. e178.

Clinical markers to allergen immunotherapy response

Umit Murat Sahiner, MD, Prof of Pediatrics, Pediatric Allergist [1,2],
Jasper H. Kappen, MD, PhD, MSc [1,3,4,5], **Omursen Yildirim, MD, Specialist ENT** [1,6],
Mohamed H. Shamji, PhD, FAAAAI [1,3,4]

[1]*Allergy and Clinical Immunology, Immunomodulation and Tolerance Group, Imperial College London, London, United Kingdom;* [2]*Hacettepe University School of Medicine, Pediatric Allergy Department, Ankara, Turkey;* [3]*MRC & Asthma UK Centre in Allergic Mechanisms of Asthma, London, United Kingdom;* [4]*Allergy and Clinical Immunology, National Heart and Lung Institute, Imperial College London, London, United Kingdom;* [5]*Department of Pulmonology, STZ Centre of Excellence for Asthma & COPD, Sint Franciscus Gasthuis and Vlietland Group, Rotterdam, The Netherlands;* [6]*Istanbul Bilim University, ENT department, Istanbul, Turkey*

Introduction

Although allergen immunotherapy (AIT) is an effective and disease-modifying treatment modality, some patients are not responders.[1-3] Additionally, from the perspective of personalized medicine, there is a clear need for identifying clinical biomarkers that may predict which patients are most likely to respond, when AIT can be discontinued (i.e., persistent responders), what "biomarkers" predict relapse, and who will benefit from a "booster" treatment.[4-6] Biomarkers are defined as "indicators of normal biologic processes, pathogenetic processes, and/or response to therapeutic or other interventions."[7] To date, no biomarker predictive or indicative of clinical response has been identified and validated. Despite the presence of several candidate biomarkers, there are problems of standardization, reproducibility of the results, and the definition of responders and nonresponders as well as difficulties related to laboratory assay variability.[4-6,8] The mechanisms of AIT and targets utilized to measure clinical efficacy are summarized in Fig. 10.1. According to a recent task force report, candidate biomarkers of AIT can be grouped into seven domains[5]:

1. IgE (total IgE, specific IgE, and sIgE/Total IgE ratio),
2. IgG subclasses (sIgG1, sIgG4 including sIgE/IgG4 ratio),
3. Serum inhibitory activity for IgE (IgE-FAB and IgE-BF),
4. Basophil activation tests,
5. Cytokines and chemokines,
6. Cellular markers like T regulatory cells, B regulatory cells, and dendritic cells,
7. In vivo markers

Immunotherapies for Allergic Disease. https://doi.org/10.1016/B978-0-323-54427-6.00010-9

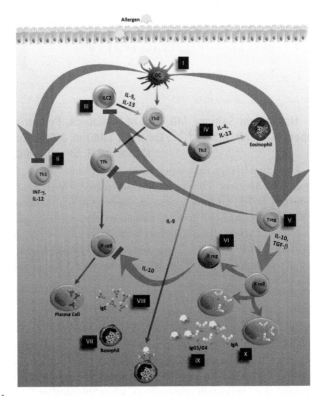

FIGURE 10.1

Mechanism of allergen immunotherapy (AIT) and targets to be measured for clinical efficacy. Pink arrows indicate the regulatory and suppressive effects of AIT. Potential biomarkers I: dendritic cells; II: Th1 cells and cytokines IL-12, INF-g; III: ILC2; IV: Th2 cells and cytokines IL-4, IL-13; V: Treg cells and cytokines IL-10, TGF-b; VI: Breg cells; VII: basophils; VIII: IgE, IX: IgG1/G4, X: IgA.

In the following sections, each group of biomarkers has been reviewed and discussed in detail with their advantages and disadvantages. A summary of different groups of biomarkers with their advantages, disadvantages, and the related studies can be found in Table 10.1.

IgE (total IgE, specific IgE, and sIgE/total IgE ratio)

Total serum IgE (tIgE) levels are often elevated in adults and children with allergy; however, its diagnostic value as an AIT biomarker is limited.[9] Serum total IgE levels

Table 10.1 Classification of clinical biomarkers to determine the clinical effect of allergen immunotherapy.[5,111]

Domain	Advantages	Disadvantages	References
1. IgE tIgE sIgE sIgE/tIgE	-Serum based, -tIgE gold standard in patient selection in AIT, -Reflect allergen exposure, -sIgE/tIgE is a promising predictor of AIT clinic response	-Early rise of sIgE does not correlate with the clinical outcomes Validity of sIgE/tIgE not confirmed -Need for equivalence studies between tIgE units and sIgE units	2,10–14,16,19–22
2. IgG and subclasses sIgG1 sIgG4 sIgE/sIgG4	-Serum based, -sIgG4 informative for allergen exposure -Presence of ISAC chip for sIgG4 -Better to use IgG4 or sIgE/IgG4	-Lack of studies showing relation between sIgG4 levels and symptom and medication scores -Insufficient data on other IgG subsets -Limited data on local antibody levels -Low sIgG4	10,13,15,16,26,29 –36,38
3. Serum inhibitory activity IgE-FAB IgE-BF ELIFAB	-Serum based -High reproducibility for IgE-FAB -Association between clinical scores and IgE-FAB and IgE-BF in several studies	-IgE-BF is not on the market -No data on IgE-FAB to discriminate responders from nonresponders -Limited data on correlation between IgE-FAB and clinical scores	10,13,25,26,29,40 –49
4. Basophil activation CD63 CD203c CD107a DAO	-Reflection of FcγRI-mediated in vivo response with basophil activation -Small amount blood needed	-Variability in basophil activation responses between studies -Limited number of studies -Difficulty of the techniques -Lack of dose response curves -Lack of basophil response to IgE-cross linking in 5%–10% of the population -Need for assay standardization	23,25,29,55–60,108 –110
5. Cytokines and chemokines ECP, Eotaxin IL-2R/IL-2 IL-4, IL-5, IL-9, IL-13, IL-17	-Useful to understand the mechanisms of AIT -Local cytokine production may relate more with clinical symptoms	-To date, no cytokine or chemokine identified to predict clinical response -Inconsistency of the results -Low frequency of specific T cells as a diluting factor for T cell originated cytokines	68–71,73,113

Continued

Table 10.1 Classification of clinical biomarkers to determine the clinical effect of allergen immunotherapy.[5,111]—cont'd

Domain	Advantages	Disadvantages	References
IFN-γ, IL-12 TGF-β, IL-10 CCR3 TARC Tryptase			
6. Cellular biomarkers Tregs Bregs Dendritic cells ILCs	-Tregs are important for the shift from Th2 to Th1 immune response -Bregs may be important in the mechanism of AIT -Newly identified DC markers can be monitored by PCR -DCs more persistent in peripheral blood compared with CD4$^+$ T cells -Treg and Breg cells may be more useful for drug development	-Technical difficulties -No specific marker for T cells -No data to show the link between Tregs and clinical efficacy -Tregs appear very early in AIT so difficult to be a predictive biomarker -Low frequency of Tregs and Bregs -Some DC markers shared with other cells -No information about myeloid or plasmacytoid dendritic cells during AIT	75,76,78,79,106 –108
7. In vivo biomarkers SPT Conjunctival provocation tests Nasal provocation tests Environmental challenge chambers	-More standardized environmental factors, avoid seasonal pollen variation -Surrogate markers of clinical response to AIT -In clinical studies decrease variability, accurate for time course and dose-response studies -EMA recommends in proof of concept and dose finding studies	-Not same as natural exposure -For conjunctival provocation test there is no standardized scoring method and outcomes mostly subjective -Need for standardization for NPT -Allergens used for provocation tests need regulatory approval -ECC are expensive, need for within or between site reproducibility -Not accepted at phase III trials as primary end points	2,82,83,85 –87,89,92,94 –97,99,100,102,114

AIT, allergen immunotherapy; CCR3, CeC chemokine receptor type 3; ECP, eosinophilic cationic protein; ELIFAB, enzyme-linked immunosorbent-facilitated antigen-binding assay; DAO, diamine oxidase; IgE-BF, IgE blocking factor; IgEFAB, IgE-facilitated antigen binding; IFN-g, interferon-gamma; ILCs, innate lymphoid cells; ISAC (ImmunoSolid Allergen Chip Assay); SPT, skin prick testing; TARC, chemokine (CeC motif) ligand 17 (CCL17); TGF-b, transforming growth factor-beta.

show a transient increase and then a gradual decrease during AIT. In published literature, the correlation of tIgE levels with AIT responses is conflicting. In different AIT studies, tIgE levels were found to be decreased,[10–12] increased,[13,14] or not changed after AIT.[15,16]

An elevated serum level of specific IgE levels, in combination with symptoms on exposure to the sensitizing allergen, is the standard for allergy diagnosis. It is also the inclusion criteria for initiating AIT.[17,18] However, sIgE does not seem to correlate with clinical responses during AIT course. Serum sIgE levels transiently increase like tIgE, but this increase in sIgE levels does not appear to be clinically relevant.[1] There is no specific sIgE level that differentiates clinical responders from nonresponders.[1,14,19]

The serum sIgE/tIgE had been shown to be a clinical biomarker in both house dust mite and grass pollen immunotherapy.[14,20–23] In a study, the serum sIgE/tIgE was evaluated to predict clinical response in patients monosensitized to either house dust mite or grass pollens. Using visual analogue scores as a clinical response marker, the ratio correlated with efficacy in sublingual and subcutaneous immunotherapy—treated patients with cutoff value of 16.2% for sIgE/tIgE was associated with a high sensitivity and specificity.[14,20,22] However, there was conflicting data on the correlation between the ratio—sIgE/tIgE—and the patients' clinical responses.[21,23]

There are advantages and disadvantages of using serum-specific antibodies as biomarkers to predict AIT response.[5] One advantage is that serum sampling methods are easy to perform. sIgE is the most clinically relevant marker for AIT patient selection.[17,18] sIgE/tIgE ratio is also a "potential" predictive biomarker in terms of AIT clinical response with some cutoff values established.[14] However, the early rise of sIgE during AIT does not appear to correlate with clinical outcomes. The validity of sIgE/tIgE ratio was not confirmed in other randomized double-blind controlled studies—in essence, the equivalence between tIgE units and sIgE units was demonstrated in only one study.[24]

IgG subtypes

AIT is associated with increased levels of allergen-specific IgG, particularly sIgG1 and sIgG4, which has an inhibitor activity.[13,25,26] This allergen-specific IgG elevation is seen not only in the serum, but also locally in nasal secretions.[27] The IgG antibodies compete with sIgE, suppress basophil histamine release, and prevent IgE-facilitated allergen presentation by B cells to T cell clones.[28,29] Despite the increase in sIgG1 and sIgG4, a clear and validated correlation between the increased allergen-specific IgG1 or IgG4 antibodies levels and clinical efficacy has not been clearly established.[15,30–33] In a grass pollen subcutaneous immunotherapy (SCIT) study, an increase in serum sIgG4 levels correlated with a decrease in allergen-IgE binding to B cells. The clinical response correlated with the serum inhibitory activity, i.e., IgE-facilitated antigen binding, but did not correlate with sIgG4 levels.[1]

In another study, that utilized grass pollen, patients were treated with 2 years of with either active immunotherapy or placebo, then followed for 2 years after AIT discontinuation. Despite significant decreases in sIgG1 and sIgG4, which approached that of preimmunotherapy levels, the inhibitory bioactivity of allergen-specific IgG antibodies was unchanged. These findings suggest the functional importance of IgG subgroups (affinity/avidity) for long-term clinical tolerance rather than the actual levels of IgG subgroups.[10]

In addition to the sIgG levels, sIgE/sIgG4 ratio was also found to be decreased in AIT and was related with reduction of the late-phase skin reactions in some studies[34−36] but not in others.[16,37]

A new method for the measurement of serum sIgG4 and sIgE levels called the ISAC (ImmunoSolid Allergen Chip Assay) chip may be useful in the future to predict clinical improvement (Fig. 10.2).[38] One of the advantages of this method is that

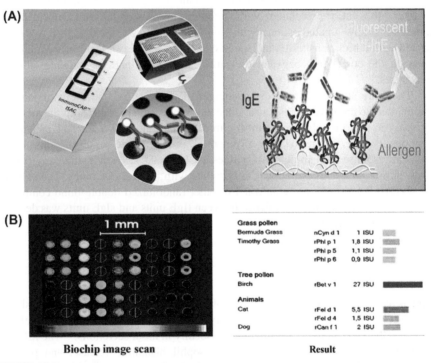

FIGURE 10.2

(A) ImmunoCAP ISAC® is an immunoassay platform. Purified natural or recombinant allergen components are immobilized on a solid support (biochip). IgE antibodies from the patient serum bind to the immobilized allergen components, and these complexes are detected by a fluorescence-labeled anti-IgE antibody. (B) ImmunoCAP ISAC® is a semiquantitative test, and results are reported in ISAC Standardized Units.

only a small amount of serum sample is needed to measure the antibody, which is particularly important for the pediatric patient.

Serum inhibitory activity for IgE

Ig-E inhibitory activity of antibodies during AIT seems to play a key role in the mechanism of the induction of tolerance.[39] These antibodies are mainly IgG and IgA subtypes and are thought to compete with IgE for allergen binding.[40] The prevention of allergen binding to IgE is assessed by a validated flow cytometry—based assay, called Ig-E FAB, which is capable of detecting IgE-allergen complexes binding to surface low-affinity IgE receptors FceRII (CD23) on B cells.[41] The elevation of IgG4 is a consistent feature of AIT.[13,25,26] Allergen-specific IgG4 antibody levels are associated with serum IgG associated inhibitory activity.[10,42] These antibodies appear to block the interaction of allergen-IgE binding to low-affinity IgE receptors on B cells preventing IgE-facilitated HLA-Class II—dependent allergen presentation and subsequent activation of effector T helper 2 cells.[42] The decrease in IgE-FAB with AIT correlates with the clinical response.[1,29,43] In a single-center study that utilized a grass pollen SCIT extract, a prominent increase in serologic blocking activity for grass pollen IgE-FAB was found after 2 years of treatment. Despite the decrease in IgG4 levels following withdrawal of immunotherapy, IgE-FAB remained strongly inhibited.[10] To date, the relationship between the levels of serum inhibitory activity for IgE-FAB in responders versus nonresponders to AIT has not been clearly established.[5]

The IgE-FAB assay is a validated and reproducible assay. However, it is highly complex and only available in a limited number of centers.[1] Recently, an alternative and simpler method called the enzyme-linked immunosorbent-facilitated antigen-binding assay (ELIFAB) has been developed. This technique uses soluble CD23 monomers bound to a solid surface instead of EBV-transformed B cell lines.[44]

Another serum inhibitory effect for IgE involves the prevention of allergen binding to IgE (IGE-blocking factor, IgE-BF). IgE-BF is the amount of IgE which is prevented from binding to its allergen which is measured by a solid-phase assay.[45,46] Wurtzen and colleagues searched the association of IgE-BF with IgE-FAB and basophil histamine release and found a significant reduction in IgE-FAB, basophil histamine release, and an increase in IgE-BF after 1 year of AIT. The effect persisted during the second year of treatment. Additionally, strong correlations were found between changes in IgE-FAB, basophil histamine release, and IgE-BF.[47] Several studies showed the increase in IgE-BF during AIT and an association between IgE-BF and clinical responses.[1,48—50] Currently, the IgE-BF assay (Advia Centaur instrument) is not commercially available.[5]

The IgE-FAB is a serum-based, reproducible assay, which has been demonstrated in several studies to be associated with clinical responses. An alternative assay, the ELIFAB, is easier to use and available for clinical practice and research. Many studies found relationship between IgE-BF and clinical outcomes. However, it is no longer available. No data concerning the comparison of responders and nonresponders is available for the IgE-FAB assay, although a recent position paper found the IgE-FAB to be a promising biomarker.[5] Thus there is a need for prospective cohort studies and clinical trials to confirm this.

Basophil activation

Basophils, which constitute about 1% of peripheral blood, are cells containing cytoplasmic secretory granules. They share common functional properties with mast cells and play an important role in systemic allergic inflammation.[51–53] After allergen exposure, the FceRI on the basophils can cross-link with the sIgE. This leads to the release of histamine and other mediators. AIT may inhibit basophil activation via allergen-specific IgG antibodies. This effect can be obtained either by competing IgG with IgE to bind allergen to prevent allergen-IgE cross-linking in basophils, or by triggering the basophil surface inhibitor IgG receptor, FcγRIIb.[29,43,54]

Basophil activation can be shown by measuring histamine release or detection of surface markers mostly CD63 and CD203c. Multicolor flow cytometry assays using whole blood is the preferred technique. Most commonly used basophil expression markers are CD63 and CD203c.[55,56] CD63 is located within granular membranes and exposed to the surface with the fusion of the granules.[55] CD203c is another marker of basophils located underneath the cell membrane and measures IL-3-dependent basophil activation, and it is highly selective for basophils in peripheral blood.[56] Some other basophil activation markers include CD164, CD13, and CD107a.[57]

The results of the studies concerning basophil activation during AIT are conflicting. While some studies showed a decrease in basophil activation after AIT, others did not.[23,25,58–60] These conflicting findings may be related with the route of application of AIT because sublingual immunotherapy (SLIT) appears to be less effective in basophil suppression compared with SCIT.[5]

One advantage of basophil activation test is small amount of blood to perform the test. Another advantage is that it involves the presentation of the FcγRI-mediated allergen in vivo response in ex vivo conditions. Current problems with the assay is the variability of the basophil responses, limited number of the studies, complexity of the technique, lack of dose response curves, and that 5%–10% of the population's basophil response is unresponsive to IgE cross-linking.[5]

Cytokines and chemokines

The mechanism by which AIT exerts its immunomodulatory effects has not been conclusively established. As allergic disorders are known to be characterized by a Th2-biased response, shift in favor of a Th1 response appears to be the pivotal "immunologic event" in AIT.[8,61] In nearly every step of the AIT "immune response," cytokines and chemokines play an important role in Th1 deviation. According to this theory, there is an upregulation of Th1-related cytokines (IFN-γ, IL-12)[62,63] and Treg response—related cytokines (IL-10 and TGF-β),[30,64] whereas, Th2 response—related cytokines (IL-4, IL-13, IL-9, IL-17, TNF-α) decrease.[63] However, not all studies have demonstrated this expected cytokine profile switch.[65,66] Several local (nasal) biomarkers for AIT response have been identified in an allergen challenge mode. This suggests immunological tolerance during AIT also takes place at a local level.[67]

Chemokines are a group of small cytokines which have chemoattractive functions playing an important role in the pathophysiology of allergic disorders. Although some studies report changes in the levels of serum chemokines associated with AIT, none of these directly correlated with clinical outcomes. Some chemokines that have been investigated as potential biomarkers are listed below:

- Increased following AIT: CCR4,[68] eotaxin,[68] complement C4a,[69] leptin,[70] apolipoprotein,[69] thymus and activation regulated protein (TARC),[68] transthyretin,[69] signaling lymphocytic activation molecule,[68] resistin[70]
- Decreased: Complement C3a, C5a,[71] aotaxin,[67] TRAIL[72]
- Unchanged: CCR3,[68] adiponectin,[73] tryptase,[67] leptin,[73] ECP,[67] soluble HLA molecules[74]

Currently, there is no validated consensus on potential cytokine or chemokine biomarkers that have a prognostic or predictive value in clinical response to AIT.

Cellular biomarkers

Potential cellular biomarkers associated with AIT response include regulatory T cells (Tregs), T helper cells (Th1, Th2), T follicular helper (Tfh) and T follicular regulatory (Tfr) cells, regulatory B cells (Bregs), and dendritic cells (DCs).[5,6] The key cells involved in reversing the inflammatory process and skewing away from the Th2 response are the natural regulatory T cells (nTreg) that express the transcription factor forkhead box P3 (FOXP3) and inducible regulatory T (iTreg) cells, that secrete regulatory cytokines, such as IL-10, IL-35, and TGF-β.[6]

One study with grass pollen—allergic patients receiving immunotherapy versus healthy controls demonstrated increased Foxp3+ CD25+ and Foxp3+ CD4+ regulatory cell numbers in the nasal mucosa. The increase was associated with a recruitment of IL-10-producing Foxp3+ CD3+ and IL-10-producing Foxp3+ CD3+1 cells, which are expected AIT outcome, i.e., Th2 response suppression.[75]

Although such changes are reported to distinguish between AIT-treated and placebo groups, they correlate with the treatment outcomes in general.[75,76] However, there is not enough data to link Treg cells with clinical efficacy. Additionally, it is rather difficult to detect them technically. Thus, they are unlikely to represent prognostic or predictive biomarkers at this time.[5]

Current evidence supports the role of Breg cells in allergen tolerance via following potential mechanisms: IL-10-mediated suppression of effector T cell, including TH2 responses, induction of TREG cells, IL-10-mediated inhibition of DC maturation, modulation of TFH responses, and production of anti-inflammatory IgG4 antibodies.[77] One study has shown remarkable similarities between bee venom—allergic patients and beekeepers in terms of allergen-specific B cell responses to high-dose venom exposure. IL-10-producing B R1 cells, phospholipase A2—specific IgG4 switched B cells, plasmablasts, and phospholipase A2—specific CCR5-expressing B cells were found to be increased in both group of allergic patients receiving venom immunotherapy or after multiple bee stings during the beekeeping season in beekeepers.[78]

Several markers associated with polarized DCs have been used in recent studies to investigate the effects of SLIT. Among these markers, component 1 (C1Q) and the receptor stabilin-1 and STAB1 were shown to be increased in the blood samples of clinically responding patients, contrary to nonresponding or control group patients.[79] At this stage, there are no validated cellular biomarkers for monitoring AIT responses. Further clinical trials are needed for a better understanding of the cellular events that impact AIT efficacy.

In vivo biomarkers

In vivo biomarkers evaluate the response to AIT directly in the involved organ by provocation with the relevant allergen. It includes:

- Skin prick tests (SPTs)
- Conjunctival provocation tests (CPTs)
- Nasal provocation tests (NPTs)
- Environmental challenge chambers (ECCs) for provocation tests

Generally, these tests are used in the clinical setting in the diagnostic process of evaluation of the relevance of an underlying IgE-mediated sensitization.[80] These tests can also be applied as *in vivo* methods for evaluating the effect of therapeutic interventions in clinical trials with AIT.[80] The current guideline of the European Medicinal Agency (EMA) states that provocation tests are recommended for proof of concept or Phase-II dose-finding trials in AIT.[81]

There are several protocols that have been published on different challenge models.[82] There is a clear unmet need for thorough harmonization and further validation of these different provocation models.[83]

Skin prick testing

Validation of SPT for research purposes was already done in 1993 by Dreborg.[84] Several studies that utilized pollen, mites, and animal dander extracts demonstrated blunted responses to the treated allergens after AIT. There was also suppression of the late phase response.[85–87] However, there was poor correlation between the SPT response and AIT clinical response. Therefore, SPT may not be clinically applicable as an AIT biomarker that can be used to monitor patient response.[86,88]

Conjunctival testing

Conjunctival testing (CPT) uses a subjective scoring system during allergen dose titration.[89] It was used in the original AIT studies conducted by Noon and Freeman.[90,91] A 10- to 30-fold decrease in immediate conjunctival allergen sensitivity was observed in a long-term trial of grass pollen. The effect persisted for 3 years after discontinuation of treatment.[2] Refinement of CPT can be achieved by a recent technique that included objective photographic assessment and scoring of conjunctival responses before/after immunotherapy.[92,93] Fig. 10.3 summarizes the procedure of conjunctival provocation testing algorithm.

Nasal provocation tests

Nasal provocation testing allows correlation of nasal symptom scores with the objective measurements of peak nasal inspiratory flow.[94] Early responses have been shown to be inhibited[95] following intralymphatic cat and epicutaneous grass AIT.[96] NPT also allows the evaluation of cells and cytokines in the nasal fluid itself. The suppression of eosinophil numbers[95,97,98] and histamine during nasal provocation after ragweed immunotherapy have been demonstrated. The use of more precise nasal allergen delivery devices[99] as well as the availability of synthetic materials for filters, sponges that enable collection of neat or minimally diluted nasal fluid directly from the nasal mucosa are recently improved.[99,100] Together with miniaturized assay systems, it allows the reproducible measurement of multiple mediators, cytokines, and antibodies in nasal fluid volumes. Nasal provocation shows an early increase in local nasal fluid tryptase at 5−30 minutes and more delayed increases in chemokines and Th2 cytokines (eotaxin, IL-4, 5, 9 and 13) and innate lymphoid 2 cells (ILC2s) that parallel the late nasal response. Grass pollen AIT was associated with blunted increases in early (5 min) tryptase and late (8 hours) eotaxin and Th2 cytokines IL-4, 5, 9, and 13 in nasal fluid compared with untreated allergic controls.[67] An algorithmic approach to nasal allergen challenges is given in Fig. 10.4.[101]

Environmental challenge chambers

An ECC represents a provocation test that closely simulates natural exposure. An EEC is a stable and reproducible allergen exposure under standardized environmental conditions.[102] Recent studies have utilized the ECC to evaluate time of onset studies of AIT.[103,104] One study even showed a correlation between symptoms in the ECC that were comparable to symptoms during natural seasonal exposure.[105]

For AIT, there is a need for further validation of treatment effect size as evaluated in EEC challenges to be correlated to effect sizes found under natural exposure in field trials.[102] Common ECCs and used allergen concentrations are given in Table 10.2.

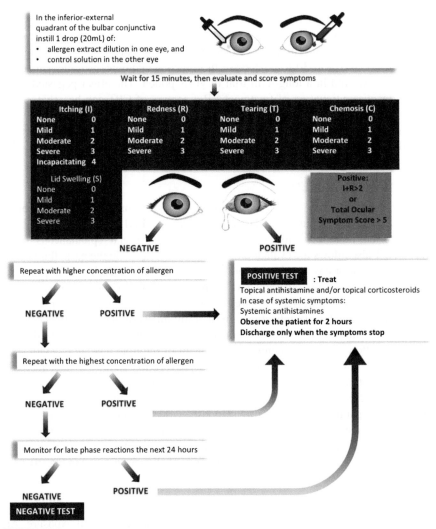

FIGURE 10.3

Schematic presentation of conjunctival provocation test.

Adapted from Fauquert JL, Jedrzejczak-Czechowicz M, Rondon C, et al. Conjunctival allergen provocation test: guidelines for daily practice. Allergy. 2017;72(1):43–54

Novel biomarkers/developments

Recently, some new biomarkers such as innate lymphoid cells (ILCs),[106,107] molecular markers of DCs,[108] and diamine oxidase (DAO) test of basophil histamine release[25] have been proposed.

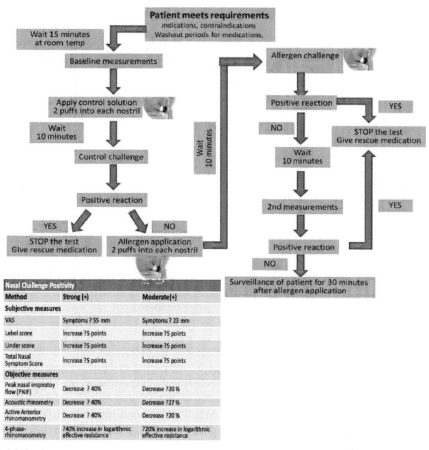

FIGURE 10.4

An algorithmic approach to the nasal allergen provocation test.

Adopted from Auge J, Vent J, Agache I, et al. EAACI position paper on the standardization of nasal allergen challenges. Allergy. 2018.

ILCs, a recently defined type of cells, might play a crucial role in allergic inflammatory diseases. Especially innate lymphoid cell type 2 (ILC2), which are important in Type 2 inflammation, produces IL-4, IL-5, IL-13 inducing basophils, eosinophils, and mast cells as well as IgE production. The contribution of ILC2s in allergic inflammation was first demonstrated in cat-allergic patients.[107] Following that, the seasonal variation of ILC2s was shown in pollen-allergic patients. Subcutaneous grass pollen immunotherapy suppressed the seasonal increase in ILC2s.[106]

Another new candidate biomarkers to assess the clinical efficacy of AIT are the molecular markers of DCs. In patients with grass pollen allergy, sublingual immunotherapy increased the tolerogenic DC markers in regulatory DCs (namely C1Q A, B, C, and Stabilin-1), and this increase correlated with clinical response.[108]

Table 10.2 Common Environmental Challenge chambers and used allergen concentrations.[102,115–122]

Device	First defined	Antigen	Max antigen concentrations	References
Vienna Challenge Chamber, Austria	1987	Der P1 Grass	40 ng/m^3 1500 ± 120 grains/m^3	Horak 1994, Horak 2002
Kinston EEU, Canada	1998	Ragweed	3500 ± 500 grains/m^3	Day 1999
Fraunhofer ECC, Germany	2003	Grass	4000 ± 300 grains/m^3	Hohlfeld 2010
Copenhagen, ECC, Denmark	1996	Der P1	50–100 ng/m^3	Ronborg 1996
Biogenics Research Chamber, Texas, USA	2011	Ragweed	3500 ± 500 grains/m^3	Jacobs 2012
Chiba ECC, Japan	2014	Japanese cedar pollen	8000 and 12,000 grains/m^3	Hamasaki 2014
Biocube, USA	2009	Ragweed	3500 ± 500 grains/m^3	Gomes 2016

ECC, environmental challenge chamber; EEU, environmental exposure unit.

Basophil activation can either be assessed by measuring surface activation markers (CD63, CD203c, and CD107a) or by measuring histamine release. A new functional assay based on the detection of intracellular expression of fluorochrome-labeled DAO in basophils has been validated and is under research as a potential biomarker of efficiency in AIT.[109] DAO binds intracellularly to histamine, and the level of DAO is proportional to that of histamine. The reduction of DAO in basophils has been shown in both SCIT and SLIT studies.[109,110] In a recent study, the reduction of basophil activation measured by DAO was shown both in SLIT and SCIT patients treated with grass pollen with the effect persisting for up to 2 years after AIT discontinuation.[25]

Further studies are needed to confirm the relationship with the clinical symptoms and DAO. The accessibility and overall clinical utility of these biomarkers are still debated.[4,5,111]

Concluding remarks

AIT is an immune-modulating treatment for allergic diseases. Although highly effective, some patients do not respond to the treatment. Although about the mechanism involved in AIT continues to be elucidated, there are no surrogate biomarkers that are reliably predictive of the clinical response to AIT. With modulation of both innate and adaptive immune responses, a reduction of ILC2s in combination with

Tregs and Bregs skews the immune response toward a Th1 response, i.e., immunological tolerance. IgG4 antibodies have the capacity to inhibit both allergen-induced basophil responsiveness and CD23-mediated IgE-facilitated allergen presentation. To date, a clear correlation with the observed immunological changes and responders versus nonresponders has not been established. The most promising biomarker is IgE-FAB as a reflection of functional IgG4. Cellular responses and cytokines give a lot of insight into the mechanisms of AIT but are not applicable as biomarkers in a clinical setting. Finally, the use of provocations testing is still limited to phase II studies. To date, they do reflect natural allergen exposure and have no correlation with clinical response. There is a need for more research for confirmation and interpretation of the possible association with biomarkers and clinical response to AIT.

Acknowledgment

We thank Neal Bradshaw from Thermo Fisher Scientific for providing the figures of ISAC.

References

1. Shamji MH, Ljorring C, Francis JN, et al. Functional rather than immunoreactive levels of IgG4 correlate closely with clinical response to grass pollen immunotherapy. *Allergy.* 2012;67(2):217−226.
2. Durham SR, Walker SM, Varga EM, et al. Long-term clinical efficacy of grass-pollen immunotherapy. *N Engl J Med.* 1999;341(7):468−475.
3. Radulovic S, Wilson D, Calderon M, Durham S. Systematic reviews of sublingual immunotherapy (SLIT). *Allergy.* 2011;66(6):740−752.
4. Kouser L, Kappen J, Walton RP, Shamji MH. Update on biomarkers to monitor clinical efficacy response during and post treatment in allergen immunotherapy. *Curr Treat Options Allergy.* 2017;4(1):43−53.
5. Shamji MH, Kappen JH, Akdis M, et al. Biomarkers for monitoring clinical efficacy of allergen immunotherapy for allergic rhinoconjunctivitis and allergic asthma: an EAACI position paper. *Allergy.* 2017;72(8):1156−1173.
6. Shamji MH, Durham SR. Mechanisms of allergen immunotherapy for inhaled allergens and predictive biomarkers. *J Allergy Clin Immunol.* 2017;140(6):1485−1498.
7. Food, Drug Administration, HHS. International Conference on harmonisation; guidance on E15 pharmacogenomics definitions and sample coding; availability. *Fed Regist.* 2008;73:19074−19076.
8. Shamji MH, Durham SR. Mechanisms of immunotherapy to aeroallergens. *Clin Exp Allergy.* 2011;41(9):1235−1246.
9. Klink M, Cline MG, Halonen M, Burrows B. Problems in defining normal limits for serum IgE. *J Allergy Clin Immunol.* 1990;85(2):440−444.
10. James LK, Shamji MH, Walker SM, et al. Long-term tolerance after allergen immunotherapy is accompanied by selective persistence of blocking antibodies. *J Allergy Clin Immunol.* 2011;127(2), 509−516 e501−505.

11. Keskin O, Tuncer A, Adalioglu G, Sekerel BE, Sackesen C, Kalayci O. The effects of grass pollen allergoid immunotherapy on clinical and immunological parameters in children with allergic rhinitis. *Pediatr Allergy Immunol.* 2006;17(6):396−407.

12. Durham SR, Yang WH, Pedersen MR, Johansen N, Rak S. Sublingual immunotherapy with once-daily grass allergen tablets: a randomized controlled trial in seasonal allergic rhinoconjunctivitis. *J Allergy Clin Immunol.* 2006;117(4):802−809.

13. Didier A, Malling HJ, Worm M, et al. Optimal dose, efficacy, and safety of once-daily sublingual immunotherapy with a 5-grass pollen tablet for seasonal allergic rhinitis. *J Allergy Clin Immunol.* 2007;120(6):1338−1345.

14. Di Lorenzo G, Mansueto P, Pacor ML, et al. Evaluation of serum s-IgE/total IgE ratio in predicting clinical response to allergen-specific immunotherapy. *J Allergy Clin Immunol.* 2009;123(5), 1103−1110, 1110 e1101−1104.

15. Gehlhar K, Schlaak M, Becker W, Bufe A. Monitoring allergen immunotherapy of pollen-allergic patients: the ratio of allergen-specific IgG4 to IgG1 correlates with clinical outcome. *Clin Exp Allergy.* 1999;29(4):497−506.

16. Rolinck-Werninghaus C, Kopp M, Liebke C, Lange J, Wahn U, Niggemann B. Lack of detectable alterations in immune responses during sublingual immunotherapy in children with seasonal allergic rhinoconjunctivitis to grass pollen. *Int Arch Allergy Immunol.* 2005;136(2):134−141.

17. Burks AW, Calderon MA, Casale T, et al. Update on allergy immunotherapy: American academy of allergy, asthma & immunology/European academy of allergy and clinical immunology/PRACTALL consensus report. *J Allergy Clin Immunol.* 2013;131(5), 1288-1296 e1283.

18. Cox L, Nelson H, Lockey R, et al. Allergen immunotherapy: a practice parameter third update. *J Allergy Clin Immunol.* 2011;127(1 Suppl). S1-55.

19. Pilette C, Nouri-Aria KT, Jacobson MR, et al. Grass pollen immunotherapy induces an allergen-specific IgA2 antibody response associated with mucosal TGF-beta expression. *J Immunol.* 2007;178(7):4658−4666.

20. Fujimura T, Yonekura S, Horiguchi S, et al. Increase of regulatory T cells and the ratio of specific IgE to total IgE are candidates for response monitoring or prognostic biomarkers in 2-year sublingual immunotherapy (SLIT) for Japanese cedar pollinosis. *Clin Immunol.* 2011;139(1):65−74.

21. Eifan AO, Akkoc T, Yildiz A, et al. Clinical efficacy and immunological mechanisms of sublingual and subcutaneous immunotherapy in asthmatic/rhinitis children sensitized to house dust mite: an open randomized controlled trial. *Clin Exp Allergy.* 2010;40(6): 922−932.

22. Li Q, Li M, Yue W, et al. Predictive factors for clinical response to allergy immunotherapy in children with asthma and rhinitis. *Int Arch Allergy Immunol.* 2014;164(3):210−217.

23. Van Overtvelt L, Baron-Bodo V, Horiot S, et al. Changes in basophil activation during grass-pollen sublingual immunotherapy do not correlate with clinical efficacy. *Allergy.* 2011;66(12):1530−1537.

24. Kober HPH. Quantitation of mouse-human chimeric allergen-specific IgE antibodies with ImmunoCAP technology. *J Allergy Clin Immunol.* 2006;117. Abstract 845.

25. Shamji MH, Layhadi JA, Scadding GW, et al. Basophil expression of diamine oxidase: a novel biomarker of allergen immunotherapy response. *J Allergy Clin Immunol.* 2015; 135(4), 913−921 e919.

26. Dahl R, Kapp A, Colombo G, et al. Sublingual grass allergen tablet immunotherapy provides sustained clinical benefit with progressive immunologic changes over 2 years. *J Allergy Clin Immunol*. 2008;121(2), 512–518 e512.
27. Reisinger J, Horak F, Pauli G, et al. Allergen-specific nasal IgG antibodies induced by vaccination with genetically modified allergens are associated with reduced nasal allergen sensitivity. *J Allergy Clin Immunol*. 2005;116(2):347–354.
28. Aalberse RC, Schuurman J. IgG4 breaking the rules. *Immunology*. 2002;105(1):9–19.
29. Wachholz PA, Soni NK, Till SJ, Durham SR. Inhibition of allergen-IgE binding to B cells by IgG antibodies after grass pollen immunotherapy. *J Allergy Clin Immunol*. 2003;112(5):915–922.
30. Bohle B, Kinaciyan T, Gerstmayr M, Radakovics A, Jahn-Schmid B, Ebner C. Sublingual immunotherapy induces IL-10-producing T regulatory cells, allergen-specific T-cell tolerance, and immune deviation. *J Allergy Clin Immunol*. 2007;120(3):707–713.
31. Gomez E, Fernandez TD, Dona I, et al. Initial immunological changes as predictors for house dust mite immunotherapy response. *Clin Exp Allergy*. 2015;45(10):1542–1553.
32. Moverare R, Elfman L, Vesterinen E, Metso T, Haahtela T. Development of new IgE specificities to allergenic components in birch pollen extract during specific immunotherapy studied with immunoblotting and Pharmacia CAP System. *Allergy*. 2002; 57(5):423–430.
33. Nelson HS, Nolte H, Creticos P, Maloney J, Wu J, Bernstein DI. Efficacy and safety of timothy grass allergy immunotherapy tablet treatment in North American adults. *J Allergy Clin Immunol*. 2011;127(1), 72–80, 80 e71–72.
34. La Rosa M, Ranno C, Andre C, Carat F, Tosca MA, Canonica GW. Double-blind placebo-controlled evaluation of sublingual-swallow immunotherapy with standardized Parietaria judaica extract in children with allergic rhinoconjunctivitis. *J Allergy Clin Immunol*. 1999;104(2 Pt 1):425–432.
35. Troise C, Voltolini S, Canessa A, Pecora S, Negrini AC. Sublingual immunotherapy in Parietaria pollen-induced rhinitis: a double-blind study. *J Investig Allergol Clin Immunol*. 1995;5(1):25–30.
36. Bahceciler NN, Arikan C, Taylor A, et al. Impact of sublingual immunotherapy on specific antibody levels in asthmatic children allergic to house dust mites. *Int Arch Allergy Immunol*. 2005;136(3):287–294.
37. Baron-Bodo V, Horiot S, Lautrette A, et al. Heterogeneity of antibody responses among clinical responders during grass pollen sublingual immunotherapy. *Clin Exp Allergy*. 2013;43(12):1362–1373.
38. Wollmann E, Lupinek C, Kundi M, Selb R, Niederberger V, Valenta R. Reduction in allergen-specific IgE binding as measured by microarray: a possible surrogate marker for effects of specific immunotherapy. *J Allergy Clin Immunol*. 2015;136(3), 806–809 e807.
39. Cooke RA, Barnard JH, Hebald S, Stull A. Serological evidence of immunity with coexisting sensitization in a type of human allergy (hay fever). *J Exp Med*. 1935;62(6): 733–750.
40. Platts-Mills TA, von Maur RK, Ishizaka K, Norman PS, Lichtenstein LM. IgA and IgG anti-ragweed antibodies in nasal secretions. Quantitative measurements of antibodies and correlation with inhibition of histamine release. *J Clin Investig*. 1976;57(4): 1041–1050.

41. Shamji MH, Wilcock LK, Wachholz PA, et al. The IgE-facilitated allergen binding (FAB) assay: validation of a novel flow-cytometric based method for the detection of inhibitory antibody responses. *J Immunol Methods*. 2006;317(1−2):71−79.

42. Nouri-Aria KT, Wachholz PA, Francis JN, et al. Grass pollen immunotherapy induces mucosal and peripheral IL-10 responses and blocking IgG activity. *J Immunol*. 2004; 172(5):3252−3259.

43. van Neerven RJ, Wikborg T, Lund G, et al. Blocking antibodies induced by specific allergy vaccination prevent the activation of CD4+ T cells by inhibiting serum-IgE-facilitated allergen presentation. *J Immunol*. 1999;163(5):2944−2952.

44. Shamji MH, Francis JN, Wurtzen PA, Lund K, Durham SR, Till SJ. Cell-free detection of allergen-IgE cross-linking with immobilized phase CD23: inhibition by blocking antibody responses after immunotherapy. *J Allergy Clin Immunol*. 2013;132(4), 1003−1005 e1001−1004.

45. Durham SR, Emminger W, Kapp A, et al. SQ-standardized sublingual grass immunotherapy: confirmation of disease modification 2 years after 3 years of treatment in a randomized trial. *J Allergy Clin Immunol*. 2012;129(3), 717-725 e715.

46. Petersen AB, Gudmann P, Milvang-Gronager P, et al. Performance evaluation of a specific IgE assay developed for the ADVIA centaur immunoassay system. *Clin Biochem*. 2004;37(10):882−892.

47. Wurtzen PA, Lund G, Lund K, Arvidsson M, Rak S, Ipsen H. A double-blind placebo-controlled birch allergy vaccination study II: correlation between inhibition of IgE binding, histamine release and facilitated allergen presentation. *Clin Exp Allergy*. 2008; 38(8):1290−1301.

48. Reich K, Gessner C, Kroker A, et al. Immunologic effects and tolerability profile of in-season initiation of a standardized-quality grass allergy immunotherapy tablet: a phase III, multicenter, randomized, double-blind, placebo-controlled trial in adults with grass pollen-induced rhinoconjunctivitis. *Clin Ther*. 2011;33(7):828−840.

49. Corzo JL, Carrillo T, Pedemonte C, et al. Tolerability during double-blind randomized phase I trials with the house dust mite allergy immunotherapy tablet in adults and children. *J Investig Allergol Clin Immunol*. 2014;24(3):154−161.

50. Blaiss M, Maloney J, Nolte H, Gawchik S, Yao R, Skoner DP. Efficacy and safety of timothy grass allergy immunotherapy tablets in North American children and adolescents. *J Allergy Clin Immunol*. 2011;127(1), 64−71, 71 e61−64.

51. Ishizaka T, De Bernardo R, Tomioka H, Lichtenstein LM, Ishizaka K. Identification of basophil granulocytes as a site of allergic histamine release. *J Immunol*. 1972;108(4): 1000−1008.

52. Schroeder JT, Kagey-Sobotka A, Lichtenstein LM. The role of the basophil in allergic inflammation. *Allergy*. 1995;50(6):463−472.

53. MacGlashan Jr D. Expression of CD203c and CD63 in human basophils: relationship to differential regulation of piecemeal and anaphylactic degranulation processes. *Clin Exp Allergy*. 2010;40(9):1365−1377.

54. Kepley CL, Cambier JC, Morel PA, et al. Negative regulation of FcepsilonRI signaling by FcgammaRII costimulation in human blood basophils. *J Allergy Clin Immunol*. 2000;106(2):337−348.

55. Knol EF, Mul FP, Jansen H, Calafat J, Roos D. Monitoring human basophil activation via CD63 monoclonal antibody 435. *J Allergy Clin Immunol*. 1991;88(3 Pt 1):328−338.

56. Buhring HJ, Streble A, Valent P. The basophil-specific ectoenzyme E-NPP3 (CD203c) as a marker for cell activation and allergy diagnosis. *Int Arch Allergy Immunol.* 2004; 133(4):317−329.

57. Hennersdorf F, Florian S, Jakob A, et al. Identification of CD13, CD107a, and CD164 as novel basophil-activation markers and dissection of two response patterns in time kinetics of IgE-dependent upregulation. *Cell Res.* 2005;15(5):325−335.

58. Kepil Ozdemir S, Sin BA, Guloglu D, Ikinciogullari A, Gencturk Z, Misirligil Z. Short-term preseasonal immunotherapy: is early clinical efficacy related to the basophil response? *Int Arch Allergy Immunol.* 2014;164(3):237−245.

59. Aasbjerg K, Backer V, Lund G, et al. Immunological comparison of allergen immunotherapy tablet treatment and subcutaneous immunotherapy against grass allergy. *Clin Exp Allergy.* 2014;44(3):417−428.

60. Ceuppens JL, Bullens D, Kleinjans H, van der Werf J, Purethal Birch Efficacy Study Group. Immunotherapy with a modified birch pollen extract in allergic rhinoconjunctivitis: clinical and immunological effects. *Clin Exp Allergy.* 2009;39(12):1903−1909.

61. Akdis CA, Akdis M. Mechanisms of allergen-specific immunotherapy and immune tolerance to allergens. *World Allergy Organ J.* 2015;8(1):17.

62. Cosmi L, Santarlasci V, Angeli R, et al. Sublingual immunotherapy with dermatophagoides monomeric allergoid down-regulates allergen-specific immunoglobulin E and increases both interferon-gamma- and interleukin-10-production. *Clin Exp Allergy.* 2006;36(3):261−272.

63. Fanta C, Bohle B, Hirt W, et al. Systemic immunological changes induced by administration of grass pollen allergens via the oral mucosa during sublingual immunotherapy. *Int Arch Allergy Immunol.* 1999;120(3):218−224.

64. Jutel M, Akdis M, Budak F, et al. IL-10 and TGF-beta cooperate in the regulatory T cell response to mucosal allergens in normal immunity and specific immunotherapy. *Eur J Immunol.* 2003;33(5):1205−1214.

65. Francis JN, Till SJ, Durham SR. Induction of IL-10+CD4+CD25+ T cells by grass pollen immunotherapy. *J Allergy Clin Immunol.* 2003;111(6):1255−1261.

66. Wachholz PA, Nouri-Aria KT, Wilson DR, et al. Grass pollen immunotherapy for hayfever is associated with increases in local nasal but not peripheral Th1:Th2 cytokine ratios. *Immunology.* 2002;105(1):56−62.

67. Scadding GW, Eifan AO, Lao-Araya M, et al. Effect of grass pollen immunotherapy on clinical and local immune response to nasal allergen challenge. *Allergy.* 2015;70(6): 689−696.

68. Plewako H, Holmberg K, Oancea I, Gotlib T, Samolinski B, Rak S. A follow-up study of immunotherapy-treated birch-allergic patients: effect on the expression of chemokines in the nasal mucosa. *Clin Exp Allergy.* 2008;38(7):1124−1131.

69. Makino Y, Noguchi E, Takahashi N, et al. Apolipoprotein A-IV is a candidate target molecule for the treatment of seasonal allergic rhinitis. *J Allergy Clin Immunol.* 2010;126(6), 1163−1169 e1165.

70. Salmivesi S, Paassilta M, Huhtala H, Nieminen R, Moilanen E, Korppi M. Changes in biomarkers during a six-month oral immunotherapy intervention for cow's milk allergy. *Acta Paediatr.* 2016;105(11):1349−1354.

71. Li H, Xu E, He M. Cytokine responses to specific immunotherapy in house dust mite-induced allergic rhinitis patients. *Inflammation.* 2015;38(6):2216−2223.

72. Casaulta C, Schoni MH, Weichel M, et al. IL-10 controls Aspergillus fumigatus- and Pseudomonas aeruginosa-specific T-cell response in cystic fibrosis. *Pediatr Res.* 2003;53(2):313−319.

73. Ciprandi G, De Amici M, Murdaca G, Filaci G, Fenoglio D, Marseglia GL. Adipokines and sublingual immunotherapy: preliminary report. *Hum Immunol.* 2009;70(1):73−78.

74. Ciprandi G, Continia P, Fenoglio D, et al. Relationship between soluble HLA-G and HLA-A,-B,-C serum levels, and interferon-gamma production after sublingual immunotherapy in patients with allergic rhinitis. *Hum Immunol.* 2008;69(7):409−413.

75. Radulovic S, Jacobson MR, Durham SR, Nouri-Aria KT. Grass pollen immunotherapy induces Foxp3-expressing CD4+ CD25+ cells in the nasal mucosa. *J Allergy Clin Immunol.* 2008;121(6), 1467−1472, 1472 e1461.

76. Scadding GW, Shamji MH, Jacobson MR, et al. Sublingual grass pollen immunotherapy is associated with increases in sublingual Foxp3-expressing cells and elevated allergen-specific immunoglobulin G4, immunoglobulin A and serum inhibitory activity for immunoglobulin E-facilitated allergen binding to B cells. *Clin Exp Allergy.* 2010; 40(4):598−606.

77. van de Veen W. The role of regulatory B cells in allergen immunotherapy. *Curr Opin Allergy Clin Immunol.* 2017;17(6):447−452.

78. Boonpiyathad T, Meyer N, Moniuszko M, et al. High-dose bee venom exposure induces similar tolerogenic B-cell responses in allergic patients and healthy beekeepers. *Allergy.* 2017;72(3):407−415.

79. Zimmer A, Bouley J, Le Mignon M, et al. A regulatory dendritic cell signature correlates with the clinical efficacy of allergen-specific sublingual immunotherapy. *J Allergy Clin Immunol.* 2012;129(4):1020−1030.

80. Bousquet J, Khaltaev N, Cruz AA, et al. Allergic rhinitis and its impact on asthma (ARIA) 2008 update (in collaboration with the World Health Organization, GA(2) LEN and AllerGen). *Allergy.* 2008;63(Suppl 86):8−160.

81. Committee for Medicinal Products for Human Use, European Medicines Agency. *Guideline on the Clinical Development of Products for Specific Immunotherapy for the Treatment of Allergic Diseases.* 2008.

82. Agache I, Bilo M, Braunstahl GJ, et al. In vivo diagnosis of allergic diseases–allergen provocation tests. *Allergy.* 2015;70(4):355−365.

83. Pfaar O, Demoly P, Gerth van Wijk R, et al. Recommendations for the standardization of clinical outcomes used in allergen immunotherapy trials for allergic rhinoconjunctivitis: an EAACI position paper. *Allergy.* 2014;69(7):854−867.

84. Dreborg SFA. Allergen standardization and skin tests. EAACI position paper. *Allergy.* 1993;48(suppl 44):49−82.

85. Francis JN, James LK, Paraskevopoulos G, et al. Grass pollen immunotherapy: IL-10 induction and suppression of late responses precedes IgG4 inhibitory antibody activity. *J Allergy Clin Immunol.* 2008;121(5), 1120−1125 e1122.

86. Des Roches A, Paradis L, Knani J, et al. Immunotherapy with a standardized dermatophagoides pteronyssinus extract. V. Duration of the efficacy of immunotherapy after its cessation. *Allergy.* 1996;51(6):430−433.

87. Bousquet J, Maasch H, Martinot B, Hejjaoui A, Wahl R, Michel FB. Double-blind, placebo-controlled immunotherapy with mixed grass-pollen allergoids. II. Comparison between parameters assessing the efficacy of immunotherapy. *J Allergy Clin Immunol.* 1988;82(3 Pt 1):439−446.

88. Cox L, Cohn JR. Duration of allergen immunotherapy in respiratory allergy: when is enough, enough? *Ann Allergy Asthma Immunol*. 2007;98(5):416−426.

89. Moller C, Bjorksten B, Nilsson G, Dreborg S. The precision of the conjunctival provocation test. *Allergy*. 1984;39(1):37−41.

90. Noon L. Prophylactic inoculation against hay fever. *Lancet*. 1911;i:1572−1573.

91. Freeman J. Further observation on the treatment of hay fever by hypodermic inoculationsof pollen vaccine. *Lancet*. 1911;ii:814−817.

92. Sarandi I, Classen DP, Astvatsatourov A, et al. Quantitative conjunctival provocation test for controlled clinical trials. *Methods Inf Med*. 2014;53(4):238−244.

93. Kruse K, Gerwin E, Eichel A, Shah-Hosseini K, Mosges R. Conjunctival provocation tests: a predictive factor for patients' seasonal allergic rhinoconjunctivitis symptoms. *J Allergy Clin Immunol Pract*. 2015;3(3):381−386.

94. Scadding G, Hellings P, Alobid I, et al. Diagnostic tools in Rhinology EAACI position paper. *Clin Transl Allergy*. 2011;1(1):2.

95. Durham SR, Ying S, Varney VA, et al. Grass pollen immunotherapy inhibits allergen-induced infiltration of CD4+ T lymphocytes and eosinophils in the nasal mucosa and increases the number of cells expressing messenger RNA for interferon-gamma. *J Allergy Clin Immunol*. 1996;97(6):1356−1365.

96. Senti G, Crameri R, Kuster D, et al. Intralymphatic immunotherapy for cat allergy induces tolerance after only 3 injections. *J Allergy Clin Immunol*. 2012;129(5): 1290−1296.

97. Creticos PS, Marsh DG, Proud D, et al. Responses to ragweed-pollen nasal challenge before and after immunotherapy. *J Allergy Clin Immunol*. 1989;84(2):197−205.

98. Furin MJ, Norman PS, Creticos PS, et al. Immunotherapy decreases antigen-induced eosinophil cell migration into the nasal cavity. *J Allergy Clin Immunol*. 1991;88(1): 27−32.

99. Scadding GW, Calderon MA, Bellido V, et al. Optimisation of grass pollen nasal allergen challenge for assessment of clinical and immunological outcomes. *J Immunol Methods*. 2012;384(1−2):25−32.

100. Scadding GW, Eifan A, Penagos M, et al. Local and systemic effects of cat allergen nasal provocation. *Clin Exp Allergy*. 2015;45(3):613−623.

101. Auge J, Vent J, Agache I, et al. EAACI position paper on the standardization of nasal allergen challenges. *Allergy*. 2018;73(8):1597−1608.

102. Rosner-Friese K, Kaul S, Vieths S, Pfaar O. Environmental exposure chambers in allergen immunotherapy trials: current status and clinical validation needs. *J Allergy Clin Immunol*. 2015;135(3):636−643.

103. Horak F, Zieglmayer P, Zieglmayer R, et al. Early onset of action of a 5-grass-pollen 300-IR sublingual immunotherapy tablet evaluated in an allergen challenge chamber. *J Allergy Clin Immunol*. 2009;124(3), 471−477, 477 e471.

104. Nolte H, Maloney J, Nelson HS, et al. Onset and dose-related efficacy of house dust mite sublingual immunotherapy tablets in an environmental exposure chamber. *J Allergy Clin Immunol*. 2015;135(6), 1494−1501 e1496.

105. Jacobs RL, Harper N, He W, et al. Responses to ragweed pollen in a pollen challenge chamber versus seasonal exposure identify allergic rhinoconjunctivitis endotypes. *J Allergy Clin Immunol*. 2012;130(1), 122−127 e128.

106. Lao-Araya M, Steveling E, Scadding GW, Durham SR, Shamji MH. Seasonal increases in peripheral innate lymphoid type 2 cells are inhibited by subcutaneous grass pollen immunotherapy. *J Allergy Clin Immunol*. 2014;134(5), 1193−1195 e1194.

107. Doherty TA, Scott D, Walford HH, et al. Allergen challenge in allergic rhinitis rapidly induces increased peripheral blood type 2 innate lymphoid cells that express CD84. *J Allergy Clin Immunol.* 2014;133(4):1203−1205.
108. Gueguen C, Bouley J, Moussu H, et al. Changes in markers associated with dendritic cells driving the differentiation of either TH2 cells or regulatory T cells correlate with clinical benefit during allergen immunotherapy. *J Allergy Clin Immunol.* 2016;137(2):545−558.
109. Ebo DG, Bridts CH, Mertens CH, Hagendorens MM, Stevens WJ, De Clerck LS. Analyzing histamine release by flow cytometry (Hista flow): a novel instrument to study the degranulation patterns of basophils. *J Immunol Methods.* 2012;375(1−2):30−38.
110. Nullens S, Sabato V, Faber M, et al. Basophilic histamine content and release during venom immunotherapy: insights by flow cytometry. *Cytometry B Clin Cytom.* 2013;84(3):173−178.
111. Pfaar O, Bonini S, Cardona V, et al. Perspectives in allergen immunotherapy: 2017 and beyond. *Allergy.* 2018;73(Suppl 104):5−23.
112. Fauquert JL, Jedrzejczak-Czechowicz M, Rondon C, et al. Conjunctival allergen provocation test : guidelines for daily practice. *Allergy.* 2017;72(1):43−54.
113. Scadding GW, Calderon MA, Shamji MH, et al. Effect of 2 Years of treatment with sublingual grass pollen immunotherapy on nasal response to allergen challenge at 3 Years among patients with moderate to severe seasonal allergic rhinitis: the GRASS randomized clinical trial. *JAMA.* 2017;317(6):615−625.
114. Position paper: Allergen standardization and skin tests. The European academy of allergology and clinical immunology. *Allergy.* 1993;48(14 Suppl):48−82.
115. Gomes PJ, Lane KJ, Angjeli E, Stein L, Abelson MB. Technical and clinical validation of an environmental exposure unit for ragweed. *J Asthma Allergy.* 2016;9:215−221.
116. Hamasaki S, Okamoto Y, Yonekura S, et al. Characteristics of the Chiba environmental challenge chamber. *Allergol Int.* 2014;63(1):41−50.
117. Jacobs RL, Ramirez DA, Andrews CP. Validation of the biogenics research chamber for Juniperus ashei (mountain cedar) pollen. *Ann Allergy Asthma Immunol.* 2011;107(2):133−138.
118. Ronborg SM, Mosbech H, Johnsen CR, Poulsen LK. Exposure chamber for allergen challenge. The development and validation of a new concept. *Allergy.* 1996;51(2):82−88.
119. Hohlfeld JM, Holland-Letz T, Larbig M, et al. Diagnostic value of outcome measures following allergen exposure in an environmental challenge chamber compared with natural conditions. *Clin Exp Allergy.* 2010;40(7):998−1006.
120. Day JH, Briscoe MP. Environmental exposure unit: a system to test anti-allergic treatment. *Ann Allergy Asthma Immunol.* 1999;83(2):83−89. quiz 89-93.
121. Horak F, Jager S, Berger U, et al. Controlled exposure to mite allergen for a dose-finding of dimethindene maleate (DMM). *Agents Actions.* 1994;41 Spec. C124−126.
122. Horak F, Stubner UP, Zieglmayer R, Harris AG. Effect of desloratadine versus placebo on nasal airflow and subjective measures of nasal obstruction in subjects with grass pollen-induced allergic rhinitis in an allergen-exposure unit. *J Allergy Clin Immunol.* 2002;109(6):956−961.

Biologics in the management of chronic obstructive pulmonary disease

11

Reynold A. Panettieri, Jr., MD

Rutgers Institute for Translational Medicine and Science, Rutgers University, New Brunswick, NJ, United States

Introduction

The Global Initiative for Obstructive Lung Disease (GOLD) defines chronic obstructive pulmonary disease (COPD) as a common preventable and treatable disease, characterized by progressive airflow limitation that occurs in response to noxious particles or fumes.[1] COPD contributes to significant morbidity and mortality with ~251 million cases of COPD accounting for an estimated three million deaths worldwide and currently is the third leading cause of death in the United States.[2,3] Although the pathogenesis of COPD remains an enigma, inhaled particulates induce airway inflammation that is associated with structural changes in the airways (chronic bronchitis) and parenchymal lung destruction (emphysema).

GOLD established a revised COPD treatment algorithm using spirometry, symptom assessment, and assessment of risk of exacerbations as shown in Fig. 11.1. Central to the success in managing COPD includes improving symptoms and reducing future exacerbations. Exacerbations of COPD significantly drive healthcare costs, contribute to decline in lung function and negatively effects quality of life associated with high mortality.[4,5] Despite some progress in the treatment of COPD, the recognition that COPD is a heterogeneous disease suggests that a "one-size-fits-all" approach to COPD management may be challenging. Although asthma phenotyping and endotyping has shed insight into the development of precision medicine approaches using biologics, such approaches in COPD remain undeveloped. Recent studies, however, have addressed whether some biomarkers can predict therapeutic responses to biologics in COPD.

Targets for biological agents in COPD

Given that COPD represents a heterogeneous disease with varying clinical traits (phenotypes) and underlying molecular mechanisms (endotypes),[6–8] the use of

Immunotherapies for Allergic Disease. https://doi.org/10.1016/B978-0-323-54427-6.00011-0

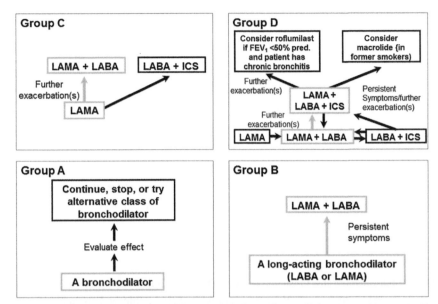

Abbreviations: FEV$_1$, forced expiratory volume in 1 second; ICS, inhaled corticosteroids; LABA, long-acting β$_2$-agonist; LAMA, long-acting muscarinic receptor antagonist.
Reproduced with permission from the Global Initiative for Obstructive Lung Disease (GOLD), Global Strategy for the Diagnosis, Management and Prevention of COPD, 2017.

FIGURE 11.1

Guideline based therapy according to GOLD criteria.

biologics could offer therapeutic value but may require biomarkers to predict clinical response. Evidence suggests that quantitative cell counts in sputum in patients with COPD can reliably assess airway inflammation, a hallmark of COPD. Based on the repertoire of cells found in the sputum, COPD phenotypes can be described as neutrophilic, eosinophilic, mixed eosinophilic and neutrophilic, or paucigranulocytic as summarized in Fig. 11.2. Unfortunately, peripheral blood counts of neutrophils may not correlate with sputum neutrophils, while blood eosinophils do correlate with sputum eosinophils in patients with eosinophilic airway disease.[9]

In COPD, neutrophilic airway inflammation is reportedly the most common type of inflammation that is mediated in part by non-T2 mechanisms and that is typically steroid insensitive. Although high T2 inflammation is characterized by activation of Helper T cells type 2 (CD4), mast cells, eosinophils, interleukin (IL)-5, IL-4, and IL-13, low-T2 inflammation mediates epithelial injury triggered by cigarette smoke, air pollution, ozone exposure, occupational exposure, and infections. This epithelial injury generates secretion of alarmins that include IL-25, thymic stromal lymphopoietin (TSLP), and IL-33.

Although commonly seen in asthma, eosinophilic airway inflammation may also occur in some COPD patients.[10] High-T2 airway inflammation that encompasses eosinophilic inflammation is propagated by adaptive and innate immune response. Alarmins including the cytokines IL-33, IL-25, and TSLP are secreted by epithelial cells in response to allergens, pollutants, or other environmental triggers. Concerning allergenic triggers, alarmins can also initiate an adaptive immune response via dendritic cells that stimulate naïve T cells to differentiate into Th2 cells that secrete IL-

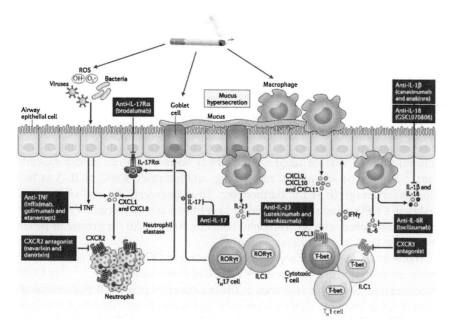

FIGURE 11.2

Proposed model of inflammation induced by environmental tobacco smoke exposure.

5, IL-13, and IL-4. Nonallergen triggers can also initiate an innate immune response by activating type 2 innate lymphoid cells (ILC-2) that also secrete type 2 effector cytokines (IL-5 and IL-13) and that in turn modulate eosinophilic airway inflammation.

To a greater degree than asthma, comorbidities are common among patients with COPD, and COPD itself may increase the risk for developing comorbidities.[2,11–14] Failure to recognize and manage comorbidities increases the risk of hospitalizations or exacerbations, worsens prognosis, increases morbidity, lowers the chances of treatment adherence, and places a greater burden on the patient, family, and healthcare resources.[12–17] Common comorbidities include cardiovascular disease, musculoskeletal dysfunction, metabolic syndrome, anxiety/depression, osteoporosis, lung cancer, and heart failure.[2,12,13] The value of effectively managing comorbidities in improving outcomes and adherence to therapy is well documented. For example, personalized management of patients with COPD and comorbid anxiety and/or depression reduces mental health symptoms and COPD-related outcomes (e.g., exercise tolerance, disability).[18–20] Given the incidence of comorbidities in COPD, systemic inflammatory targets such as IL-6, TNF-α, or CRP may also serve as predictors for therapeutic responses to some biologic agents.

Taken together, the heterogeneity of the pathogenesis of COPD suggests that components of dysfunctional high- and low-T2 inflammation can promote structural changes in the airways and the lung parenchyma, which then facilitates progressive loss of lung function. Targeted biologic therapy in COPD will be discussed within the context of high T2 airway inflammation as seen in asthma, systemic comorbidities, and those specific to parenchymal lung destruction.

High-T2 inflammation in COPD

Eosinophil levels in airways are a hallmark of high-T2 inflammation. Nearly 40% of patients with COPD manifest elevated numbers (>3%) found in sputum.[21,22] Interestingly, approximately one in five exacerbations are associated with an eosinophilic exacerbation.[23–25] Sputum and airway biopsies taken during acute exacerbations showed more eosinophil concentrations compared with stable COPD. Eosinophils release eosinophilic cationic protein and eosinophil peroxidase that induce necrosis of bronchial epithelial cells and increase levels of cytokines that perpetuates airway inflammation.[21] Evidence suggests that airway eosinophilia can predict exacerbations,[22] lung tissue and airway remodeling, and increased levels of IL-5 in bronchoalveolar lavage (BAL).[23] Furthermore, large interventional and observational studies in COPD using stratified analyses confirmed that an increased exacerbation risk was associated with an eosinophil count of 300 cells/µL or greater in patients with a history of frequent exacerbations.[26]

Biologics that target eosinophilic inflammation in COPD: Reducing eosinophilic airway inflammation in asthma reduces the risk of acute exacerbation.[24,25,27] In COPD, an eosinophilic phenotype is defined as the presence of a peripheral blood eosinophil count of 3% or more or >150 cells per cubic millimeter. Recent advances in targeting eosinophilic inflammation demonstrated the efficacy of monoclonal antibodies in the management of eosinophilic disease especially in the treatment of severe asthma.[28,29]

Interleukin 5 (IL-5), a cytokine involved in eosinophil differentiation, recruitment, maturation, activation and degranulation,[30] activates the IL-5 receptor (IL-5R) that is necessary for eosinophil survival. IL-5- and IL-5R-driven allergic and inflammatory immune responses contribute to the pathogenesis of numerous diseases, such as asthma, atopic dermatitis, chronic obstructive pulmonary disease, eosinophilic gastrointestinal diseases, hypereosinophilic syndrome, eosinophilic granulomatosis with polyangiitis, and eosinophilic nasal polyposis. Sputum levels of IL-5 correlate with the degree of eosinophilia and response to inhaled corticosteroids for patients with stable COPD as soluble IL-5Rα is increased during virus-induced COPD exacerbations.[31]

Biologics targeting IL-5 include monoclonal antibodies against circulating IL-5 (mepolizumab, reslizumab) or the IL-5 receptor α (benralizumab). Mepolizumab is a humanized, IgG1 monoclonal antibody that targets circulating IL-5, inhibiting the binding of IL-5 to IL-5R.[32,33] Mepolizumab has been approved as an add-on maintenance treatment of severe eosinophilic asthma.[34] In an exploratory study, mepolizumab was evaluated in a randomized clinical trial in COPD with eosinophilic bronchitis.[35] The primary objective was to determine if mepolizumab could decrease sputum eosinophil percentage in COPD patients with sputum eosinophilia. Other secondary outcomes included blood eosinophilia, lung function, exacerbation rate, symptoms and quality of life, and sputum hyaluronan and versican. In a study of 18 subjects, mepolizumab 750 mg given once intravenously markedly reduced sputum eosinophil counts from 11% to 0.5% after 6 months versus the placebo (7%−2% ($P < .05$)). Blood eosinophils decreased from 0.7 ± 0.5 cells mm^{-3} to

0.03 ± 0.05 cells mm^{-3} ($P < .05$). However, there was no significant difference in pre- and postbronchodilator spirometry measures, residual volume, total lung capacity, diffusion capacity, sputum hyaluronan, versican or radiological evidence of remodeling or patient-related outcomes at 3 and 6 months. Collectively, this exploratory study confirmed that mepolizumab profoundly decreases sputum and blood eosinophils (a pharmacodynamic biomarker) but had little effect on lung function parameters, exacerbation rates, or sputum markers of remodeling and health-related quality of life scores.

In two multicenter, Phase 3 randomized, placebo-controlled, double-blinded clinical trials, for the prevention of exacerbation, the therapeutic effect of mepolizumab was evaluated for patients with eosinophilic COPD. The mepolizumab versus placebo as add-on treatment for frequently exacerbating COPD patients characterized by eosinophil level trial (METREO) Phase 3 study (NCT02105961) evaluated two dosages of mepolizumab administered subcutaneously (100 and 300 mg, every 4 weeks) versus placebo ($n = 674$) for 62 weeks for patients with two or more exacerbations, or with one or more severe exacerbation in the previous year while they were on triple therapy (including inhaled corticosteroids, LABA and LAMA) and with an eosinophilic phenotype ($\geq$150 cells/μL at screening or $\geq$300 cells/μL during the previous year).[36,37] The mepolizumab versus placebo as add-on treatment for frequently exacerbating COPD patients trial (METREX) Phase 3 study (NCT02105948) compared mepolizumab 100 mg administered subcutaneously every 4 weeks with placebo ($n = 837$) over 52 weeks for patients with COPD who had two or more moderate exacerbations (i.e., treated with systemic glucocorticoids, antibiotics, or both in association with worsening of COPD) or one or more severe exacerbations (i.e., requiring a hospitalization) in the previous year. Patients with eosinophilic ($\geq$150 cells/μL at screening or $\geq$300 cells/μL during the previous year) or noneosinophilic ($<$150 cells/μL at screening and no evidence of $\geq$300 cells/μL in the previous year) phenotypes were included; outcomes were analyzed for those with baseline blood eosinophil counts $\geq$150 cells/μL versus $<$150 cells/μL. The primary endpoint for both studies was the annual rate of moderate or severe exacerbations. Secondary endpoints included time to first exacerbation, rate of exacerbations requiring emergency department visit, hospitalization or both, mean change from baseline at week 52 in St. George's Respiratory Questionnaire (SGRQ-C), and COPD assessment test score (CAT score).

In the METREO study, the exacerbation rate ratios in the 100 and 300 mg mepolizumab groups compared with placebo were 0.80 and 0.86 ($P = .07$ and $P = .14$, respectively). In the METREX study, mepolizumab reduced the mean annual exacerbation rate for patients with eosinophilia ($n = 462$) (1.40 vs. 1.71 exacerbations/year; $P = .04$), but no significant benefit over placebo was observed in the overall population. In these studies, there were no statistically significant differences observed between the two groups in patient-reported outcomes.

A post hoc analysis of the eosinophilic patient populations ($\geq$300 cells/μL at screening or during the previous year) from the combined trials demonstrated that the rate of moderate or severe exacerbations was 23% lower for patients treated with mepolizumab 100 mg compared with placebo (rate ratio, 0.77). The meta-analysis also demonstrated greater treatment effects with mepolizumab versus placebo with increasing screening blood eosinophil counts for exacerbations treated with systemic glucocorticoids but not in patients whose exacerbations were treated with antibiotics. The differential therapeutic response to mepolizumab in potentially noninfectious causes of exacerbations as compared with those requiring antibiotics was surprising. Collectively, these data support the notion that acute exacerbations of COPD are heterogeneous with some but not all being responsive to maintenance antiinflammatory agents. No significant differences in adverse events were observed. Despite a post hoc analysis showing efficacy in diminishing annual exacerbation rates in a select cohort of eosinophilic COPD subjects, the drug was not approved by the FDA.

Benralizumab, a humanized anti—IL-5Rα monoclonal antibody, prevents IL-5 signaling by binding to the IL-5Rα receptor. Furthermore, benralizumab promotes natural killer cells to induce rapid and direct depletion of eosinophils and basophils via enhanced antibody-dependent cell-mediated cytotoxicity.[29] Currently, benralizumab has been approved for severe eosinophilic asthma based on two successful Phase 3 clinical trials.[38,39] Benralizumab was the first anti-IL5 to be evaluated in COPD. In a Phase 2a clinical trial, Brightling et al.[40] conducted a randomized, double-blinded, placebo-controlled study in adults 40—85 years old, with moderate-to-severe COPD, at least one acute exacerbation of COPD, and a sputum eosinophil count of 3.0% or more within the previous year (NCT01227278). Benralizumab (100 mg) was given subcutaneously every 4 weeks (three doses), then every 8 weeks (five doses) over 48 weeks. One hundred and one patients were randomized to receive benralizumab versus placebo and 88 patients completed the study. Benralizumab did not reduce the annualized rate of exacerbations compared to placebo in the overall population (0.95 vs. 0.92) but was associated with significant improvement in prebronchodilator FEV1 compared with placebo (0.13 L vs. −0.06 L; $P = .014$) as early as week 4. In subanalysis, there was a 31% reduction in exacerbations with benralizumab versus placebo for patients with baseline blood eosinophils ≥ 200 cells/μL. Patients with blood eosinophils ≥ 200 cells/μL also exhibited significant improvement in FEV1 ($P = .035$), but patients with lower eosinophil counts did not. Adverse events were similar in the two groups.

Recently, two Phase 3 studies (GALATHEA and TERRANOVA, NCT02138916 and NCT02155660), randomized, double-blinded, 56-week placebo-controlled multicenter trials assessed the safety and efficacy of benralizumab as an add-on therapy to dual or triple inhaled therapy compared to placebo in patients with moderate-to-severe COPD with a history of exacerbation across a range of blood eosinophils. Preliminary data from GALATHEA[41] and TERRANOVA[42] revealed that these trials failed to meet the primary endpoint of statistically significant reduction of exacerbations in patients with COPD.

In sum, eosinophil numbers in peripheral blood and in sputum can identify some COPD patients who manifest frequent exacerbations and progressive decrements in lung function. Recent studies, however, suggest that eliminating eosinophils in the peripheral blood had little effect on improving COPD clinical outcomes. Further studies are needed to address whether higher eosinophil numbers may predict therapeutic response or other inflammatory biomarkers in tandem with eosinophil counts improve therapeutic responses to anti-IL5 therapies.

Systemic comorbidities in COPD

COPD typically manifests as a chronic systemic illness associated with comorbidities.[1] A variety of biological agents has been studied within the context of systemic inflammatory mediators, comorbidities, and neutrophilic inflammation. These biological agents include monoclonal antibodies to TNF-α, IL-1β, or IL-6.

TNF-α, a pleotropic cytokine, mediates systemic and localized inflammation and is secreted by activated macrophages that orchestrate and perpetuate cigarette-induced airway and alveolar inflammation. Levels of TNF-α are increased in the peripheral blood, sputum, and BAL fluid of COPD patients.[12,13,43] Genetic studies confirmed that TNF-α polymorphisms are associated with the pathogenesis of COPD.[43] Given the compelling evidence that TNF-α levels are associated with COPD severity, a number of anti-TNF-α trials in COPD were initiated. In a small Phase 2 trial, infliximab was compared to placebo for improvement in lung function, exacerbation frequency, and quality of life. In this study, infliximab had little effect on any clinical outcome and in fact showed a trend toward inducing pneumonia and cases of cancer.[15] In contrast, a study of etanercept for rheumatoid arthritis patients with concomitant COPD serendipitously manifested a 50% decrease in COPD exacerbations.[16] Other clinical trials using either etanercept or infliximab targeting acute COPD exacerbations or cachexia/muscle mass loss in small COPD cohorts were disappointing, showing no significant effects over placebo.[18] Whether anti-TNF-α agents may be more effective in COPD patients with multiple comorbidities warrants further investigation.

Trials with other biologics targeting IL-1β have also been performed in COPD. IL-1β is associated with systemic or neutrophilic inflammation. Using cakinumab, an anti-IL-1β antibody, or a blocking antibody of the IL-1β receptor, investigators addressed whether either agent improved exacerbation rates or other clinical outcomes. Neither study showed value in improving lung function or decreasing exacerbation rates.[19,44] In neither study were patients enrolled for treatment using pharmacodynamic biomarkers that could improve the prediction for therapeutic responsiveness. Other biologic agents that could target systemic and neutrophilic inflammation such as tocilizumab (anti-IL-6) or anti-TH17 antibodies hold promise in rheumatoid arthritis and psoriasis, respectively. Whether such agents would be effective in COPD remains unknown.

Targets specific to parenchymal lung destruction in COPD

Parenchymal destruction of lung tissue manifests as airspace enlargement in some but not all patients with COPD. Intuitively, the imbalance of proteases and antiproteases could promote lung destruction as seen in hereditary antiprotease deficiencies. Significant research effort has focused on modulating this balance. The neutrophil, with an array of secreted proteases, may contribute to this diathesis. Unfortunately, clinical trials of biologics targeting the neutrophil are limited. ABX-IL-8, a blocking CXCR2 antibody, versus placebo showed only modest improvements in a dyspnea index but demonstrated no benefit in lung function or exacerbation rates in COPD patients.[45] Several studies using small molecule inhibitors of chemokine receptors have been performed in COPD but had no significant clinical value when compared to placebo.[14] Whether other biologics could target active proteases or serve as antiproteases remains to be determined.

Table 11.1 Current and investigational biologics in the treatment of asthma and COPD.

Cytokine target	Inhibitor	Delivery	Patients	Effects	Associated diseases	Biomarkers	Refs
IL-5	Mepolizumab	Subcutaneous administration every 4 wks	Severe type 2 asthma	• Reduced exacerbations • Reduced need for oral steroids	Nasal polyps, EGPA and (possibly) rhinitis	Blood and sputum eosinophils	28-30, 46-51
	Mepolizumab	Subcutaneous administration every 4 wks	COPD	Small reduction in exacerbations	ND	Blood eosinophils	36, 52
	Reslizumab	Intravenous administration every 4 wks	Severe type 2 asthma	Reduced exacerbations	ND	Blood eosinophils	31, 53-56
IL-5Rα	Benralizumab	Subcutaneous administration every 4 or 8 wks	Severe type 2 asthma	• Reduced exacerbations • Reduced need for oral steroids	Nasal polyps	Blood eosinophils	32-33, 57-61
	Benralizumab	Subcutaneous administration every 4 wks	COPD	Small effect on FEV1	ND	Blood eosinophils	62
IL-13	Lebrikizumab	Subcutaneous administration every 4 wks	Severe type 2 asthma	Small effect on FEV1	ND	Serum periostin	63-64
	Tralokinumab	Subcutaneous administration every 2 wks	Severe type 2 asthma	No effect on exacerbations	ND	FeNO	65-66
IL-4Rα	Dupilumab	Subcutaneous administration every 4 wks	Severe asthma	• Reduced exacerbations • Reduced symptoms • Increased FEV1	Atopic dermatitis, rhinosinusitis and nasal polyps	Blood eosinophils and FeNO	34, 67-70
TSLP	Tezepelumab	Subcutaneous administration every 4 wks	Severe asthma	• Reduced exacerbations • Reduced symptoms • Increased FEV1	Atopic dermatitis and rhinosinusitis	Blood eosinophils and FeNO	35
TNF	Golimumab and infliximab	Subcutaneous administration every 4 wks	Severe asthma	No effects or side effects	ND	ND	17, 71-72
	Infliximab	Subcutaneous administration every 4 wks	Severe COPD	No effects or side effects	ND	ND	16, 73
IL-1β	Canakinumab	Subcutaneous administration every 8 wks	COPD	No effect	ND	ND	19
CXCR2	Navarixin	Oral administration once a day	Neutrophilic asthma	No effect	ND	Sputum neutrophils	74
	AZD5069	Oral administration once a day	Neutrophilic asthma	No effect	ND	ND	75
	Navarixin	Oral administration once a day	COPD	Minor effect on FEV1	ND	ND	14
IL-17Rα	Brodalumab	Subcutaneous administration every 2 wks	Severe asthma	No effect	ND	ND	76

Yellow shading denotes COPD clinical trials; gray shading denotes failed clinical trials

Conclusions

Given the heterogeneous nature of COPD and its associated comorbidities, it is unlikely that a one-size-fits-all therapy will improve lung destruction, progressive loss of lung function, and morbidity. The era of precision medicine that espouses the use of biomarkers to serve as pharmacodynamic indicators of target engagement may identify and predict therapeutic responses in specific patients. The cost of biologics mandates a fiscally sound approach to improve outcomes in COPD. The disproportionate increases in the incidence of COPD is alarming, especially in vulnerable populations. Extending the use of biologics into COPD that are effective in other chronic diseases such as asthma, rheumatoid arthritis, and psoriasis offers promise but as of yet has not been successful. A better understanding of the pathogenesis of COPD and the characterization of patient subtypes may offer promise for improving the therapeutic success of biologics in COPD (Table 11.1).

References

1. The Global Strategy for the Diagnosis, M. a. P. o. C.. *Global Initiative for Chronic Obstuctive Lung Disease (GOLD)*. 2017.
2. Guarascio AJ, Ray SM, Finch CK, Self TH. The clinical and economic burden of chronic obstructive pulmonary disease in the USA. *Clinicoecon Outcomes Res.* 2013;5:235−245.
3. Lozano R, Naghavi M, Foreman K, et al. Global and regional mortality from 235 causes of death for 20 age groups in 1990 and 2010: a systematic analysis for the Global Burden of Disease Study 2010. *Lancet.* 2012;380(9859):2095−2128.
4. Barnes PJ. Cellular and molecular mechanisms of asthma and COPD. *Clin Sci (Lond).* 2017;131(13):1541−1558.
5. Celli BR, Thomas NE, Anderson JA, et al. Effect of pharmacotherapy on rate of decline of lung function in chronic obstructive pulmonary disease: results from the TORCH study. *Am J Respir Crit Care Med.* 2008;178(4):332−338.
6. Lange P, Celli B, Agusti A, et al. Lung-function trajectories leading to chronic obstructive pulmonary disease. *N Engl J Med.* 2015;373(2):111−122.
7. Suissa S, Patenaude V, Lapi F, Ernst P. Inhaled corticosteroids in COPD and the risk of serious pneumonia. *Thorax.* 2013;68(11):1029−1036.
8. Wedzicha JA, Calverley PM, Seemungal TA, et al. The prevention of chronic obstructive pulmonary disease exacerbations by salmeterol/fluticasone propionate or tiotropium bromide. *Am J Respir Crit Care Med.* 2008;177(1):19−26.
9. Pavord ID, Beasley R, Agusti A, et al. After asthma: redefining airways diseases. *Lancet.* 2018;391(10118):350−400.
10. Agusti A, Bel E, Thomas M, et al. Treatable traits: toward precision medicine of chronic airway diseases. *Eur Respir J.* 2016;47(2):410−419.
11. Han MK, Agusti A, Calverley PM, et al. Chronic obstructive pulmonary disease phenotypes: the future of COPD. *Am J Respir Crit Care Med.* 2010;182(5):598−604.
12. Keatings VM, Collins PD, Scott DM, Barnes PJ. Differences in interleukin-8 and tumor necrosis factor-alpha in induced sputum from patients with chronic obstructive pulmonary disease or asthma. *Am J Respir Crit Care Med.* 1996;153(2):530−534.

13. Matera MG, Calzetta L, Cazzola M. TNF-alpha inhibitors in asthma and COPD: we must not throw the baby out with the bath water. *Pulm Pharmacol Ther.* 2010;23(2):121−128.

14. Rennard SI, Dale DC, Donohue JF, et al. CXCR2 antagonist MK-7123. A phase 2 proof-of-concept trial for chronic obstructive pulmonary disease. *Am J Respir Crit Care Med.* 2015;191(9):1001−1011.

15. Rennard SI, Fogarty C, Kelsen S, et al. The safety and efficacy of infliximab in moderate to severe chronic obstructive pulmonary disease. *Am J Respir Crit Care Med.* 2007; 175(9):926−934.

16. Suissa S, Ernst P, Hudson M. TNF-alpha antagonists and the prevention of hospitalisation for chronic obstructive pulmonary disease. *Pulm Pharmacol Ther.* 2008;21(1): 234−238.

17. Berry MA, Hargadon B, Shelley M, et al. Evidence of a role of tumor necrosis factor alpha in refractory asthma. *N Engl J Med.* 2006;354(7):697−708.

18. Aaron SD, Vandemheen KL, Maltais F, et al. TNFalpha antagonists for acute exacerbations of COPD: a randomised double-blind controlled trial. *Thorax.* 2013;68(2): 142−148.

19. Rogliani P, Calzetta L, Ora J, Matera MG. Canakinumab for the treatment of chronic obstructive pulmonary disease. *Pulm Pharmacol Ther.* 2015;31:15−27.

20. Dentener MA, Creutzberg EC, Pennings HJ, Rijkers GT, Mercken E, Wouters EF. Effect of infliximab on local and systemic inflammation in chronic obstructive pulmonary disease: a pilot study. *Respiration.* 2008;76(3):275−282.

21. Bafadhel M, Pavord ID, Russell REK. Eosinophils in COPD: just another biomarker? *Lancet Respir Med.* 2017;5(9):747−759.

22. Brusselle GG, Maes T, Bracke KR. Eosinophils in the spotlight: eosinophilic airway inflammation in nonallergic asthma. *Nat Med.* 2013;19(8):977−979.

23. Bafadhel M, Davies L, Calverley PM, Aaron SD, Brightling CE, Pavord ID. Blood eosinophil guided prednisolone therapy for exacerbations of COPD: a further analysis. *Eur Respir J.* 2014;44(3):789−791.

24. Berry MA, Shaw DE, Green RH, Brightling CE, Wardlaw AJ, Pavord ID. The use of exhaled nitric oxide concentration to identify eosinophilic airway inflammation: an observational study in adults with asthma. *Clin Exp Allergy.* 2005;35(9):1175−1179.

25. Hanania NA, Wenzel S, Rosen K, et al. Exploring the effects of omalizumab in allergic asthma: an analysis of biomarkers in the EXTRA study. *Am J Respir Crit Care Med.* 2013;187(8):804−811.

26. Green RH, Brightling CE, McKenna S, et al. Asthma exacerbations and sputum eosinophil counts: a randomised controlled trial. *Lancet.* 2002;360(9347):1715−1721.

27. Staton TL, Choy DF, Arron JR. Biomarkers in the clinical development of asthma therapies. *Biomark Med.* 2016;10(2):165−176.

28. Bel EH, Wenzel SE, Thompson PJ, et al. Oral glucocorticoid-sparing effect of mepolizumab in eosinophilic asthma. *N Engl J Med.* 2014;371(13):1189−1197.

29. Pavord ID, Korn S, Howarth P, et al. Mepolizumab for severe eosinophilic asthma (DREAM): a multicentre, double-blind, placebo-controlled trial. *Lancet.* 2012; 380(9842):651−659.

30. Ortega HG, Liu MC, Pavord ID, et al. Mepolizumab treatment in patients with severe eosinophilic asthma. *N Engl J Med.* 2014;371(13):1198−1207.

31. Castro M, Mathur S, Hargreave F, et al. Res-5- Study, G., Reslizumab for poorly controlled, eosinophilic asthma: a randomized, placebo-controlled study. *Am J Respir Crit Care Med.* 2011;184(10):1125−1132.

32. Bleecker ER, FitzGerald JM, Chanez P, et al. Efficacy and safety of benralizumab for patients with severe asthma uncontrolled with high-dosage inhaled corticosteroids and long-acting beta2-agonists (SIROCCO): a randomised, multicentre, placebo-controlled phase 3 trial. *Lancet*. 2016;388(10056):2115−2127.

33. FitzGerald JM, Bleecker ER, Nair P, et al. Benralizumab, an anti-interleukin-5 receptor alpha monoclonal antibody, as add-on treatment for patients with severe, uncontrolled, eosinophilic asthma (CALIMA): a randomised, double-blind, placebo-controlled phase 3 trial. *Lancet*. 2016;388(10056):2128−2141.

34. Wenzel S, Ford L, Pearlman D, et al. Dupilumab in persistent asthma with elevated eosinophil levels. *N Engl J Med*. 2013;368(26):2455−2466.

35. Corren J, Parnes JR, Wang L, et al. Tezepelumab in adults with uncontrolled asthma. *N Engl J Med*. 2017;377(10):936−946.

36. Pavord ID, Chanez P, Criner GJ, et al. Mepolizumab for eosinophilic chronic obstructive pulmonary disease. *N Engl J Med*. 2017;377(17):1613−1629.

37. Ortega HG, Yancey SW, Mayer B, et al. Severe eosinophilic asthma treated with mepolizumab stratified by baseline eosinophil thresholds: a secondary analysis of the DREAM and MENSA studies. *Lancet Respir Med*. 2016;4(7):549−556.

38. Bafadhel M, McCormick M, Saha S, et al. Profiling of sputum inflammatory mediators in asthma and chronic obstructive pulmonary disease. *Respiration*. 2012;83(1):36−44.

39. Pavord ID, Lettis S, Locantore N, et al. Blood eosinophils and inhaled corticosteroid/long-acting beta-2 agonist efficacy in COPD. *Thorax*. 2016;71(2):118−125.

40. Bafadhel M, McKenna S, Terry S, et al. Acute exacerbations of chronic obstructive pulmonary disease: identification of biologic clusters and their biomarkers. *Am J Respir Crit Care Med*. 2011;184(6):662−671.

41. Bafadhel M, McKenna S, Terry S, et al. Blood eosinophils to direct corticosteroid treatment of exacerbations of chronic obstructive pulmonary disease: a randomized placebo-controlled trial. *Am J Respir Crit Care Med*. 2012;186(1):48−55.

42. Brightling CE, Monteiro W, Ward R, et al. Sputum eosinophilia and short-term response to prednisolone in chronic obstructive pulmonary disease: a randomised controlled trial. *Lancet*. 2000;356(9240):1480−1485.

43. Sakao S, Tatsumi K, Igari H, Shino Y, Shirasawa H, Kuriyama T. Association of tumor necrosis factor alpha gene promoter polymorphism with the presence of chronic obstructive pulmonary disease. *Am J Respir Crit Care Med*. 2001;163(2):420−422.

44. Calverley P SS, Dawson M, Ward C, Newbold P, Van der Merwe R. A phase 2 study of MED18968, an anti-interleukin 1 receptor-1 monoclonal antibody in adults with moderate to severe COPD (abstract). *Am J Respir Crit Care Med*. 2015;191:A3964.

45. Mahler DA, Huang S, Tabrizi M, Bell GM. Efficacy and safety of a monoclonal antibody recognizing interleukin-8 in COPD: a pilot study. *Chest*. 2004;126(3):926−934.

46. Chupp GL, Bradford ES, Albers FC, et al. Efficacy of mepolizumab add-on therapy on health-related quality of life and markers of asthma control in severe eosinophilic asthma (MUSCA): a randomised, double-blind, placebo-controlled, parallel-group, multicentre, phase 3b trial. *Lancet Respir Med*. 2017;5(5):390−400.

47. Flood-Page P, Swenson C, Faiferman I, et al. A study to evaluate safety and efficacy of mepolizumab in patients with moderate persistent asthma. *Am J Respir Crit Care Med*. 2007;176(11):1062−1071.

48. Haldar P, Brightling CE, Hargadon B, et al. Mepolizumab and exacerbations of refractory eosinophilic asthma. *N Engl J Med*. 2009;360(10):973−984.

49. Leckie MJ, ten Brinke A, Khan J, et al. Effects of an interleukin-5 blocking monoclonal antibody on eosinophils, airway hyper-responsiveness, and the late asthmatic response. *Lancet*. 2000;356(9248):2144–2148.
50. Nair P, Pizzichini MM, Kjarsgaard M, et al. Mepolizumab for prednisone-dependent asthma with sputum eosinophilia. *N Engl J Med*. 2009;360(10):985–993.
51. Powell C MS, Dwan K, Bax K, Walters N. Mepolizumab versus placebo for asthma. *Cochrane Database Syst Rev*. 2015;7.
52. Dasgupta A, Kjarsgaard M, Capaldi D, et al. A pilot randomised clinical trial of mepolizumab in COPD with eosinophilic bronchitis. *Eur Respir J*. 2017;49(3).
53. Bjermer L, Lemiere C, Maspero J, Weiss S, Zangrilli J, Germinaro M. Reslizumab for inadequately controlled asthma with elevated blood eosinophil levels: a randomized phase 3 study. *Chest*. 2016;150(4):789–798.
54. Brusselle G, Germinaro M, Weiss S, Zangrilli J. Reslizumab in patients with inadequately controlled late-onset asthma and elevated blood eosinophils. *Pulm Pharmacol Ther*. 2017;43:39–45.
55. Castro M, Zangrilli J, Wechsler ME, et al. Reslizumab for inadequately controlled asthma with elevated blood eosinophil counts: results from two multicentre, parallel, double-blind, randomised, placebo-controlled, phase 3 trials. *Lancet Respir Med*. 2015;3(5):355–366.
56. Corren J, Weinstein S, Janka L, Zangrilli J, Garin M. Phase 3 study of reslizumab in patients with poorly controlled asthma: effects across a broad range of eosinophil counts. *Chest*. 2016;150(4):799–810.
57. Castro M, Wenzel SE, Bleecker ER, et al. Benralizumab, an anti-interleukin 5 receptor alpha monoclonal antibody, versus placebo for uncontrolled eosinophilic asthma: a phase 2b randomised dose-ranging study. *Lancet Respir Med*. 2014;2(11):879–890.
58. Ferguson GT, FitzGerald JM, Bleecker ER, et al. Benralizumab for patients with mild to moderate, persistent asthma (BISE): a randomised, double-blind, placebo-controlled, phase 3 trial. *Lancet Respir Med*. 2017;5(7):568–576.
59. Khorasanizadeh M, Eskian M, Assa'ad AH, Camargo Jr CA, Rezaei N. Efficacy and safety of benralizumab, a monoclonal antibody against IL-5Ralpha, in uncontrolled eosinophilic asthma. *Int Rev Immunol*. 2016;35(4):294–311.
60. Nair P, Wenzel S, Rabe KF, et al. Oral glucocorticoid-sparing effect of benralizumab in severe asthma. *N Engl J Med*. 2017;376(25):2448–2458.
61. Nowak RM, Parker JM, Silverman RA, et al. A randomized trial of benralizumab, an antiinterleukin 5 receptor alpha monoclonal antibody, after acute asthma. *Am J Emerg Med*. 2015;33(1):14–20.
62. Brightling CE, Bleecker ER, Panettieri Jr RA, et al. Benralizumab for chronic obstructive pulmonary disease and sputum eosinophilia: a randomised, double-blind, placebo-controlled, phase 2a study. *Lancet Respir Med*. 2014;2(11):891–901.
63. Corren J, Lemanske RF, Hanania NA, et al. Lebrikizumab treatment in adults with asthma. *N Engl J Med*. 2011;365(12):1088–1098.
64. Hanania NA, Noonan M, Corren J, et al. Lebrikizumab in moderate-to-severe asthma: pooled data from two randomised placebo-controlled studies. *Thorax*. 2015;70(8):748–756.
65. Brightling CE, Chanez P, Leigh R, et al. Efficacy and safety of tralokinumab in patients with severe uncontrolled asthma: a randomised, double-blind, placebo-controlled, phase 2b trial. *Lancet Respir Med*. 2015;3(9):692–701.

66. Piper E, Brightling C, Niven R, et al. A phase II placebo-controlled study of tralokinumab in moderate-to-severe asthma. *Eur Respir J.* 2013;41(2):330−338.

67. Bachert C, Mannent L, Naclerio RM, et al. Effect of subcutaneous dupilumab on nasal polyp burden in patients with chronic sinusitis and nasal polyposis: a randomized clinical trial. *J Am Med Assoc.* 2016;315(5):469−479.

68. Blauvelt A, de Bruin-Weller M, Gooderham M, et al. Long-term management of moderate-to-severe atopic dermatitis with dupilumab and concomitant topical corticosteroids (LIBERTY AD CHRONOS): a 1-year, randomised, double-blinded, placebo-controlled, phase 3 trial. *Lancet.* 2017;389(10086):2287−2303.

69. Kraft M, Worm M. Dupilumab in the treatment of moderate-to-severe atopic dermatitis. *Expert Rev Clin Immunol.* 2017;13(4):301−310.

70. Wenzel S, Castro M, Corren J, et al. Dupilumab efficacy and safety in adults with uncontrolled persistent asthma despite use of medium-to-high-dose inhaled corticosteroids plus a long-acting beta2 agonist: a randomised double-blind placebo-controlled pivotal phase 2b dose-ranging trial. *Lancet.* 2016;388(10039):31−44.

71. Erin EM, Leaker BR, Nicholson GC, et al. The effects of a monoclonal antibody directed against tumor necrosis factor-alpha in asthma. *Am J Respir Crit Care Med.* 2006;174(7):753−762.

72. Howarth PH, Babu KS, Arshad HS, et al. Tumour necrosis factor (TNFalpha) as a novel therapeutic target in symptomatic corticosteroid dependent asthma. *Thorax.* 2005;60(12):1012−1018.

73. Wenzel SE, Barnes PJ, Bleecker ER, et al. A randomized, double-blind, placebo-controlled study of tumor necrosis factor-alpha blockade in severe persistent asthma. *Am J Respir Crit Care Med.* 2009;179(7):549−558.

74. Lazaar AL, Sweeney LE, MacDonald AJ, Alexis NE, Chen C, Tal-Singer R. SB-656933, a novel CXCR2 selective antagonist, inhibits ex vivo neutrophil activation and ozone-induced airway inflammation in humans. *Br J Clin Pharmacol.* 2011;72(2):282−293.

75. Nair P, Gaga M, Zervas E, et al. Safety and efficacy of a CXCR2 antagonist in patients with severe asthma and sputum neutrophils: a randomized, placebo-controlled clinical trial. *Clin Exp Allergy.* 2012;42(7):1097−1103.

76. McKinley L, Alcorn JF, Peterson A, et al. TH17 cells mediate steroid-resistant airway inflammation and airway hyperresponsiveness in mice. *J Immunol.* 2008;181(6):4089−4097.

Allergen immunotherapy (AIT) and allergen immunomodulatory (AIM) therapies

Breakthroughs in subcutaneous allergy immunotherapy

12

Harold S. Nelson, MD

Professor of Medicine, National Jewish Health and University of Colorado Denver School of Medicine, Denver, CO, United States

Introduction

In 1911, Noon and Freeman combined to describe a method for and the results of subcutaneous injections of timothy grass extract for the prophylactic relief of hay fever due to grass pollen.[1] Noon described a gradual increase in dose, adjusted to the patients' tolerance of the injections, which were typically given weekly preceding the arrival of the grass pollen season. The basic principles of this treatment continue to the present day. However, the original approach was empiric and much has been learned through carefully conducted studies to better define the practice of subcutaneous allergy immunotherapy (SCIT) and how to achieve maximal benefit. The attributes of SCIT that have been demonstrated are listed in Table 12.1, while important practical considerations for practicing SCIT are listed in Table 12.2. This chapter will discuss sentinel papers that have established this body of knowledge.

Table 12.1 Favorable attributes of subcutaneous immunotherapy.

(1) Proven efficacy in allergic rhinitis, allergic asthma, hymenoptera venom sensitivity, and selected cases of atopic dermatitis.
(2) Effective when administered as multiple allergen mixtures.
(3) Specific for the allergen administered.
(4) Established effective and ineffective doses for many allergens
(5) Clinical evidence of disease modification
    a. Reducing new sensitizations in monosensitized individuals.
    b. Reducing the development of asthma in patients with only allergic rhinitis
    c. Persisting benefit following an adequate course of treatment
    d. Possible protective effect for development of allergies on fetus
(6) Evidence of modification of underlying immunologic derangement.
(7) Established optimal duration for disease modification

Immunotherapies for Allergic Disease. https://doi.org/10.1016/B978-0-323-54427-6.00012-2

Table 12.2 Subcutaneous immunotherapy: other important considerations.

(1) Safety
- **a.** Asthma
- **b.** Large local reactions
- **c.** Seasonal dosing
- **d.** Concomitant autoimmune disease
- **e.** Cluster/rush schedules

(2) Compounding allergen mixtures

(3) Adjuvants

(4) Relative efficacy versus sublingual immunotherapy.

Proven efficacy in allergic diseases

For decades, SCIT was accepted as an effective treatment for allergic diseases based on patient and physician clinical experience. The first of many controlled clinical trials establishing efficacy in allergic rhinitis was conducted with grass pollen extract in 1954 by Frankland and Augustine in England[1] followed by studies with ragweed pollen extract in 1965 and 1967 in the United States by Lowell and Franklin.[1] Frankland and Augustine compared the response to grass pollen extract, its purified proteins, the protein-free ultrafiltrate, and phenol saline. The two protein-containing extracts provided significantly better relief for the symptoms of both allergic rhinitis and asthma. Lowell and Franklin improved upon their methods by ensuring that the placebo was indistinguishable from the active extract. They identified patients symptomatic during the ragweed pollen season who were receiving immunotherapy with a mixture of multiple allergens including ragweed. They removed the ragweed from the extract of half the patients replacing it with a caramelized-sugar saline that ensured similar color to the mixture, while the other allergens in the mixture ensured a similar occurrence of local reactions. They demonstrated in two studies that complete removal or 95% reduction in the ragweed content in the patients' treatment resulted in significantly worse symptom/medication scores during the ensuing ragweed pollen season. Meanwhile, Douglas Johnstone in the United States demonstrated efficacy of SCIT in allergic asthma in a 14-year controlled trial in children reported in 1968.[1] All children with asthma and positive skin prick tests to inhalant allergens were randomly assigned to treatment with saline, a very weak allergen extract, and extract with maximum strength of 1:5000 w/v or one with each allergen at 1:250 w/v. The outcome, freedom from asthma for the previous year, significantly favored the two strongest extracts at both 4 years and on the patients reaching age 16 years and those receiving a top dose of 1:250 w/v fared better than those receiving one of 1:5000 w/v. Recent systematic reviews of the medical literature have confirmed the efficacy of SCIT for the treatment of allergic rhinitis and allergic asthma.[2,3]

For years, the accepted treatment for hymenoptera venom allergy was SCIT with a whole body extract. In 1978, allergists at Johns Hopkins reported on a study in 59 subjects in which patients received 6–10 weeks of immunotherapy with either the venom of the hymenoptera to which they were allergic, an extract of the whole body of that insect, or placebo.[1] They were then subjected to a sting challenge by the implicated insect. Systemic reactions occurred in 7/11 and 7/12 subjects receiving WBE and placebo respective, but only 1/18 of those who had received venom immunotherapy, which subsequently became the standard of care. A Cochran systematic review published in 2012 identified seven controlled trials of SCIT for ant, bee, or wasp venom allergy.[4] Systemic allergic reactions to subsequent stings occurred in 2.7% of those who had received active treatment and 39.8% of the untreated.

Following a number of anecdotal reports of improvement of atopic dermatitis with SCIT, a randomized dose-response study was performed in 89 adults with chronic atopic dermatitis employing three doses of house dust mite (HDM) extract.[5] The highest dose compared to the lowest significantly reduced disease severity, and the two highest doses significantly reduced use of topical steroids. However, the most recent Cochran systematic review found no consistent evidence that immunotherapy is effective for treating atopic dermatitis, noting that the overall quality of the evidence was low.[6]

Evidence for efficacy of SCIT with mixtures of unrelated allergens

Most of the controlled studies of SCIT have been conducted with a single allergen. Single allergen SCIT is recommended by European guidelines[7] and continues to predominate in Europe. In one large French study, in which all patients were polysensitized, 86% were prescribed a single allergen extract, 12.8% a mixture of two allergens, and only 1.1% to receive a mixture of three or more allergens.[7] US allergists, in contrast, typically administer SCIT with mixtures of multiple unrelated allergens.[8] The evidence supporting this practice is not recent, but is of good quality all studies being randomized and blinded. They consist of the two studies in ragweed pollen induced allergic rhinitis by Lowell and Frankland[1], referred to in the section on proof of efficacy in allergic diseases, the study in allergic asthmatic children by Johnstone,[1] referred to in that same section, and a study in adults with allergic rhinitis and allergic asthma due to grass pollen by Michael Reid.[9]

Evidence for allergen specificity of SCIT

The problem of SCIT in polysensitized patients would be solved, if immunotherapy provided symptom improvement that extended beyond the allergen administered. This possibility was effectively ruled out by a study by Phillip Normal and Larry

Lichenstein.[1] They identified a group of patients symptomatically allergic to both grass and ragweed pollen. They treated half with 2 years of ragweed pollen extract SCIT and the other half with placebo. In the final ragweed pollen season there was marked improvement in symptom/medication scores in those who received the ragweed extract compared to the placebo recipients, but in the final grass pollen season there was no difference in symptoms between the two groups.

Determination of optimal dosing of SCIT

The response to SCIT is clearly dose related. This was demonstrated by the loss of protection against ragweed pollen in the second Frankland and Lowell study when the dose of ragweed extract was reduced by 95%[1] and in the Johnstone study by the superior benefit from a maintenance dose of each extract of 1:250 w/v rather than 1:5000 w/v.[1] Subsequent randomized, double-blind studies have established effective and in many cases ineffective doses expressed in the major allergen of grasses, birch, short ragweed, house dust mites, cat and dog dander, and *Alternaria*.[10] These major allergen doses have been translated into FDA potency nomenclature in the Immunotherapy Practice Parameters, Third Update.[11]

Evidence of disease modification

Three lines of clinical evidence have demonstrated that SCIT induces a persisting alteration in the pathological processes underlying allergic respiratory diseases. First is the reduction in development of new sensitivities in monosensitized recipients of SCIT that was described first by Des Roches,[1] and confirmed in larger populations and with evidence of persistence 3 years after discontinuation of SCIT by both Pajno[1] and Purello-D; Ambrosio.[12] Second is the reduction in the development of asthma in SCIT recipients who only had allergic rhinitis at its initiation. The outstanding study here is the Preventative Allergy Treatment (PAT) study of 3 years of SCIT with grass and/or birth extracts in children who only demonstrated allergic rhinitis during an observational season.[13] Importantly, the reduction in development of asthma in the active treatment group showed no evidence of diminution at 10-year follow-up. This protection against the development of asthma was again demonstrated in a large study employing data from the German National Health Insurance beneficiaries.[14] Patients with allergic rhinitis who initiated SCIT in 2006 were at reduced risk of developing asthma over the next 5 years compared to those with allergic rhinitis not receiving SCIT (Relative Risk 0.69, 95% CI 0.42–0.84). The third line of evidence is the persistence of clinical improvement following completion of a course of SCIT. Two studies demonstrate the continuing improvement following completion of 3 or 4 years of SCIT with grass pollen extract.[1] Ebner followed 108 patients who were asymptomatic after 3–4 years of SCIT with grass pollen extract for evidence of exacerbation of rhinitis symptoms during subsequent grass pollen seasons. In the first grass pollen season 2.7% relapsed, in the second 16.7%, and in the third 30.6%. Durham brought the power of a double-blind study to this question.[1] In a group who had received 3–4 years of SCIT, half were continued on maintenance injections of grass pollen extract and half received injections of placebo. Over the ensuing three grass pollen seasons, there was no difference between the two groups in rhinitis symptoms, indicating persistent benefit for those who had received placebo.

Long-term effect on offspring

There is a strong hereditary component to allergic diseases. Is it possible that a fetus, in utero, could benefit from SCIT being administered to the mother? A report by Bozek compared the allergic outcome in 176 children who had at least one parent with allergy who had received SCIT compared with 181 children of similarly allergic parents who did not receive SCIT.[15] The odds risks for development of any allergic disease or asthma were significantly lower in the children of SCIT recipients (Odds Risk 0.73) compared to the children of parents who had not received SCIT (Odds Risk 1.85). The risk was further reduced if both parents had received SCIT, rather than just one.

Evidence of modification of underlying immunologic derangement

The fundamental abnormality underlying allergy appears to be an imbalance of type-2 over type-1 cytokine responses and an inadequate regulatory response.[16] SCIT is known to increase the threshold of the skin and nasal mucosa to allergen challenge and Bousquet demonstrated that both changes correlated with symptoms during natural pollen exposure.[1] The first identified immunologic response to SCIT was the development of blocking antibody described by Robert Cooke in 1935.[1] Later, blocking antibody was identified as belonging to the IgG_4 subclass. Levels of IgG_4 have not correlated with clinical improvement, but levels of functional assays of IgG_4, such as IgE blocking factor and IgE-facilitated allergen binding to B cells, have shown modest correlations with clinical outcome (spearmen $r = -0.28$ and -0.25, respectively).[17] The discovery of IgE in 1967 was followed by demonstration that clinical response to SCIT did not correlate with specific IgE levels.[1]

In 1976, Evans reported that immunotherapy suppressed allergen-specific T-cell proliferation[1] and, in 1980, Rocklin demonstrated that this was due to the generation of allergen-specific suppressor cells.[1] The suppressor activity was shown to reside in inducible regulatory T lymphocytes, which secreted IL-10 and transforming growth factor-β.[16] These cells suppressed both Th_1 and Th_2 cytokine responses and induced a shift in B cells from IgE to IgG_4 and IgA production.[16] The generation of regulatory T cells occurred early in the administration of SCIT.[16] Hamid demonstrated that, when subjects who had been on grass immunotherapy for 3–4 years were injected intradermally with grass pollen extract and the site biopsied 24 hours later, there were more cells expressing mRNA for IL-12, a driver of Th_1 responses.[1] The number of IL-12+ cells in the biopsies correlated positively with cells expressing mRNA for the Th_1 cytokine interferon-γ and negatively with cells expressing mRNA for the Th_2 cytokine IL-4, thus demonstrating immune deviation from Th_2 to Th_1 in the response to grass pollen extract. Studies employing ex vivo peptide-MHC class II tetramers suggested that preferential allergen-specific Th_2 cell deletion is an independent mechanism in restoring tolerance to the allergens administered in SCIT.[18] Recent studies have demonstrated the breadth of the immune response to SCIT including restoration of IFN-α expression in dendritic cells on toll-like receptor-9 stimulation by CpG DNA,[19] increase in regulatory B cells secreting Il-10, TGFβ, and IL-35,[20] inhibition of the seasonal increases in peripheral innate lymphoid type 2 cells,[21] and suppression of plasma levels of Il-17, IL-6, and IL-23 in patients with allergic rhinitis receiving HDM sublingual immunotherapy (SLIT).[22]

Necessary duration of SCIT to achieve disease modification

In the studies reported by Ebner[1] and Durham,[1] subjects had received 3 or 4 years of SCIT. Other studies have sought to determine if this duration of SCIT is necessary and optimal. Des Roches followed, for 3 years after discontinuation, 40 patients with asthma who had become asymptomatic, off medication, while receiving house dust mite SCIT for variable periods of time.[1] Approximately half of the patients relapsed. A predictor of persistent remission was having received SCIT for at least 36 months. The inadequacy of 2 years of SCIT was confirmed in a study in which grass pollen SCIT was given for 2 years with follow-up the next grass pollen season off treatment.[23] There was highly significant improvement, compared to placebo, in subjects' symptoms during the two grass pollen seasons while on treatment, but no significant difference 1 year after stopping SCIT. Two studies have examined whether there is additional benefit continuing SCIT with house dust mite extract for 5 years rather than stopping after 3 years.[24,25] Stelmach found few differences in asthma remission or inhaled corticosteroid dose between the two treatment durations.[24] Tabar found significant improvement in symptoms of rhinitis and asthma as well as quality of life after 3 years of SCIT with some further improvement in rhinitis symptoms after 5 years.[25] The investigators concluded that 3 years of SCIT may be sufficient.

Safety of subcutaneous immunotherapy

The issue of safety of SCIT was addressed in two retrospective surveys of deaths following skin testing or immunotherapy injections that were conducted by the

Committee on Immunotherapy of the American Academy of Allergy, Asthma and Immunology.[26,27] These surveys documented 34 fatal reactions to immunotherapy in the United States between 1985 and 2001. Eighty-eight percent occurred in patients with asthma, even though it was assumed that they constituted a minority of patients receiving SCIT. Furthermore, the patients' asthma was often characterized as severe or not well controlled. At about this same time, a report by Bousquet on systemic reactions in patients undergoing rush SCIT with HDM extract identified a low FEV_1 (presumably indicating poorly controlled asthma) as a major risk for bronchoconstrictive systemic reactions.[1] Perhaps due to increased attention to the risk of SCIT in patients with poorly controlled asthma, a subsequent online survey of fatalities with SCIT covering the years 2008—13 reported a reduction in the rate of fatal reactions from 1 per 2 or 2.5 million injections in the first two surveys to 1 per 14.5 million injections during this most recent period.[28]

It is common practice to reduce the subsequent dose of SCIT if the previous injection had resulted in a large local reaction. At Wilford Hall Air Force Base allergy clinic the rate of systemic reactions was not significantly different when local reactions to immunotherapy resulted in adjustment of the subsequent dose or when no adjustment was made for large or late local reactions.[29] These investigators concluded that dose adjustment for most local reactions is unnecessary and may delay therapy, increase cost, and put the patient at increased risk of dosing errors. Another common practice is to reduce the dose of SCIT during the patient's pollen season. An academic practice in Pittsburg prospectively assessed the occurrence of systemic reactions to over 500,000 immunotherapy injections.[30] They specifically addressed the question of seasonal increase in the risk of systemic reactions and found no increase in the incidence during grass or ragweed pollination seasons in those patients who received grass or ragweed extract injections. A systematic review of eight studies comparing the safety of initiating SCIT during or out of the patient's season found no increase in adverse events with coseasonal initiation.[31] Finally, some recommend avoidance of SCIT in patients with autoimmune diseases; however, in a Danish study population, SCIT was associated with a lower risk of development of autoimmune disease than conventional allergy therapy.[32]

Alternative injection schedules

In 1930, John Freeman described rush immunotherapy, achieving maintenance in 2—4 days in an attempt to provide the patients with more rapid relief.[1] However, his experience as well as that of those subsequently employing rush SCIT was a high rate of systemic reactions. Cluster SCIT achieves maintenance dosing by administering more than one injection per day on nonconsecutive days. Tabar randomized 239 HDM patients with rhinitis and/or asthma to a 6-week cluster schedule or a 12-week conventional study using an alum precipitated D pteronyssinus extract.[33] There was no difference in adverse reactions, but the cluster group achieved more rapid onset of symptom relief. In a US private practice, which used dosing consistent with Practice Parameter recommendations, administered 30–40 injections for standard and 22 for cluster to reach maintenance, and administering premedication with oral prednisone, an antihistamine and an antileukotriene before each cluster, systemic reactions were recorded in 2.8% receiving standard and 2.5% receiving cluster dosing.[34] On the other hand, 11.9% of patients receiving rush build-up experienced systemic reactions.

Compounding allergen mixtures

Fungal and cockroach allergen extracts have been shown to contain protease-like activity that can breakdown the allergens in pollen, dander and HDM extracts.[35] The best practice is to not mix pollen, dander, or mite extracts with either fungal or cockroach extracts and to not mix the two latter groups with each other.[36]

Adjuvants

Attempts have been made to use adjuvants to enhance the response to SCIT. Efforts this far with CpG DNA or MPL have resulted in disappointing results. Vitamin D has shown some promise. In a retrospective analysis of children treated for 1 year with SCIT, children with a higher serum level of 25(OH)D experienced more significant reduction in asthma symptoms scores and steroid-sparing effect and had higher TGF-α production and higher Fox f 3 induction.[37] In a prospective study SCIT plus vitamin D resulted in a significantly lower asthma symptom score after 6 months that did SCIT alone, however, there was no difference in outcomes after 1 year.[38] Thus far, the most impressive, but not yet replicated, enhancement of the response to SCIT was a Chinese study with the probiotic *Clostridium butyricum*.[39] Subjects, monosensitized to HDMs, were randomized to placebo, SCIT with HDM, twice daily oral probiotic, or SCIT plus probiotic for 6 months, with a 6-month follow-up. SCIT-alone produced 50% reduction in symptoms that was not sustained on follow-up. SCIT plus probiotics produced a sustained 80% reduction in symptoms, marked and sustained increase in IgG4 and regulatory B cells, and decrease in IgE, skin prick tests, and Th$_2$ cytokine levels.

Comparative efficacy of subcutaneous versus sublingual immunotherapy

The relative efficacy of SCIT and SLIT have been compared by meta-analyses of each versus placebo and by direct head-to-head studies. Both approaches suffer from the variable quality of and limited number of subjects in many of the studies. One study compared the response to commercially employed doses of timothy pollen extract from the same company, one by depot injection and the other by SLIT tablets.[40] The primary outcomes, over the 15-month study, were the symptoms on nasal allergen challenge and the IgG_4 and IgG_4 functional assays. Only SCIT significantly reduced symptoms on nasal challenge, although there was a trend for improvement with SLIT. Both resulted in favorable humeral responses, but those to SCIT were more than twice as great as with SCIT. As the best available comparison, this study suggests that at least in the short term, the response to SCIT is superior to that to SLIT.

References

1. Nelson HS. Some highlights of the first century of immunotherapy. *Ann Allergy Asthma Immunol.* 2011;107(5):417–421.
2. Meadows A, Kaambwa B, Novielli N, et al. A systematic review and economic evaluation of subcutaneous and sublingual allergen immunotherapy in adults and children with seasonal allergic rhinitis. *Health Technol Assess.* 2013;17(27):1–322. vi,xi-xiv.
3. Lin SY, Erekosima N, Suarez-Cuervo C, et al. Allergen-specific immunotherapy for the treatment of allergic rhinoconjunctivitis and/or asthma: comparative effectiveness review. In: *Comparative Effectiveness Review No. 111. (Prepared by the Johns Hopkins University Evidence-Based Practice Center under Contract No. 290-2007-10061-1.) AHRQ Publication No. 13-Ehc061-EF.* Rockville, MD: Agency for Healthcare Research and Quality; 2013. www.effectivehealthcare.ahrq.gov/reports/final.cfm.
4. Boyle RJ, Elremeli M, Hockenhull J, et al. Venom immunotherapy for preventing allergic reactions to insect stings. *Cochrane Database Syst Rev.* 2012;10:CD008838. https://doi.org/10.1002/14651858.
5. Werfel T, Breuer K, Rueff F, et al. Usefulness of specific immunotherapy in patients with atopic dermatitis and allergic sensitization to house dust mites: a multi-center, randomized, dose-response study. *Allergy.* 2006;61(2):202–205.
6. Tam HH, Calderon MA, Manikam L, et al. Specific allergen immunotherapy for the treatment of atopic eczema: a Cochrane systematic review. *Allergy.* 2016;71(9):1345–1356.
7. Demoly P, Passalacqua G, Pfaar O, et al. Management of the polyallergic patient with allergy immunotherapy: a practice-based approach. *Allergy Asthma Clin Immunol.* 2016;12:2. https://doi.org/10.1186/s13223-015-0109-6.
8. Blume SW, Yeomans K, Allen-Ramey F, et al. Administration and burden of subcutaneous immunotherapy for allergic rhinitis in U.S. and Canadian clinical practice. *J Manag Care Spec Pharm.* 2015;21(11):982–990.
9. Reid M, Moss RB, Hsu YP, et al. Seasonal asthma in northern California: allergic causes and efficacy of immunotherapy. *J Allergy Clin Immunol.* 1986;78(4 pt. 1):590–600.
10. Nelson HS. Subcutaneous injection immunotherapy for optimal effectiveness. *Immunol Allergy Clin N AM.* 2011;31(2):211–226.
11. Cox L, Nelson H, Lockey R, et al. Allergen immunotherapy: practice parameter third update. *J Allergy Clin Immunol.* 2011;127(suppl 1):S1–S55.
12. Purello-D'Ambrosio F, Gangemi S, Merendino RA, et al. Prevention of new sensitizations in monosensitized subjects submitted to specific immunotherapy or not. A retrospective study. *Clin Exp Allergy.* 2001;31(8):1295–1302.

13. Jacobsen L, Niggemann B, Dreborg S, et al. Specific immunotherapy has long-term preventive effect of seasonal and perennial asthma: 10-year follow-up on the PAT study. *Allergy.* 2007;62(8):943−948.

14. Schmitt J, Schwarz K, Stadler E, Wustenberg EG. Allergy immunotherapy for allergic rhinitis effectively prevents asthma: results from a large retrospective cohort study. *J Allergy Clin Immunol.* 2015;136(6):1511−1516.

15. Bozek A, Jarzab J, Bednarski P. The effect of allergen-specific immunotherapy on offspring. *Allergy Asthma Proc.* 2016;37(4):59−63.

16. Jutel M, Akdis M, Budak F, et al. IL-10 and TGFβ cooperate in the regulatory T cell response to mucosal allergen in normal immunity and specific immunotherapy. *Eur J Immunol.* 2003;33(5):1205−1214.

17. Shamji MH, Ljorring C, Francis JN, et al. Functional rather than immunoreactive levels of IgG$_4$ correlate closely with clinical response to grass pollen immunotherapy. *Allergy.* 2012;67(2):217−226.

18. Wambre E, DeLong JH, James EA, et al. Specific immunotherapy modifies allergen-specific CD4+ T-cell responses in an epitope-dependent manner. *J Allergy Clin Immunol.* 2014;133(3):872−879.

19. Tversky JR, Bieneman AP, Chichester KL, et al. Subcutaneous allergen immunotherapy restores human dendritic cell innate immune function. *Clin Exp Allergy.* 2010;40(1):94−102.

20. Van de Veen W, Stanic B, Wirz OF, et al. Role of regulatory B cells in immune tolerance to allergen and beyond. *J Allergy Clin Immunol.* 2016;138(3):654−665.

21. Lao-Amaya M, Steveling E, Scadding GW, et al. Seasonal increases in peripheral innate lymphoid type 2 cells are inhibited by subcutaneous grass pollen immunotherapy. *J Allergy Clin Immunol.* 2014;134(5):1193−1195.

22. Li CW, LU HG, Chen DH, et al. In vivo and in vitro studies of the Th$_{17}$ response to specific immunotherapy in house dust mite-induced allergic rhinitis patients. *PLoS One.* 2014;9(3):e91950.

23. Scadding GW, Calderon MA, Shamji HM, et al. Effect of 2 years of treatment with sublingual grass pollen immunotherapy on nasal response to allergen challenge at 3 years among patients with moderate to severe seasonal allergic rhinitis. *J Am Med Assoc.* 2017;317(6):615−625.

24. Stelmach I, Sobocinska A, Majak P, et al. Comparison of the long-term efficacy of 3- and 5-year house dust mite allergen immunotherapy. *Ann Allergy Asthma Immunol.* 2012;109(4):274−278.

25. Tabar A, Arrobarren E, Echechipia S, et al. Three years of specific immunotherapy may be sufficient in house dust mite respiratory allergy. *J Allergy Clin Immunol.* 2011;127(1):57−63.

26. Reid MJ, Lockey RF, Turkeltaub PC, Platts-Mills TA. Survey of fatalities from skin testing and immunotherapy 1985-1989. *J Allergy Clin Immunol.* 1993;92(1 pt. 1):6−15.

27. Bernstein DI, Wanner M, Borish L, Liss GM. Twelve-year survey of fatal reactions to allergen injections and skin testing: 1990-2001. *J Allergy Clin Immunol.* 2004;113(6):1129−1136.

28. Epstein TG, Liss GM, Murphy-Berendts K, Bernstein DI. Risk factors for fatal and nonfatal reactions to subcutaneous immunotherapy: National Surveillance Study on Allergen Immunotherapy (2008-2013). *Ann Allergy Asthma Immunol.* 2016;116(4):354−359.

29. Tankersley M, Butler KK, Butler WK, Goetz DW. Local reactions during allergen immunotherapy do not require dose adjustment. *J Allergy Clin Immunol.* 2000;106(5): 840–843.

30. Lin MS, Tanner E, Lynn J, Friday Jr GA. Nonfatal systemic allergic reactions induced by skin testing and immunotherapy. *Ann Allergy.* 1993;71(6):557–562.

31. Creticos PS, Bernstein DI, Casale TB, et al. Coseasonal initiation of allergen immunotherapy: a systematic review. *J Allergy Clin Immunol Pract.* 2016;4(6):1194–1204.

32. Linneberg A, Jacobsen RK, Jespersen L, Abildstrom SZ. Association of subcutaneous allergen-specific immunotherapy with incidence of autoimmune disease, ischemic heart disease and mortality. *J Allergy Clin Immunol.* 2012;129(2):413–419.

33. Tabar AI, Echechipia S, Garcia BE, et al. Double-blind comparative study of cluster and conventional immunotherapy schedules with Dermatophagoides pteronyssinus. *J Allergy Clin Immunol.* 2005;116(1):109–118.

34. Winslow AW, Turbyville JC, Sublett JW, et al. Comparison of systemic reactions in rush, cluster and standard-build aeroallergen immunotherapy. *Ann Allergy Asthma Immunol.* 2016;117(5):542–545.

35. Esch RE. Role of proteases on the stability of allergenic extracts. *Arb Paul Ehrlich Inst Bundesamt Sera Impfstoffe Frankf A M.* 1992;85:171–177.

36. Esch RE, Grier TJ. Allergen compatibilities in extract mixtures. *Immunol Allergy Clin N AM.* 2011;31:227–239.

37. Majak P, Jerzynska J, Smejda K, et al. Correlation of vitamin D with Foxp3 induction and steroid-sparing effect of immunotherapy in asthmatic children. *Ann Allergy Asthma Immunol.* 2012;109(5):329–335.

38. Baris S, Kiykim A, Ozen A, et al. Vitamin D as an adjunct to subcutaneous allergen immunotherapy in asthmatic children sensitized to house dust mite. *Allergy.* 2014; 69(2):246–253.

39. Xu L-Z, Yang LT, Qiu SQ, et al. Combination of specific allergen and probiotics induces specific regulatory B cells and enhances specific immunotherapy effect on allergic rhinitis. *Oncotarget.* 2016;7(34):54360–54369.

40. Aasbjerg K, Backer V, Lund G, et al. Comparison of allergen immunotherapy tablet treatment and subcutaneous immunotherapy against grass allergy. *Clin Exp Allergy.* 2014;44(3):417–428.

Breakthroughs in sublingual immunotherapy

13

Stefania Nicola, MD [1], Giovanni Rolla, MD [1], Enrico Heffler, MD, PhD [2,3],
Francesca Puggioni, MD [2,3], Giorgio Walter Canonica, MD [2,3], Luisa Brussino, MD [1]

[1]*Università degli Studi di Torino, Dipartimento di Scienze Mediche, AO Ordine Mauriziano Umberto I, Torino, Italy;* [2]*Department of Biomedical Sciences, Humanitas Univeristy, Pieve Emanuele (MI), Italy;* [3]*Personalized Medicine, Asthma and Allergy, Humanitas Research Hospital IRCCS, Rozzano (MI), Italy*

Allergen immunotherapy (AIT) is the only disease-modifying treatment for allergic rhinitis, conjunctivitis, and asthma, which provides added symptom control on top of pharmacotherapy.[1]

The rationale for AIT is the modification of the underlying allergic disease mechanisms. AIT disease modification involves several immunological events that result in allergen-specific tolerance and suppression of inflammation.[2,3] Ths translates into multicomponent clinical improvement (e.g., improved asthma or nasal symptoms) and sustained clinical efficacy after discontinuation.

The first commonly used and approved AIT was the subcutaneous immunotherapy (SCIT) followed by sublingual immunotherapy (SLIT), although other administration routes are emerging, including the oral, intralymphatic, and epicutaneous ones.[1]

SLIT, in its liquid and tablet forms, has been known and used for years, but only in 2015 the European Medicines Agency (EMA) approved the first SLIT tablets for the treatment of allergic rhinitis and asthma in patients sensitized to specific aeroallergens. Up to now, two products for grass pollen, one for house dust mites (HDM), and one for ragweed pollen treatment are marketed.[4−8]

In contrast to SCIT, which can be associated with severe adverse events and may be responsible for severe and sometimes fatal systemic reactions,[9−13] SLIT offers a better safety profile. However, sublingual immunotherapy does have adverse reactions, although no fatal reactions have been described. Adverse events (AEs) after SLIT administration are usually local, mild, and self-limiting. There have been some reports of patients experiencing asthma exacerbations and reactions deemed "anaphylaxis" that requiring hospital care after SLIT administration.[14,15]

AIT contraindications

Based on the European Academy of Allergy and Clinical Immunology (EAACI) guidelines for rhinoconjunctivitis, published in 2018, contraindications to allergen

Immunotherapies for Allergic Disease. https://doi.org/10.1016/B978-0-323-54427-6.00013-4

immunotherapy were uncontrolled or severe asthma, the presence of an active systemic autoimmune disorder or an active malignant neoplasia, and the AIT initiation during pregnancy.[16] However, the same document states that the evidence of risk with uncontrolled asthma, active systemic autoimmune disease, and malignancy is weak and derives mainly from case reports or case series of adverse events with AIT. Moreover, although initiation of AIT is considered as contraindicated during pregnancy, an ongoing AIT is permissible when having been well tolerated by the patient in the past.

On the other hand, if benefits outweigh potential risks in an individual patient, AIT could be carefully used in case of partially controlled asthma, severe cardiovascular diseases, systemic autoimmune disorders in remission or organ specific, severe psychiatric disorders, poor adherence, primary and secondary immunodeficiencies, and in case of a history of serious systemic reactions to AIT.[16]

Novel AIT approaches in asthma

Asthma represents a major health burden, currently affecting around 350 million people globally, and it is responsible for considerable morbidity and mortality. Treatment of asthma is mainly based on inhaled corticosteroids and bronchodilators, to achieve and maintain a disease control preventing exacerbations and improving quality of life.[17,18] In this setting of disease, even if an adequate asthma control is not achieved, the prescription and administration of allergen immunotherapy are extremely limited, in both children and adults, probably because asthmatic patients were excluded from AIT clinical trials and due to the increased risk of exacerbations after AIT administration in case of uncontrolled asthma.[19]

House dust mites allergic asthma

The exposure to indoor allergens, including HDM, such as *Dermatophagoides (D.) pteronyssinus* or *D. farinae*, is known to be associated with asthma worldwide, and it leads to the development of high-titer allergen-specific IgE.[20,21]

In the past, allergic asthma was a contraindication to AIT. However, in 2016, a worldwide survey[22] about the safety of AIT in pollen and HDM sensitized patients with allergic rhinitis and asthma, showed an excellent safety profile of AIT in asthmatic patients.

Thus, for the first time, the Global Initiative of Asthma (GINA) 2019 guidelines listed AIT as add-on therapy for step 3 asthma, in patients sensitized to HDM presenting FEV1 >70% predicted.[23]

In addition, EAACI has recently developed new guidelines providing evidence-based recommendations for the use of AIT as add-on treatment for HDM-driven allergic asthma. AIT for HDM should be considered in patients sensitized to HDM, with AR and persistent asthma despite Step 2 therapy, with FEV1 >70% predicted.[24]

The EAACI guidelines formulated different recommendations for adults and children, based on both available routes of SLIT administration, drops, and tablets, remarking the need of regularly assessing lung function tests.

HDM SLIT drops are recommended for children with controlled HDM-driven allergic asthma as an add-on treatment, to decrease symptoms and medication use. However, due to lack of evidence, no recommendations can be provided for the use of HDM SLIT drops in adults with HDM-driven allergic asthma in reducing exacerbations, improving asthma control, or in decreasing specific and nonspecific AHR.[24]

On the other hand, HDM SLIT-tablets are recommended for adults with controlled and partially controlled HDM-driven allergic asthma as an add-on treatment to regular therapy to reduce exacerbations and to improve asthma control. However, there are not enough evidences as to recommend the use of HDM SLIT-tablets for children or for adults to improve asthma lung function or quality of life or to decrease specific and nonspecific AHR.[24]

Concerning treatment duration, it is widely accepted that, whether efficacy is proven after 1 year, AIT should be continued for at least 3 years to achieve long-term efficacy,[25,26] otherwise cessation of AIT therapy should be considered after the first year.[23,27,28]

Birch pollen allergic asthma

Allergic rhinitis is estimated to affect up to 25% of the global population, with a considerable impact on patients' quality of life.[29,30] Moreover, allergic rhinitis is one of the major risk factors for asthma development.[31−33] Tree pollen−induced allergic rhinoconjunctivitis is commonly caused by allergens from the birch-homologous group, which includes birch, alder, hornbeam, hazel, and oak, which all have Bet v 1-homologous allergens with high sequence identity.[34,35]

Between 2014 and 2016, a multicenter, randomized, double-blind, placebo-controlled (DBPC), phase III study in adults with birch pollen allergy aimed to evaluate the efficacy of birch pollen SLIT drops in patients affected by allergic rhinitis and mild-to-moderate controlled asthma (NCT02231307)[36] and in 2016 a similar study aimed to evaluate clinical efficacy on birch pollen tablet SLIT (EudraCT 2015-004,821-15).[37]

In both studies, the primary endpoint, corresponding to the difference in combined symptoms and medications scores, was achieved. On the other hand, among the secondary endpoints, no differences were found between the active group and the placebo, concerning the Asthma Control Questionnaire evaluation[36] and the Asthma Control Test.[37] This lack in significance could be linked, according to the authors, with the adequate control of asthma during the trial.[36]

Emerging approaches for food allergy

Food allergy incidence is progressively increasing and it currently affects about 5% of adults and 8% of children in the United States,[38–40] the most common foods responsible for anaphylaxis being peanut and tree nut.[41]

Up to now, no treatments for food allergy are approved by FDA or EMA, and the only safe approach is the strict avoidance. However, several ongoing phase II and III clinical trials are evaluating both clinical efficacy and safety of Food Allergen Immunotherapy.

AIT for peanut allergy

As mentioned earlier, the risk of peanut allergens-induced anaphylaxis in allergic patients is extremely high. However, several immunotherapy clinical trials with different administration routes are ongoing, supporting the evidence that repeated and progressively increasing exposure to a specific peanut allergen can reduce sensitivity toward the allergen.[42]

Among the different administration routes, SLIT seems to be the easiest and safest one, in both its tablet and liquid form, although its efficacy needs to be further analyzed.

Tolerability of peanut SLIT is well described, and AEs were reported in 11.5% of patients, with nobody needing epinephrine administration. Nevertheless, its efficacy is extremely variable, ranging from complete to partial desensitization, although many subjects did not show any differences compared to the placebo group.[43] However, lower baseline peanut Ara h 2 and Ara h 3 specific IgE seemed to predict successful desensitization in children after 1 year of AIT.[44]

More recently, a long-term study analyzed the response to peanut ingestion (from 2 mg to 5 g) in 37 patients after 3–5 years of peanut immunotherapy. The results showed a good response in the double-blind placebo-controlled food challenge (DBPCFC) during the immunotherapy, but a lack in efficacy, that is, sustained unresponsiveness, in 27% of patients after 2–4 weeks off therapy.[45]

Despite a good safety profile and overall ease of administration, peanut SLIT is limited by its variable efficacy. Higher maintenance doses and a longer duration of therapy may, in fact, address some of these concerns. In addition, alternative strategies, such as the use of SLIT in combination with adjuvants or, possibly, in combination with other forms of immunotherapy (e.g., OIT or EPIT) represent areas for future research.

AIT for cow's milk allergy

Allergy to cow's milk (CM) is a relevant cause of immediate-type food hypersensitivity among children under 3 years old. The self-reported prevalence of milk allergy is up to 17%, but the one confirmed with double-blind placebo-controlled food-challenge or open-challenge varied between 0% and 3%.[46] As for peanut allergy, the most common approach to cow's milk allergy is allergen avoidance until clinical tolerance is induced.

Conversely to what happens with peanuts allergy, about 50% of children can tolerate CM by 5 years old, and up to 75% by their early teenage years.[46] Nevertheless, some children experience persistent allergic reactions[47] and many oral immunotherapy (OIT) studies showed to be effective but not risk free. Many adverse effects requiring parenteral epinephrine were actually reported.[48–51]

In contrast to the numerous studies examining milk OIT, only one trial has examined the use of SLIT in milk allergy. In 2006, de Boissieu published a proof-of-concept study, in which eight children with confirmed milk allergy underwent milk SLIT to a goal dose of 1 mL/day of cow's milk over 6 months.[52] Six of the eight children completed the protocol, but only three (38%) were able to consume 200 mL of milk without symptoms at the final DBPCFC.

AIT in other foods allergy

Hazelnut

In 2005, a DBPC randomized trial aimed to assess SLIT in hazelnut allergy, analyzing the response of 29 individuals randomized to active treatment with hazelnut extract ($n = 12$) or a placebo ($n = 11$).[53] After 8–12 weeks of treatment with 25 drops daily (66,25 mg), 11/12 individuals reached the target dose, and 5 of them (42%) were able to ingest 20 g of hazelnut in a DBPCFC without symptoms. On the other hand, only 1 of the 11 individuals in the placebo group was able to ingest 20 g.

Peach

In 2009, the use of SLIT for treatment of peach allergy using a Pru p3 extract[53] was assessed in 56 individuals randomized to active treatment ($n = 37$) or a placebo ($n = 19$). After 6 months of active treatment, with a goal of 10 µg of Pru p3 three times weekly, 33 individuals completed the therapy, and 32 individuals were able to tolerate the maintenance dose. Compared to the placebo, this group was able to tolerate 3–9-fold higher doses of peach after therapy.[54]

Key points

- Allergen immunotherapy (AIT) is the only disease-modifying treatment for allergic rhinitis, conjunctivitis, and asthma, which provides added symptom control to medications and a sustained clinical effect based on allergen-specific tolerance.
- Contraindications to allergen immunotherapy are uncontrolled or severe asthma, the presence of an active systemic autoimmune disorder or an active malignant neoplasia, and the AIT initiation during pregnancy.

- AIT in asthma. EAACI has recently developed new guidelines providing evidence-based recommendations for the use of AIT as add-on treatment for HDM-driven allergic asthma, in patients sensitized to HDM, with AR and persistent asthma requiring Inhaled CorticoSteroids (ICS), with FEV1 >70% predicted, and with exacerbations despite taking Step 2 therapy.
- AIT in food allergy. At the moment, no treatments for food allergy have been approved by FDA or EMA, and the only safe approach is strictly avoidance.
- AIT trials in peanut allergy. DBPCFC after 3—5 years of peanut immunotherapy showed a good response during the immunotherapy, but a lack in efficacy in 27% of patients after 2—4 weeks off therapy.
- AIT trials in other food allergy. Milk: although 6/8 patients completed the protocol, only 3 were able to consume 200 mL of milk without symptoms at the final DBPCFC. Hazelnut: after 8—12 weeks of treatment, 11/12 individuals reached the target dose, but only 5 were able to ingest 20 g of hazelnut in a DBPCFC without symptoms. Peach:

($n = 37$) or a placebo ($n = 19$). After 6 months of active treatment, 33/37 patients completed the therapy, and 32 individuals were able to tolerate the maintenance dose of 10 μg of Pru p3 three times weekly.

References

1. Heffler E, et al. New drugs in early-stage clinical trials for allergic rhinitis. *Expert Opin Investig Drugs*. 2019;28(3):267—273. https://doi.org/10.1080/13543784.2019.1571581.
2. Jutel M, Agache I, Bonini S, et al. International consensus on allergy immunotherapy. *J Allergy Clin Immunol*. 2015;136:556—568.
3. Jutel M, Agache I, Bonini S, et al. International consensus on allergen immunotherapy II: mechanisms, standardization, and pharmacoeconomics. *J Allergy Clin Immunol*. 2016; 137:358—368.
4. Pepper AN, et al. Sublingual immunotherapy for the polyallergic patient. *J Allergy Clin Immunol Pract*. 2017;5(1):41—45.
5. Content available to: https://www.ema.europa.eu/en/documents/psusa/allergen-therapy-dactylis-glomerata-l-phleum-pratense-l-anthoxanthum-odoratum-l-lolium-perenne-l-poa/00010465/201612_en.pdf.
6. Content available to: https://www.ema.europa.eu/en/documents/psusa/allergen-therapy-phleum-pratense-oromucosal-use-product-authorised-mutually-recognition-procedure/00010475/201607_en.pdf.
7. Content available to: https://www.ema.europa.eu/en/documents/pip-decision/p/0056/2018-ema-decision-16-march-2018-acceptance-modification-agreed-paediatric-investigation-plan/dermatophagoides-farinae-allergen-extract-acarizax-asso_en.pdf.
8. Content available to: https://www.ema.europa.eu/en/documents/additional-monitoring/list-medicinal-products-under-additional-monitoring_en-0.pdf.
9. Makatsori M, Calderon MA. Anaphylaxis: still a ghost behind immunotherapy. *Curr Opin Allergy Clin Immunol*. 2014;14(4):316—322.

10. Epstein TG, Liss GM, Murphy-Berendts K, Bernstein DI. "AAAAI/ACAAI surveillance study of subcutaneous immunotherapy, years 2008–2012: an update on fatal and nonfatal systemic allergic reactions. *J Allergy Clin Immunol: In Pract*. 2014;2(2), 161.e3–167.e3.

11. Cook PR, Bryant II JL, Davis WE, Benke TT, Rapoport AS. Systemic reactions to immunotherapy: the American Academy of Otolaryngic Allergy Morbidity and Mortality Survey. *Otolaryngol Head Neck Surg*. 1994;110(6):487–493.

12. Davis WE, Cook PR, McKinsey JP, Templer JW. Anaphylaxis in immunotherapy. *Otolaryngol Head Neck Surg*. 1992;107(1):78–83.

13. Lockey RF, Benedict LM, Turkeltaub PC, Bukantz SC. Fatalities from immunotherapy (IT) and skin testing (ST). *J Allergy Clin Immunol*. 1987;79(4):660–677.

14. Calderon MA, Simons FER, Malling H-J, Lockey RF, Moingeon P, Demoly P. Sublingual allergen immunotherapy: mode of action and its relationship with the safety profile. *Allergy*. 2012;67(3):302–311.

15. Saporta D. *Sublingual Immunotherapy: Useful Tool for the Allergist in Private Practice*. Hindawi Publishing Corporation, BioMed Research International; 2016. Article ID 9323804.

16. Roberts G, et al. EAACI guidelines on allergen immunotherapy: allergic rhinoconjunctivitis. *Allergy*. 2018;73:765–798.

17. Bucca C, et al. Effect of iron supplementation in women with chronic cough and iron deficiency. *Int J Clin Pract*. 2012;66(11):1095–1100.

18. Brussino L, et al. Eosinophils target therapy for severe asthma: critical points. *BioMed Res Int*. 2018;2018:7582057.

19. Bousquet J, Hejjaoui A, Dhivert H, Clauzel AM, Michel FB. Immunotherapy with a standardized Dermatophagoides pteronyssinus extract. Systemic reactions during the rush protocol in patients suffering from asthma. *J Allergy Clin Immunol*. 1989;83:797–802.

20. Sylvestre L, Jégu J, Metz-Favre C, Barnig C, Qi S, de Blay F. Component-based allergenmicroarray: Der p 2 and Der f 2 dust mite sensitization is more common in patients with severe asthma. *J Investig Allergol Clin Immunol*. 2016;26:141–143.

21. Dzoro S, Mittermann I, Resch-Marat Y, et al. House dust mites as potential carriers for IgE sensitization to bacterial antigens. *Allergy*. 2018;73(1):115–124.

22. Calderón MA, et al. European survey on adverse systemic reactions in allergen immunotherapy (EASSI): a real-life clinical assessment. *Allergy*. 2017;72(3):462–472.

23. Global Initiative for Asthma. Pocket guide for asthma management and prevention. https://ginasthma.org/wp-content/uploads/2019/04/GINA-2019-main-Pocket-Guidewms.pdf.

24. Agache I, et al. EAACI Guidelines on Allergen Immunotherapy: house dust mite-driven allergic asthma. *Allergy*. 2019;7 4:855–873.

25. Stelmach I, Sobocińska A, Majak P, Smejda K, Jerzyńska J, Stelmach W. Comparison of the long-term efficacy of 3- and 5-year house dust mite allergen immunotherapy. *Ann Allergy Asthma Immunol*. 2012;109:274-278.

26. Arroabarren E, Tabar AI, Echechipía S, Cambra K, García BE, Alvarez- Puebla MJ. Optimal duration of allergen immunotherapy in children with dust mite respiratory allergy. *Pediatr Allergy Immunol*. 2015;26(1):34-41.

27. Reddel H, Taylor DR, et al. An official American Thoracic Society/European Respiratory Society statement: asthma control and exacerbations: standardizing endpoints for clinical asthma trials and clinical practice. *Am J Respir Crit Care Med*. 2009; 180(1):59-99.

28. Cox L, Nelson H, Lockey R, et al. Allergen immunotherapy: a practice parameter third update. *J Allergy Clin Immunol.* 2011;127(1 suppl):S1–S55.

29. Bousquet J, Khaltaev N, Cruz AA, et al. Allergic rhinitis and its impact on asthma (ARIA) 2008 update (in collaboration with the World Health Organization, GA(2) LEN and AllerGen). *Allergy.* 2008;63(suppl 86):8–160.

30. Canonica GW, Bousquet J, Mullol J, Scadding GK, Virchow JC. A survey of the burden of allergic rhinitis in Europe. *Allergy.* 2007;62(suppl 85):17–25.

31. Bacharier LB, Boner A, Carlsen KH, et al. Diagnosis and treatment of asthma in childhood: a PRACTALL consensus report. *Allergy.* 2008;63:5–34.

32. Burgess JA, Walters EH, Byrnes GB, et al. Childhood allergic rhinitis predicts asthma incidence and persistence to middle age: a longitudinal study. *J Allergy Clin Immunol.* 2007;120:863–869.

33. Schmitt J, Schwarz K, Stadler E, Wustenberg EG. Allergy immunotherapy for allergic rhinitis effectively prevents asthma: results from a large retrospective cohort study. *J Allergy Clin Immunol.* 2015;136:1511–1516.

34. Smith M, Jager S, Berger U, et al. Geographic and temporal variations in pollen exposure across Europe. *Allergy.* 2014;69:913–923.

35. Heath MD, Collis J, Batten T, Hutchings JW, Swan N, Skinner MA. Molecular, proteomic and immunological parameters of allergens provide inclusion criteria for new candidates within established grass and tree homologous groups. *World Allergy Organ J.* 2015;8:21.

36. Pfaar O, et al. Sublingual allergen immunotherapy with a liquid birch pollen product in patients with seasonal allergic rhinoconjunctivitis with or without Asthma. *J Allergy Clin Immunol.* 2019;143(3).

37. Biedermann T, et al. The SQ tree SLIT-tablet is highly effective and well tolerated: results from a randomized, double-blind, placebo-controlled phase III trial. *J Allergy Clin Immunol.* 2019;143(3):1058–1066. e6.

38. Sampson HA, Aceves S, Bock SA, et al. Food allergy: a practice parameter update-2014. *J Allergy Clin Immunol.* 2014;134:1016–1025.e43.

39. Sicherer SH. Epidemiology of food allergy. *J Allergy Clin Immunol.* 2011;127:594–602.

40. Sicherer SH, Munoz-Furlong A, Godbold JH, Sampson HA. US prevalence of self-reported peanut, tree nut, and sesame allergy: 11-year follow-up. *J Allergy Clin Immunol.* 2010;125:1322–1326.

41. Samady W, Trainor J, Smith B, Gupta R. Food-induced anaphylaxis in infants and children. *Ann Allergy Asthma Immunol.* 2018;121:360–365.

42. Anagnostou K, Clark A. Oral immunotherapy for peanut allergy. *Annu Rev Med.* 2016; 67(1):375–385. https://doi.org/10.1146/annurev-med-061014-094943.

43. Kim EH, Bird JA, Kulis M, et al. Sublingual immunotherapy for peanut allergy: clinical and immunologic evidence of desensitization. *J Allergy Clin Immunol.* 2011;127: 640–646.e1.

44. Burk CM, Kulis M, Leung N, Kim EH, Burks AW, Vickery BP. Utility of component analyses in subjects undergoing sublingual immunotherapy for peanut allergy. *Clin Exp Allergy.* 2016;46(2):347–353.

45. Yang L, Steele PH, Hamilton DK, et al. Sustained unresponsiveness after sublingual immunotherapy for peanut-allergic children. *J Allergy Clin Immunol.* 2017;139(suppl): AB175.

46. Rona RJ, Keil T, Summers C, et al. *J Allergy Clin Immunol.* 2007;120(3):638–646.

47. Spergel JM. Natural history of cow's milk allergy. *J Allergy Clin Immunol*. 2013;131(3): 813−814.
48. Longo G, Barbi E, Berti I, et al. Specific oral tolerance induction in children with very severe cow's milk-induced reactions. *J Allergy Clin Immunol*. 2008;121:343−347.
49. Martorell A, De la Hoz B, Ibáñez MD, et al. Oral desensitization as a useful treatment in 2-year-old children with cow's milk allergy. *Clin Exp Allergy*. 2011;41:1297−1304.
50. Pajno GB, Caminiti L, Ruggeri P, et al. Oral immunotherapy for cow's milk allergy with a weekly up-dosing regimen: a randomized single-blind controlled study. *Ann Allergy Asthma Immunol*. 2010;105:376−381.
51. Skripak JM, Nash SD, Rowley H, et al. A randomized, double blind, placebo-controlled study of milk oral immunotherapy for cow's milk allergy. *J Allergy Clin Immunol*. 2008; 122:1154−1160.
52. De Boissieu D, Dupont C. Sublingual immunotherapy for cow's milk protein allergy: a preliminary report. *Allergy*. 2006;61:1238−1239.
53. Enrique E, Pineda F, Malek T, et al. Sublingual immunotherapy for hazelnut food allergy: a randomized, double-blind, placebo-controlled study with a standardized hazelnut extract. *J Allergy Clin Immunol*. 2005;116:1073−1079.
54. Fernandez-Rivas M, Garrido Fernandez S, Nadal JA, et al. Randomized double-blind, placebo-controlled trial of sublingual immunotherapy with a Pru p 3 quantified peach extract. *Allergy*. 2009;64:876−883.

Food immunotherapy

Wenyin Loh, MBBS, MRCPCH [1,2,*],
Mimi L.K. Tang, MBBS, PhD, FRACP, FRCPA, FAAAAI [1,3,4,*]

[1]*Allergy and Immune Disorders, Murdoch Children's Research Institute, Melbourne, VIC, Australia;* [2]*Allergy Service, Department of Paediatrics, KK Women's and Children's Hospital, Singapore, Singapore;* [3]*Department of Allergy and Immunology, The Royal Children's Hospital, Melbourne, VIC, Australia;* [4]*Department of Paediatrics, University of Melbourne, Melbourne, VIC, Australia*

Introduction

Food allergy is a growing public health problem in both developed and developing countries.[1,2] Current management involves allergen avoidance and administration of emergency medications. Despite careful attention to food avoidance, accidental exposures are inevitable and food-allergic patients are faced with the ever present risk of life-threatening reactions or fatal anaphylaxis. The constant vigilance required to maintain allergen avoidance and unpredictability of reactions results in a significantly impaired quality of life (QOL).[3] There is a pressing and unmet need for a curative treatment that can reduce or remove the risk of reaction, which has driven intense research in the area of food allergen immunotherapy over the past decade.

Food allergen immunotherapy holds much promise, given the success of allergen immunotherapy in desensitizing patients with venom and environmental allergy. However, high rates of systemic reactions in patients receiving subcutaneous immunotherapy (SCIT) for peanut allergy in the 1990s led to the search for alternative routes of delivery, use of modified allergens and/or cotreatment with adjuvants to improve safety and efficacy. This chapter will focus on oral immunotherapy (OIT), OIT together with adjuvants, sublingual immunotherapy (SLIT), epicutaneous immunotherapy (EPIT), and other novel approaches currently undergoing active investigation for treatment of food allergy.

Understanding the clinical outcomes that can be achieved with food immunotherapy

Food allergen immunotherapy may be administered by oral, sublingual or epicutaneous routes and typically involves administering increasing doses of allergen in an

---

* Both authors contributed equally to the preparation and writing of this chapter.

Immunotherapies for Allergic Disease. https://doi.org/10.1016/B978-0-323-54427-6.00014-6

attempt to induce desensitization, sustained unresponsiveness (SU), or ideally oral tolerance.[4] **Desensitization** is defined as a temporary increase in the reaction threshold to an allergen that is only maintained while receiving active therapy. **SU** refers to the lack of clinical reaction to a food allergen after active therapy has been discontinued for a period of time, although currently it is considered that SU requires some level of continued allergen exposure to sustain the unresponsive state.[5] The length of time that active treatment is withheld to demonstrate SU remains poorly defined, but a period of 4—8 weeks withdrawal of allergen exposure has been applied in published studies. **Oral tolerance** describes a complete lack of reactivity to an ingested food allergen that is maintained without the need for continued food allergen exposure and is expected to persist in the face of ad libitum allergen ingestion, which is how an individual who is not allergic might ingest the allergen.[5]

These definitions have aided in bringing greater consistency to reporting of trial outcomes; however, there remain several important areas of ambiguity regarding SU and tolerance that require delineation. One important shortcoming with the current definition of SU is that there is no distinction made in regard to the level of protection that is sustained over time. For example, there is a substantial difference between sustained protection against low-level exposure to peanut (e.g., 300—600 mg peanut protein/one to two peanuts/accidental exposure to peanut) and the sustained ability to tolerate a large amount of peanut such as might be found in a peanut-containing meal (e.g., 5g of peanut protein/20 peanuts/>two slices of peanut butter on toast). At this time, the term SU would be equally applicable to both situations, yet these are undoubtedly very different outcomes for the patient. Moreover, protection against one to two peanuts would still require avoidance of peanut other than some limited intermittent exposure to maintain the SU state, while the ability to ingest more than two standard serves of a peanut meal would effectively allow the patient to incorporate peanut into their diet ad libitum just like a person who is not allergic. A recent review article suggested that "remission" and "sustained unresponsiveness" could be used interchangeably[5]; however, it may be more appropriate to apply the term "remission" to the latter situation where the level of sustained protection allows incorporation of the allergen into the diet ad libitum and to retain the term "sustained unresponsiveness" or "sustained desensitization" for situations where an increase in reaction threshold is maintained after withdrawal of active treatment for a period of time. Further consideration of how these distinct situations might be identified and defined is necessary. A second issue requiring clarification is how to identify the presence of true oral tolerance. One pragmatic approach would be to demonstrate the persistence of SU after a prolonged period of ad libitum allergen intake, which mimics the way in which a nonallergic person would ingest the allergen. The applicability of such an approach is supported by findings of a recent study in which subjects who maintained their SU status (defined as passing a 4 g peanut protein challenge after 8 weeks peanut elimination) at 4 years after discontinuation of active treatment had not experienced any allergic reactions in the intervening 4 years while continuing ad libitum peanut intake.[6] Absence of any reactions with ad libitum allergen ingestion while remaining off active treatment together with demonstration of SU by food challenge following 8 weeks of secondary elimination years after stopping active treatment would arguably suggest the presence of true tolerance. In order to progress the development of effective food allergy treatments, it will be imperative to establish clear guidance on how the various clinical outcomes achieved with food immunotherapy might be differentiated from each other, as well as a pragmatic approach to demonstrate oral tolerance in the setting of a clinical trial.

Oral immunotherapy

OIT involves daily consumption of an allergen which is commenced at low doses then incrementally increased over weeks to months. While protocols may vary in terms of dose and duration of treatment, most include an initial rapid dose escalation over one or more days followed by a more gradual dose build-up over months and a prolonged maintenance phase over months to years.[4] Although OIT with various food allergens have been studied, the majority of randomized controlled trials (RCTs) have focused on peanut, milk, and egg. OIT trials for food allergy show considerable heterogeneity with respect to study design, dosing protocol, and outcomes measured. While this limits the generalizability of findings, there is cumulative evidence that OIT can induce desensitization in the majority of treated subjects but is less effective at inducing SU. How OIT induces desensitization is still incompletely understood; however, an increase in food-specific IgG4 levels, decrease in basophil and mast cell activity,[7,8] and generation of regulatory T cells[9,10] have all been suggested to play a role. The critical immune mechanisms that determine SU as distinct from desensitization alone remain unknown. Changes in sIgG4, basophil or mast cell activity and T regulatory cells do not appear to be reliable biomarkers to distinguish between SU and desensitisation.

Peanut Oral immunotherapy

One of the first trials of peanut OIT was published in 2009.[8] Of 29 subjects who successfully completed the OIT protocol, 27 (93%) passed a 3.9 g peanut protein challenge after 4−22 months of maintenance therapy, confirming desensitization. This was followed by the first randomized, double-blind, placebo-controlled trial (DBPCT) of peanut OIT in 2011.[11] Varshney et al. presented data on 28 peanut allergic patients randomized to receive OIT (n = 19) or placebo (n = 9). A double-blind placebo-controlled food challenge (DBPCFC; cumulative dose 5g peanut protein) to assess for desensitization was conducted at 48 weeks. Sixteen of 19 (84%) OIT-treated subjects passed compared with 0 of 9 placebo-treated subjects. Subsequent studies reported similar desensitization rates ranging from 49% to 87%; however, few trials have assessed for SU (Table 14.1). The first study assessing SU enrolled 39 children aged 1−16 years with peanut allergy.[7] SU was assessed by DBPCFC with 5 g of peanut protein performed 4 weeks after stopping OIT once peanut IgE levels were less

Table 14.1 Peanut oral immunotherapy (OIT) studies.

Reference	Year	Design	Sample size	Maintenance dose (mg peanut protein)	Duration of OIT	DS: Intention to treat analysis	SU: Intention to treat analysis
Jones et al.[8]	2009	Open label	39	300–1800	36 mo	3.9g peanut protein OFC: 69% (27/39)	—
Blumchen et al.[14]	2010	Open label	23	125	8 wk	61% (14/23)	4g peanut protein DBPCFC after 2 weeks elimination: 13% (3/23)
Varshney et al.[11]	2011	Randomized, placebo-controlled	OIT n = 19; Placebo n = 9	4000	48 wk	5g peanut protein DBPCFC: OIT 84% (16/19) versus placebo 0% (0/9)	—
Anagnostou et al.[15]	2011	Open label	22	800	32 wk	6.6g peanut protein OFC: 64% (14/22)	—
Anagnostou et al.[16]	2014	Randomized controlled	OIT n = 49; avoidance n = 50	800	26 wk	1.4g peanut protein DBPCFC: OIT 49% (24/49) versus avoidance 0% (0/50)	—
Vickery et al.[7]	2014	Open label	39	1800–4000	Up to 5 yr	—	5g peanut protein DBPCFC after 4 weeks elimination: 31% (12/39)
Syed et al.[12]	2014	Age-matched controlled	OIT n = 23; avoidance n = 20	4000	24 mo	3.9g peanut protein OFC: OIT 87% (20/23) versus avoidance 0% (0/20)	3.9g peanut protein OFC after 3 months elimination: 30% (7/23); after 6 months elimination: 13% (3/23)

Study	Year	Design	n	Dose (mg)	Duration	Desensitization	Sustained unresponsiveness
Narisety et al.[17]	2015	Randomized OIT versus SLIT	OIT n = 11; SLIT n = 10	OIT 2g, SLIT 3.7 mg	16–22 mo	10g peanut protein OFC: 16 mo OIT 9% (1/11), 22mo OIT + 6mo SLIT 45% (5/11) vs 16mo SLIT 0% (0/10), 22mo SLIT + 6mo OIT 50% (5/10)	10g peanut protein OFC after 4 weeks elimination: 16 mo OIT 9% (1/11), 22 mo OIT + 6 mo SLIT 27% (3/11) 16 mo SLIT 0% (0/10), 22 mo SLIT + 6 mo OIT 10% (1/10)
Vickery et al.[13]	2016	2 doses of OIT	Low dose n = 20; high dose n = 17	300 (low dose); 3000 (high dose)	Up to 48 mo	5g peanut protein DBPCFC: low dose 85% (17/20) versus high dose 76% (13/17)	5g peanut protein DBPCFC after 4 weeks elimination: low dose 85% (17/20) versus high dose 71% (12/17)
Kukkonen et al.[18]	2017	Randomized controlled	OIT n = 39; avoidance n = 21	800	8 mo	1.255g peanut protein DBPCFC: OIT 67% (26/39) versus avoidance 0% (0/21)	—

DS, desensitization; SU, sustained unresponsiveness; OFC, open food challenge; DBPCFC, double-blind placebo-controlled food challenge; SLIT, sublingual immunotherapy.

than 2kU/L (the protocol was later amended to offer DBPCFC to subjects with peanut IgE levels less than 15kU/L, skin prick wheal of less than 5 mm and no peanut-related reaction in the previous 6 months). All remaining subjects underwent DBPCFC to assess for SU at the end of 5 years of OIT after stopping OIT for 4 weeks regardless of their immune parameters. SU was attained in 31% (12 of 39) subjects by intention to treat analysis (50% by per protocol analysis), and SU was associated with lower IgE levels for peanut, Ara h1, Ara h2, smaller skin prick wheal size and lower ratios of peanut-specific IgE/total IgE compared with subjects who failed challenges. Of note, the SU achieved with OIT appears to be transient. In a recent controlled study by Syed et al., of 23 peanut-allergic subjects who completed 24 months of OIT, 20 (87%) were successfully desensitized compared with 0 of 20 age-matched controls.[12] Desensitized subjects went on to avoid peanut for 3 months following which they underwent open food challenges (OFCs). SU was achieved 7 of 23 (30%) subjects; however, only 3 (13%) passed a second OFC after avoiding peanut for a further 3 months. Therefore OIT was highly effective at inducing desensitization but had a lesser ability to induce SU, and SU was lost by 6 months in approximately half of the subjects who initially achieved SU.

Higher rates of SU were reported in a more recent randomized trial comparing OIT with 300 mg peanut protein versus 3000 mg peanut protein in young children less than 36 months of age.[13] A caveat of this study is that there was no parallel control group to account for natural resolution of peanut allergy. Nevertheless, the findings suggest that the ability for OIT to induce SU may be enhanced by commencing treatment in the first years of life when there is greater plasticity of immune responses. Given the potential for natural resolution of allergy in this early period, the appropriateness of commencing OIT in the first years of life will ultimately depend upon an ability to identify those children who would not be expected to outgrow their peanut allergy naturally.

Egg oral immunotherapy

The first report of egg OIT used to treat a child with egg anaphylaxis was published in 1908.[19] Since then, studies have reported desensitization rates of 57%–94% with egg OIT (Table 14.2). The first double blind placebo controlled trial evaluating for SU randomized egg-allergic patients to receive OIT (n = 40) or placebo (n = 15).[20] Desensitization was assessed with a DBPCFC at 10 months in all subjects, following which placebo was stopped while OIT was continued in the active group on an open-label basis. OIT was discontinued at 22 months following which a DBPCFC was performed after 2 months egg elimination to assess for SU in all active participants and selected placebo-treated subjects with egg-specific IgE less than 2kU/L (applicable to 1 of 15 placebo participants). SU was achieved in 11 of 40 (28%) subjects receiving OIT compared with 0 of 15 placebo-treated children. Given that only 1 placebo-treated subject underwent the OFC to assess for SU while all OIT-treated subjects completed SU food challenges, this finding should be interpreted with caution. OIT was continued in OIT-treated children who failed to achieve SU at

Table 14.2 Egg Oral immunotherapy (OIT).

Reference	Year	Design	Sample size	Maintenance dose (g egg white protein)	Duration	DS: Intention to treat analysis	SU: Intention to treat analysis
Buchanan et al.[22]	2007	Open label	7	0.3	24 mo	8g egg protein DBPCFC: 57% (4/7);	8g egg protein DCPFC after 4 months elimination: 29% (2/7)
Vickery et al.[23]	2010	Open label	8	0.3–3.6	18–50 mo	10g egg protein DBPCFC: 75% (6/8)	10g egg protein DBPCFC after 4 weeks elimination: 75% (6/8)
Burks et al.[20]	2012	Randomized, placebo-controlled	OIT n = 40, placebo n = 15	2	22 mo	10g egg protein DBPCFC: OIT 75% (30/40) versus placebo 0% (0/15)	10g egg protein DBPCFC after 2 months elimination: OIT 28% (11/40) placebo not tested
Jones et al.[21]	2016	Open label follow-up study of Burks et al. 2012[19]	55	2	Up to 4 yr	10g egg protein OFC: 78% (31/40)	10g egg protein OFC after 4 weeks elimination: 50% (20/40) after 4 years
Escudero et al.[24]	2015	Randomized controlled	OIT n = 30, avoidance n = 31	1 undercooked egg every 48h	3 mo	2.8 g EW protein DBPCFC: OIT 93% (28/30)	2.8 g EW protein DBPCFC after 4 weeks elimination: OIT 37% (11/30) versus avoidance 3% (1/31)
Caminiti et al.[25]	2015	Randomized placebo-controlled	OIT n = 17, placebo n = 14	4	10 mo	3.7 g EW protein DBPCFC: OIT 94% (16/17) versus placebo 0% (0/14);	3.7 g EW protein DBPCFC after 3 months elimination: OIT 29% (5/17) versus placebo 7% (1/14)

DS, desensitization; SU, sustained unresponsiveness; EW, egg white; OFC, open food challenge; DBPCFC, double-blind placebo-controlled food challenge.

24 months in a follow-up study.[21] SU was achieved in 20 of 40 (50%) subjects after up to 4 years of treatment. However, lack of a parallel placebo-treated group to control for natural resolution of egg allergy again makes this finding difficult to interpret—one is unable to assess whether the increased rate of SU over time related to an increased duration of OIT or to natural resolution of egg allergy over time.

Milk Oral immunotherapy

As with egg OIT, cow's milk OIT consistently induces desensitization in 36%—90% of treated subjects (Table 14.3). However, few studies have evaluated for SU following milk OIT. In an RCT by Keet et al. comparing milk OIT with SLIT,[26] 30 milk allergic patients were randomized to SLIT alone or SLIT followed by OIT. Desensitization rates were greater with SLIT/OIT compared with SLIT/SLIT (70% in the SLIT-/OIT-treated group compared to 10% in the SLIT/SLIT group). SU, as assessed by OFC 6 weeks after stopping treatment, was only achieved in 8 of 20 (40%) of OIT-treated subjects compared to 1 of 10 (10%) in the SLIT group. Of the 8 OIT-treated subjects who achieved SU, 2 regained reactivity after just 1 additional week off therapy.

Safety and tolerability of oral immunotherapy
Reactions during oral immunotherapy

Adverse events related to OIT are frequent, and reactions requiring adrenaline occur more frequently when compared with other forms of immunotherapy[26] or dietary avoidance.[33] In a recent retrospective analysis of data pooled from three peanut OIT trials, it was reported that 80% of subjects experienced OIT-related adverse events with 72% occurring during build-up and 47% during maintenance.[34] Of the 104 subjects included in the study, 42% experienced systemic reactions and 49% experienced gastrointestinal symptoms. It has also been reported that up to 36% of participants discontinue OIT because of adverse events.[35] While cofactors such as infection, exercise, or allergen exposure have been reported to increase the risk of reaction,[36,37] these have been identified in only the minority of adverse reactions and a major concern with OIT is that reactions remain unpredictable.

There have also been reports of eosinophilic esophagitis (EoE) developing while on OIT.[38–41] EoE, a chronic esophageal disorder characterized by esophageal dysfunction and eosinophil-predominant inflammation, is considered a form of food allergy because food avoidance can induce remission in up to 90% of patients.[42] In an RCT comparing egg OIT (n = 40) with avoidance (n = 32), 1 subject in the active group was withdrawn because of EoE development while none were reported in the avoidance group.[40] A recent metaanalysis reported that new onset EoE after OIT occurs in up to 2.7% of patients undergoing OIT for an IgE-mediated food allergy.[41] However, significant publication bias was noted with a

Table 14.3 Milk Oral immunotherapy (OIT).

Reference	Year	Design	Sample size	Maintenance dose (g milk protein)	Duration	DS: Intention to treat analysis	SU: Intention to treat analysis
Meglio et al.[27]	2004	Open label	21	3.2	6 mo	8g milk protein DBPCFC: 71% (15/21)	–
Longo et al.[28]	2008	Randomized controlled	OIT n = 30, Avoidance = 30	4.8	1 yr	4.8g milk protein DBPCFC: OIT 36% (11/30) versus avoidance 0% (0/30)	–
Skripak et al.[29]	2008	Randomized placebo controlled	OIT n = 13, placebo n = 7	0.5	23 wk	Median eliciting dose increased from 40 to 5140 mg in OIT versus no change in placebo ($P = 0.0003$)	–
Narisety et al.[30]	2009	Open label follow-up study of Skripal et al. 2008	15	1–16	17 wk	Median eliciting dose increased from 40 mg to 10 000 mg	–
Pajno et al.[31]	2010	Randomized placebo-controlled	OIT n = 15, Soy n = 15	6.4	18 wk	4.6g milk protein DBPCFC: OIT 67% (10/15) versus Soy 0% (0/15)	–
Martorell et al.[32]	2011	Randomized placebo-controlled	OIT n = 30, Placebo n = 30	6.4	1 yr	4.4g milk protein DBPCFC: OIT 90% (27/30) versus placebo 23% (7/30)	–
Keet at al.[26]	2012	Randomized OIT versus SLIT	OIT n = 20, SLIT n = 10	OIT: 1–2g, SLIT: 7 mg	60 wk	8g milk protein OFC: OIT 70% (14/20) versus SLIT 10% (1/10);	8g milk protein OFC after 1 week elimination: OIT 60% (12/20) versus SLIT 10% (1/10)

DS, desensitization; SU, sustained unresponsiveness; OFC, open food challenge; DBPCFC, double-blind placebo-controlled food challenge; SLIT, sublingual immunotherapy.

trend toward reporting a positive association between OIT and EoE. Furthermore, the prevalence of EoE in patients with IgE-mediated food allergy is reported to be higher than the general population (4.7% vs. 0.04%).[43] This raises the intriguing possibility that OIT leads to EoE because of repeated exposure to the offending food rather than OIT being a risk factor for EoE per se. In other words, the underlying allergic response to food allergen which initially manifested as an IgE-mediated phenotype when food allergen is encountered infrequently may instead shift toward a chronic inflammatory response, which manifests as EoE, when there is frequent and regular or repeated exposure to food allergen that induces downregulation of the immediate allergic response to allergen.

Long-term safety of desensitization following oral immunotherapy

Since desensitization does not modify the underlying allergy, desensitized subjects remain allergic to their food allergen and must continue regular (usually daily) ingestion of the allergen to maintain the level of protection that has been achieved by the OIT protocol. However, in the desensitized state, an individual's reaction threshold (i.e., level of protection) can fluctuate over time, so reactions to the continuing allergen ingestion that is required to maintain desensitization are not uncommon, even to previously tolerated doses. In a 5-year follow-up of 32 milk-allergic children desensitized following OIT,[44] 16 (50%) were limiting cow's milk intake because of symptoms. Additionally, 6 of 27 participants who continued regular cow's milk intake experienced at least one episode of anaphylaxis in the preceding 12 months and intramuscular adrenaline was required at least twice a month for one subject. Another study[45] reported similar findings among 132 children desensitized to cow's milk. Of those on daily doses of cow's milk, 64% experienced one or more reactions up to 7 years after discharge with 35% reporting 5 or more reactions. A nationwide questionnaire-based survey looking at the use and practice of OIT in Japan found that during a median follow-up period of 4 years, immediate allergic reactions occurred in 68% of patients while hospitalized and 56% following discharge.[46] Allergic reactions requiring adrenaline at home were reported in 2% of patients. Furthermore, 16 of 7973 patients treated with OIT reported adverse reactions other than immediate allergic reactions with eosinophilic gastroenteritis being the most common diagnosis. This frequency of reactions, particularly severe reactions, is higher than what has been reported with allergen avoidance. There have been no studies comparing the long-term safety of desensitization and SU.

Additional follow-up studies evaluating the long-term safety and impact of OIT-induced desensitization on QOL are necessary. Although studies suggest that desensitization is associated with some improvement in QOL,[47,48] it remains to be determined whether this improvement is maintained over time as individuals experience unexpected and frequent reactions to continuing regular allergen exposure that is required to maintain the desensitized state.

Oral immunotherapy with adjuvant therapy

In order to reduce adverse events associated with OIT and improve efficacy in inducing tolerance, the use of an adjuvant together with food immunotherapy has been explored with varying success. One such adjuvant is the anti-IgE monoclonal antibody, omalizumab, which was previously shown to increase the threshold of reactivity during peanut challenges.[49,50] Omalizumab has been used in combination with OIT for various foods including peanut,[51] egg,[31] and milk.[52–54] In one of the first trials evaluating rapid OIT to milk using omalizumab, 11 children received omalizumab for 9 weeks prior to starting OIT.[52] This was discontinued after 16 weeks while daily milk intake was continued. Desensitization was confirmed by DBPCFC at 25 weeks in 9 of 11 (82%) children although 1 subject dropped out because of abdominal pain.

While omalizumab appears effective in facilitating faster attainment of higher maintenance OIT doses with fewer reactions, this protection is not sustained once omalizumab is discontinued. Lafuente et al.[31] described recurrence of gastrointestinal symptoms 3–4 months after omalizumab was stopped in three children desensitized with omalizumab-egg OIT which resolved once omalizumab was restarted. Furthermore, studies indicate that administration of omalizumab with OIT does not improve the likelihood of achieving desensitization or SU. In a double blind placebo controlled randomised trial by Wood et al.,[54] 57 milk-allergic children were randomized to receive omalizumab or placebo 4 months prior to initiation of OIT. This was stopped at month 28 when a DBPCFC to assess for desensitization was performed. Those who were successfully desensitized continued OIT for a further 8 weeks, following which a second DBPCFC to assess for SU was performed 2 months after stopping OIT. While omalizumab-assisted OIT was associated with fewer allergic reactions, decreased subject withdrawal rate, and faster time to reach maintenance dose, it had no beneficial effect on desensitization or SU rates.

There has been growing interest in the use of bacterial adjuvants to enhance immunotherapy based on their ability to support Th1 and/or tolerance responses. Tang et al.[55] performed a double blind placebo controlled randomized trial of probiotic *Lactobacillus rhamnosus* CGMCC 1.3724 and peanut OIT (probiotic and peanut oral immunotherapy (PPOIT)) in 62 children with peanut allergy. Participants were randomized to receive PPOIT (n = 31) or placebo (n = 31) for 18 months, following which a DBPCFC to assess for SU was conducted 2–6 weeks after treatment was discontinued. Of PPOIT-treated subjects, 23 of 31 (74%) achieved SU compared 1 of 31 (3%) placebo-treated subjects. Persistent SU was demonstrated 4 years after completing treatment in a long-term follow-up study.[6] Among those subjects who were enrolled in the follow-up study, 67% (16/24) of PPOIT-treated subjects were still eating peanut compared with 4% (1/24) of placebo-treated subjects. Challenge-proven 8-week SU was confirmed in 58% (7/12) of the PPOIT group compared with 7% (1/15) of the placebo group (95% CI 21–82, P = .012) 4 years after stopping treatment. Among initial treatment responders who achieved SU at end of treatment, 80% (16/20) were still eating peanut and 70% (7/10) had challenge-confirmed 8-week SU 4 years after stopping treatment. Reactions to peanut were uncommon and similar in both PPOIT and placebo-treated groups, and there were no episodes of anaphylaxis. Of note, those subjects who were shown to have persistent SU at 4 years after stopping treatment reported no allergic reactions to ad libitum peanut intake in the intervening 4 years, suggesting that they had indeed achieved true oral tolerance. A limitation of this study was that it did not include an OIT-only group to confirm whether the addition of probiotic was important for enhancing tolerance acquisition. A larger multicentre RCT comparing PPOIT, placebo-peanut OIT, and placebo-placebo is currently underway to address this question.

Sublingual immunotherapy

SLIT for food allergy involves daily application of a food allergen extract under the tongue which is held for 2–3 minutes and then swallowed. The immunological effects of SLIT are thought to be mediated by the high numbers of tolerogenic antigen-presenting cells present in the sublingual space.[56] However, efficacy may be limited by the low concentrations of allergen in available extracts and the volume of liquid that can be held sublingually.

Sublingual immunotherapy efficacy

The first double blind placebo controlled randomized trial was conducted in adults with hazelnut allergy.[57] Hazelnut-allergic patients with either oral allergy syndrome (n = 12) or acute IgE-mediated reactions (n = 10) were randomized to receive SLIT (n = 12) or placebo (n = 11). DBPCFCs were conducted between 8 and 12 weeks of therapy to assess for desensitization. SLIT-treated subjects demonstrated an increase in dose of tolerated protein from 2.29 to 11.56g ($P = 0.02$) while no change in tolerated dose was noted among placebo-treated subjects.

Subsequent studies of peanut and milk SLIT also demonstrated increase in tolerated doses of allergen after therapy. In a DBPCT of peanut SLIT,[58] 40 subjects were randomized to receive SLIT with a maximum dose of 1.4 mg (n = 20) or placebo (n = 20). All subjects underwent an OFC after 44 weeks of treatment, of which 14 of 20 (70%) SLIT subjects were considered responders with desensitization (tolerated 5g or more than 10-fold increase in peanut protein) compared with 3 of 20 (15%) in the placebo group. After the 44-week OFC, participants in the placebo group crossed over to a dose of 3.7 mg and treatment in both groups was continued for 3 years in an open label study.[59] Responders showed a significant decrease in peanut-specific basophil activation and skin prick test wheal size compared with nonresponders. SU, as determined by an OFC with 10g of peanut protein following 8 weeks of elimination, was then assessed and was achieved in 4 of 37 (11%) subjects, and the authors concluded that "peanut SLIT safely induced a modest level of desensitization in a majority of subjects compared with placebo."

Three studies compared OIT and SLIT, and one of them was a retrospective comparison.[17,26,60] Keet et al. compared OIT against SLIT for milk allergy, and the results are as reported in a previous section.[26] In a randomized double-blind study of peanut-allergic children, 21 participants were randomized to receive SLIT/placebo OIT (n = 10) or OIT/placebo SLIT (n = 11).[17] DBPCFCs were conducted at 6 and 12 months of therapy. Of the 16 subjects who completed 12 months of treatment, all had a greater than 10-fold increase in the tolerated dose with the increase being significantly greater in the OIT group (21 −7246 mg, $P < 0.001$) compared to the SLIT group (21 −496 mg, $P = 0.01$). Similarly, a greater decrease in skin prick test results, reduction in peanut-specific IgE, and increase in peanut-specific IgG4 levels were noted among OIT-treated subjects. SU was assessed with a 10g peanut protein OFC performed 4 weeks after stopping therapy. Only 3 of 11 (27%) OIT subjects and 1 of 10 (10%) SLIT subjects achieved SU. It appears that while SLIT is moderately effective in inducing desensitization, it has little ability to induce SU.

Sublingual immunotherapy safety

SLIT is well tolerated in the majority of individuals with most allergic reactions limited to oropharyngeal itching. In the study by Fleischer et al.,[58] of 5825 peanut SLIT doses given in the first phase (baseline to week 44 challenge), 40.1% were associated with symptoms. However, on exclusion of oropharyngeal symptoms, 94.7% were symptom free. The majority (86%) of adverse events were assessed to be mild in severity and only one dose of adrenaline was given in a patient who initially complained of oropharyngeal symptoms but went on to develop urticaria and coughing during the build-up stage. A dose of adrenaline was given at home following which the decision was made to stop SLIT. In the follow-up study by Burks et al.,[59] 98% of doses were tolerated without adverse reactions beyond oropharyngeal symptoms and there were no severe symptoms that required adrenaline. However, only 16 of 40 (40%) participants completed the full 3 years of therapy and among those who chose to withdraw for reasons other than dosing symptoms or noncompliance, most subjects found the daily dosing "too difficult to maintain."

Studies that compared OIT and SLIT also show that SLIT is generally better tolerated than OIT. Keet et al.[26] noted that while OIT was more effective at inducing desensitization, it was associated with more multisystem (IRR 11.5, $P < 0.001$), upper respiratory tract (IRR 4.7, $P = 0.004$), gastrointestinal (IRR 3.3, $P = 0.01$), and lower respiratory tract (IRR 8.9, $P < 0.001$) symptoms compared with SLIT. Similar findings were reported by Narisety et al.[17] with more adverse reactions, doses requiring adrenaline and study discontinuation due to gastrointestinal symptoms reported with OIT (Table 14.4).

Epicutaneous immunotherapy

EPIT involves applying an allergen-containing patch to different locations on the back or upper arm every 24 hours for 1 year or longer. It is designed to activate skin Langerhans cells and lead to systemic downregulation of effector cell responses.[63]

Table 14.4 Sublingual immunotherapy studies.

Reference	Year	Food	Design	Sample size	Maintenance dose	Duration	DS	SU
Enrique et al.[57]	2005	Hazelnut	Randomized placebo-controlled	SLIT n = 12, placebo n = 11	13.25 mg	8–12 wk	Mean tolerated dose increased from 2.29 to 11.56g ($P = 0.02$) in SLIT versus no change in placebo	
Kim et al.[61]	2011	Peanut	Randomized placebo-controlled	SLIT n = 11, placebo n = 7	2 mg	12 mo	Median tolerated dose: SLIT 1710 mg versus placebo 85 mg ($P = 0.011$)	
Fleischer et al.[58]	2012	Peanut	Randomized placebo-controlled	SLIT n = 20, placebo n = 20	1.4 mg	44 wk	5g peanut protein or 10-fold increase in tolerated dose: SLIT 70% (14/20) versus placebo 15% (3/20)	
Burks et al.[59]	2015	Peanut	Open label	37	1.4 mg, 3.7 mg	3 yr		10g peanut protein OFC after 8 weeks elimination: 11% (4/37)
Narisety et al.[17]	2015	Peanut	Double-blind randomized OIT versus SLIT	OIT n = 11, SLIT n = 10	OIT: 2000 mg, SLIT: 3.7 mg	6 mo	Median-tolerated dose increased from 21 to 7246 mg ($P < 0.001$) in OIT versus 21 –496 mg ($P = 0.01$) in SLIT	10g peanut protein OFC after 4 weeks elimination: OIT 27% (3/11) versus SLIT 10% (1/10)
Boissieu et al.[62]	2006	Milk	Open label	8	1 mL	6 mo	Mean-eliciting dose increased from 1.2 to 4.6g ($P < 0.01$)	
Keet at al.[26]	2012	Milk	Randomized OIT versus SLIT	OIT n = 20, SLIT n = 10	OIT: 1–2g, SLIT: 7 mg	60 wk	8g milk protein OFC: OIT 70% (14/20) versus SLIT 10% (1/10);	8g milk protein OFC after 1 week elimination: OIT 60% (12/20) versus SLIT 10% (1/10)

Epicutaneous immunotherapy efficacy

A pilot study of milk EPIT[64] in 19 children randomized to receive EPIT (n = 10) or placebo (n = 9) for 3 months reported a 12-fold increase in the mean cumulative tolerated dose from $1.77 + 2.98$ mL to $23.61 + 28.61$ mL ($P = .18$) in the EPIT group compared with no change ($4.36 + 5.87$ mL to $5.44 + 5.88$ mL) in the placebo group.

Jones et al.[65] evaluated the efficacy of EPIT in peanut allergy. In a Phase II clinical trial, 74 children and young adults with peanut allergy were randomized to receive either Viaskin Peanut 100 mcg (VP100, n = 24), Viaskin Peanut 250 mcg (VP250, n = 25), or placebo (n = 25). Treatment success was defined as passing a DBPCFC with 5g of peanut protein or achieving a 10-fold increase in tolerated dose from baseline OFC after 52 weeks of treatment. Treatment success was achieved in 12 of 25 (48%) subjects receiving 250mcg, 11 of 24 (46%) receiving 100mcg, and 3 of 25 (12%) receiving placebo ($P = 0.003$ and $P = 0.005$ respectively, compared with placebo). However, all except one placebo-treated participant met the treatment success criteria by achieving a 10-fold increase in tolerated dose and none of the actively treated subjects passed the 5g peanut protein challenge. Post hoc analysis of patients who tolerated at least 1044 mg of peanut protein and a 10-fold increase from baseline revealed that only 4 VP250-treated subjects, 2 VP100-100-treated subjects, and 2 placebo-treated subjects met this definition of success (P = not significant for all comparisons). Successful outcomes were noted to be more common in subjects less than 11 years: 11 of 18 (61%) in VP250 group versus 10/17 (59%) in VP100 group versus 1/18 (6%) in placebo group. Treatment with peanut EPIT was associated with increases in peanut-specific IgG4 levels and IgG4/IgE ratios as well as trends toward reduced basophil activation.

EPIT appears to be more effective in inducing desensitization in younger age groups. In the VIPES trial,[66] 221 peanut allergic individuals were randomized to receive patches (Viaskin peanut) containing 50 mcg (n = 53), 100 mcg (n = 56), or 250 mcg (n = 56) of peanut protein or placebo (n = 56) for 12 months. Treatment responders were defined if the OFC eliciting dose was 1000 mg or more than 10-fold increase from baseline. A significant difference in response rates was noted between the 250 mcg and placebo groups (50% vs. 25%). There was no significant difference between the 100 mcg and placebo groups. A significant difference was noted in the 6-to-11 years stratum between those who received 250 mcg and placebo patches (53.6% vs. 19.4%) while no difference was found in adolescents/adults. Following the first year of treatment, 171 subjects were enrolled in a 2-year, open label extension where they were transitioned to the 250-mcg patch for the remainder of the study. Response rates at 12 and 24 months were 59.7% (89/149) and 64.5% (80/124), respectively. Again higher response rates were noted in children compared with adolescents/adults. In the PEPITES study, a Phase III double blind placebo controlled randomized trial, 356 peanut-allergic children aged 4–11 years with a baseline eliciting dose (ED) of <300 mg peanut protein on DBPCFC were randomized 2:1 to receive VP250mcg or placebo-patch for 12 months.[67] Response was defined as an increase in ED to >300 mg (if baseline ED <10 mg) or >1000 mg (if baseline ED > 10 mg) at the 12-month DBPCFC. Response rates were 35.3% in the VP250 group compared to 13.6% in the placebo group ($P = .00,001$). The median cumulative reactive dose increased from median 144 mg in both groups to 444 mg in the VP250 group and 144 mg in the placebo group ($P < .001$).

Epicutaneous immunotherapy safety

As the epidermis is not vascularized, the risk of systemic reactions to EPIT is expected to be low, and studies have confirmed this.[64-68] EPIT is generally well tolerated with the majority of reactions being mild and limited to the patch site. In the study by Jones et al.,[65] non–patch site reactions were uncommon (0.1% of VP250 doses, 0.2% of VP100 doses, and 0.2% of placebo). The most frequent treatment was topical corticosteroids followed by oral antihistamines while adrenaline was not used for any dosing symptoms. Local skin reactions may decrease over time[67] but still remain the most common adverse event reported in the second year of treatment (Table 14.5).

Other novel approaches

Other approaches to food immunotherapy, including DNA vaccines,[69,70] recombinant vaccines,[71] tolerogenic peptides,[72,73] and Chinese herbal formula (FAHF-2),[74,75] have been explored in animal models and preclinical trials with varying results. Use of attenuated bacteria as carriers of recombinant allergens to induce Th1 responses and thereby enhance immunogenicity was found to protect peanut allergic mice from anaphylaxis.[76] This study was followed by a Phase I trial of heat/phenol filled *Escherichia coli* encapsulated recombinant modified peanut proteins Ara h 1, Ara h 2, and Ara h 3 (EMP-123) in peanut allergic human subjects and healthy controls.[71] However, treatment in allergic subjects had to be discontinued because 5 of 10 peanut allergic patients experienced unexpected severe adverse reactions. Similarly, a recent Phase 2 trial[75] evaluating the efficacy of a traditional Chinese herbal medication (food allergy herbal formula, FAHF-2) failed to demonstrate efficacy in allergic subjects despite promising results in preclinical trials.[74,77] These findings emphasize that murine models do not fully replicate the physiology of human disease and efficacy in preclinical studies may not translate to successful outcomes in human clinical trials. Future studies are being pursued to determine if these novel strategies will be safe and effective for treatment of food allergy in human subjects.

Conclusion

There are several potential outcomes that an effective food allergy treatment may offer: desensitization, SU, or tolerance. Tolerance is the preferred outcome for

Table 14.5 Epicutaneous immunotherapy (EPIT) studies.

Reference	Year	Food	Design	Sample size	Maintenance dose	Duration	Primary outcome
Dupont et al.[64]	2010	Milk	Randomized placebo-controlled	EPIT n = 10, placebo n = 9	1 mg	3 mo	Mean tolerated dose increased from 1.77 to 23.61 mL (P = 0.18) in EPIT versus no change in placebo
Jones et al.[65]	2016	Peanut	Randomized placebo-controlled	VP100 n = 24, VP250 n = 25, Placebo n = 25	100 mcg 250 mcg	52 wk	5g peanut protein or 10-fold increase in tolerated dose: VP100 46% (11/24) versus VP250 48% (12/25) versus placebo 12% (3/25)
Sampson et al.[66] VIPES trial	2017	Peanut	Randomized placebo-controlled	EPIT n = 165, placebo n = 56	50, 100, 250 mcg	12 mo	1g peanut protein or 10-fold increase in eliciting dose: 250 mcg 50% (28/56) versus placebo 25% (14/56)
Fleischer et al.[67] PEPITES trial	2018	Peanut	Randomized placebo-controlled	n = 356	250 mcg	12 mo	Median reactive dose increased from 144 to 444 mg in EPIT versus no change in placebo (P < 0.001)

patients as this provides continuing protection against reactions without the need for ongoing regular allergen exposure and allows the individual to incorporate the food into their diet ad libitum if they so desire. SU also offers substantial protection, providing sustained ability to tolerate the allergen without reaction, although it is expected that some degree of continuing exposure is required to maintain this protection. The level of protection that is provided with SU can vary widely, and improved definitions are necessary to ensure that clear messages can be given to patients regarding their level of protection and whether this might only be to low levels of allergen thus requiring continued allergen avoidance or to higher amounts of allergen that allow them to incorporate their allergen into their diet. Clear guidance in this regard is vital for patient safety. Desensitization offers some benefit to patients; however, the level of benefit is diminished by the need for continued regular allergen ingestion to maintain protection and unpredictable fluctuations in the level of this protection such that the individual remains at risk of reaction to a previously tolerated dose of allergen. Yet, the majority of treatments currently under investigation are only able to induce desensitization and fail to induce SU in more than a minority of subjects. OIT appears to be more effective at inducing desensitization than SLIT or EPIT; however, it is associated with the highest rate and severity of treatment-related side effects and is more heath resource−intensive compared with SLIT and EPIT. SLIT is moderately effective at inducing desensitization and safer than OIT although adherence is a potential limiting factor. EPIT has the most favorable safety profile, but efficacy in inducing desensitization appears to be limited. The combination of a probiotic immune modifying adjuvant with OIT is the only treatment that has been shown to induce high rates of SU and to provide sustained benefit years after stopping active treatment suggesting the possibility of true tolerance; this approach may enhance the acquisition of SU and tolerance that can achieved with OIT as a stand-alone treatment and warrants further investigation. Major issues requiring further examination before any treatments can be recommended in clinical practice are whether it is safe or feasible to remain desensitized in the longer term and a greater understanding of the long-term efficacy and safety outcomes for potential interventions.

Competing Interests

MLK Tang is a past member of the Medical Advisory Board Oceania for Nestle Nutrition Institute; a past member of Global Scientific Advisory Board, Danone Nutricia; consultant to Abbott Nutrition and Bayer Pharmaceuticals; employee of and holding share options/interest in Prota Therapeutics; inventor on a patent owned by The Murdoch Children's Research Institute; presenter at seminars sponsored by Danone Nutricia and Nestle Health Science. W. Loh has no conflicts of interest to disclose.

References

1. Sampson HA, Aceves S, Bock SA, et al. Food allergy: a practice parameter update-2014. *J Allergy Clin Immunol*. 2014;134:1016–1025.
2. Leung ASY, Wong GWK, Tang MLK. Food allergy in the developing world. *J Allergy Clin Immunol*. 2018;141:76–78.
3. Flokstra-de Blok BM, Dubois AE. Quality of life measures for food allergy. *Clin Exp Allergy*. 2012;42:1014–1020.
4. Wood RA. Food allergen immunotherapy: current status and prospects for the future. *J Allergy Clin Immunol*. 2016;137:973–982.
5. Burks AW, Sampson HA, Plaut M, Lack G, Akdis C. Treatment for food allergy. *J Allergy Clin Immunol*. 2018;141:1–9.
6. Hsiao K-C, Posonby A-L, Axelrad C, Pitkin S, Tang MLK. Long-term clinical and immunological effects of probiotic and peanut oral immunotherapy after treatment cessation: 4-year follow-up of a randomised, double-blind, placebo-controlled trial. *Lancet Child Adolesc Health*. 2017;1:97–105.
7. Vickery BP, Scurlock AM, Kulis M, et al. Sustained unresponsiveness to peanut in subjects who have completed peanut oral immunotherapy. *J Allergy Clin Immunol*. 2014;133:468–475.
8. Jones SM, Pons L, Roberts JL, et al. Clinical efficacy and immune regulation with peanut oral immunotherapy. *J Allergy Clin Immunol*. 2009;124:292–300.
9. Vickery BP, Scurlock AM, Jones SM, Burks AW. Mechanisms of immune tolerance relevant to food allergy. *J Allergy Clin Immunol*. 2011;127:576–584.
10. Bedoret D, Singh AK, Shaw V, et al. Changes in antigen-specific T-cell number and function during oral desensitization in cow's milk allergy enabled with omalizumab. *Mucosal Immunol*. 2012;5:267–276.
11. Varshney P, Jones SM, Scurlock AM, et al. A randomized controlled study of peanut oral immunotherapy: Clinical desensitization and modulation of the allergic response. *J Allergy Clin Immunol*. 2011;127:654–660.
12. Syed A, Garcia MA, Lyu S, et al. Peanut oral immunotherapy results in increased antigen-induced regulatory T-cell function and hypomethylation of forkhead box protein 3 (FOXP3). *J Allergy Clin Immunol*. 2014;133:500–510.
13. Vickery BP, Berglund JP. Early oral immunotherapy in peanut allergic preschool children is safe and highly effective. *J Allergy Clin Immunol*. 2017;139:173–181.
14. Blumchen K, Ulbricht H, Staden U, et al. Oral peanut immunotherapy in children with peanut anaphylaxis. *J Allergy Clin Immunol*. 2010;126:83–91.
15. Anagnostou K, Clark A, King Y, Islam S, Deighton J, Ewan P. Efficacy and safety of high-dose peanut oral immunotherapy with factors predicting outcome. *Clin Exp Allergy*. 2011;41:1273–1281.
16. Anagnostou K, Islam S, King Y, et al. Assessing the efficacy of oral immunotherapy for the desensitisation of peanut allergy in (STOP II): a phase 2 randomised controlled trial. *Lancet*. 2014;383:1297–1304.
17. Narisety SD, Frischmeyer-Guerrerio PA, Keet CA, et al. A randomized, double-blind, placebo-controlled pilot study of sublingual versus oral immunotherapy for the treatment of peanut allergy. *J Allergy Clin Immunol*. 2015;135:1275–1282.
18. Kukkonen AK, Uotila R, Malmberg LP, Pelkonen AS, Makela MJ. Double-blind placebo-controlled challenge showed that peanut oral immunotherapy was effective

for severe allergy without negative effects on airway inflammation. *Acta Paediatr*. 2017; 106:274–281.

19. Schofield AT. A case of egg poisoning. *Lancet*. 1908;171:716.

20. Burks AW, Jones SM, Wood RA, et al. Oral immunotherapy for treatment of egg allergy in children. *N Engl J Med*. 2012;367:233–243.

21. Jones SM, Burks AW, Keet C, et al. Long-term treatment with egg oral immunotherapy enhances sustained unresponsiveness that persists after cessation of therapy. *J Allergy Clin Immunol*. 2016;137:1117–1127.

22. Buchanan AD, Green TD, Jones SM, et al. Egg oral immunotherapy in nonanaphylactic children with egg allergy. *J Allergy Clin Immunol*. 2007;119:199–205.

23. Vickery BP, Pons L, Kulis M, et al. Individualized IgE-based dosing of egg oral immunotherapy and the development of tolerance. *Ann Allergy Asthma Immunol*. 2010;105: 444–450.

24. Escudero C, Rodriguez Del Rio P, Sanchez-Garcia S, et al. Early sustained unresponsiveness after short-course egg oral immunotherapy: a randomized controlled study in egg-allergic children. *Clin Exp Allergy*. 2015;45:1833.

25. Caminiti L, Pajno GB, Crisafulli G, et al. Oral Immunotherapy for egg allergy: a double-blind placebo-controlled study, with post desensitization follow-up. *J Allergy Clin Immunol Pract*. 2015;3:532–539.

26. Keet CA, Frischmeyer-Guerrerio PA, Thyagarajan A, et al. The safety and efficacy of sublingual and oral immunotherapy for milk allergy. *J Allergy Clin Immunol*. 2012; 129:448–455.

27. Meglio P, Giampietro PG, Gianni S, Galli E. Oral desensitization in children with immunoglobulin E-mediated cow's milk allergy—follow-up at 4 yr and 8 months. *Pediatr Allergy Immunol*. 2008;19:412–419.

28. Longo G, Barbi E, Berti I, et al. Specific oral tolerance induction in children with very severe cow's milk-induced reactions. *J Allergy Clin Immunol*. 2008;121:343–347.

29. Skripak JM, Nash SD, Rowley H, et al. A randomized, double-blind, placebo-controlled study of milk oral immunotherapy for cow's milk allergy. *J Allergy Clin Immunol*. 2008; 122:1154–1160.

30. Narisety SD, Skripak JM, Steele P, et al. Open-label maintenance after milk oral immunotherapy for IgE-mediated cow's milk allergy. *J Allergy Clin Immunol*. 2009;124: 610–612.

31. Lafuente I, Mazon A, Nieto M, Uixera S, Pina R, Nieto A. Possible recurrence of symptoms after discontinuation of omalizumab in anti-IgE-assisted desensitization to egg. *Pediatr Allergy Immunol*. 2014;25:717–719.

32. Martorell A, De la Hoz B, Ibanez MD, et al. Oral desensitization as a useful treatment in 2-year-old children with cow's milk allergy. *Clin Exp Allergy*. 2011;41:1297–1304.

33. Brozek JL, Terracciano L, Hsu J, et al. Oral immunotherapy for IgE-mediated cow's milk allergy: a systematic review and metaanalysis. *Clin Exp Allergy*. 2012;42:363–374.

34. Yamini V, Burks AW, Steele PH, et al. Novel baseline predictors of adverse events during oral immunotherapy in children with peanut allergy. *J Allergy Clin Immunol*. 2017;139: 882–888.

35. Staden U, Rolinck-Werninghaus C, Brewe F, Wahn U, Niggemann B, Beyer K. Specific oral tolerance induction in food allergy in children: efficacy and clinical patterns of reaction. *Allergy*. 2007;62:1261–1269.

36. Varshney P, Steele PH, Vickery BP, et al. Adverse reactions during peanut oral immunotherapy home dosing. *J Allergy Clin Immunol*. 2009;124:1351–1352.

37. Sato S, Yanagida N, Ogura K, et al. Clinical studies in oral allergen-specific immuno-therapy: differences among allergens. *Int Arch Allergy Immunol.* 2014;164:1−9.
38. Ridolo E, De Angelis GL, Dall'Aglio P. Eosinophilic esophagitis after specific oral toler-ance induction for egg protein. *Ann Allergy Asthma Immunol.* 2011;106:73−74.
39. Sánchez-García S, Rodríguez Del Río P, Escudero C, Martínez-Gómez MJ, Ibáñez MD. Possible eosinophilic esophagitis induced by milk oral immunotherapy. *J Allergy Clin Immunol.* 2012;129:1155−1157.
40. Fuentes-Aparicio V, Alvarez-Perea A, Infante S, Zapatero L, D'Oleo A, Alonso-Lebrero E. Specific oral tolerance induction in paediatric patients with persistent egg allergy. *Allergol Immunopathol.* 2013;41:143−150.
41. Lucendo AJ, Angel A, Tenias JM. Relation between eosinophilic esophagitis and oral immunotherapy for food allergy: a systemic review with meta-analysis. *Ann Allergy Asthma Immunol.* 2014;113:624−629.
42. Greenhawt M, Aceves SS, Spergel JM, Rothenberg ME. The manangement of eosi-nophlic esophagitis. *J Allergy Clin Immunol Pract.* 2013;1:332−340.
43. Hill DA, Dudley JW, Spergel JM. The prevalence of eosinophilic esophagitis in pediatric patients with IgE-mediated food allergy. *J Allergy Clin Immunol Pract.* 2017;5: 369−375.
44. Keet CA, Seopaul S, Knorr S, Narisety S, Skripak J, Wood RA. Long-term follow-up of oral immunotherapy for cow's milk allergy. *J Allergy Clin Immunol.* 2013;132:737−739.
45. Barbi E, Longo G, Berti I, et al. Adverse effects during specific oral tolerance induction: in home phase. *Allergol Immunopathol.* 2012;40:41−50.
46. Sato S, Sugizaki C, Yanagida N, et al. Nationwide questionnaire-based survey of oral immunoterhapy in Japan. *Allergol Int.* 2018;1−6.
47. Carraro S, Frigo AC, Perin M, et al. Impact of oral immunotherapy on quality of life in children with cow milk allergy: a pilot study. *Int J Immunopathol Pharmacol.* 2012;25: 793−798.
48. Factor JM, Mendelson L, Lee J, Nouman G, Lester MR. Effect of oral immunotherapy to peanut on food-specific quality of life. *Ann Allergy Asthma Immunol.* 2012;109: 348−352.
49. Sampson HA, Leung DY, Burks AW, et al. A phase II, randomized, double-blind, parallel-group, placebo-controlled oral food challenge trial of xolair (omalizumab) in peanut allergy. *J Allergy Clin Immunol.* 2011;127:1309−1310.
50. Savage JH, Courneya JP, Sterba PM, Macglashan DW, Saini SS, Wood RA. Kinetics of mast cell, basophil, and oral food challenge responses in omalizumab-treated adults with peanut allergy. *J Allergy Clin Immunol.* 2012;130:1123−1129.
51. Schneider LC, Rachid R, LeBovidge J, Blood E, Mittal M, Umetsu DT. A pilot study of omalizumab to facilitate rapid oral desensitization in high-risk peanut allergic patients. *J Allergy Clin Immunol.* 2013;132:1368−1374.
52. Nadeau KC, Schneider LC, Hoyte L, Borras I, Umetsu DT. Rapid oral desensitization in combination with omalizumab therapy in patients with cow's milk allergy. *J Allergy Clin Immunol.* 2011;127:1622−1624.
53. Takahasi M, Taniuchi S, Soejima K, et al. Successful desensitisation in a boy with severe cow's milk allergy by combination therapy using omalizumab and rush oral immunotherapy. *Allergy Asthma Clin Immunol.* 2015;11:18.
54. Wood RA, Kim JS, Lindblad R, et al. A randomized, double-blind, placebo-controlled study of omalizumab combined with oral immunotherapy for the treatment of cow's milk allergy. *J Allergy Clin Immunol.* 2016;137:1103−1110.

55. Tang ML, Ponsonby AL, Orsini F, et al. Administration of a probiotic with peanut oral immunotherapy: a randomized trial. *J Allergy Clin Immunol*. 2015;135:737–744.

56. Akdis CA, Barlan IB, Bahceciler N, Akdis M. Immunological mechanisms of sublingual immunotherapy. *Allergy*. 2006;61:11–14.

57. Enrique E, Pineda F, Malek T, et al. Sublingual immunotherapy for hazelnut food allergy: a randomized, double-blind, placebo controlled study with a standardized hazelnut extract. *J Allergy Clin Immunol*. 2005;116:1073–1079.

58. Fleischer DM, Burks AW, Vickery BP, et al. Sublingual immunotherapy for peanut allergy: a randomized, double-blind, placebo-controlled multicenter trial. *J Allergy Clin Immunol*. 2013;131:119–127.

59. Burks AW, Wood RA, Jones SM, et al. Sublingual immunotherapy for peanut allergy: long-term follow-up of a randomized multicenter trial. *J Allergy Clin Immunol*. 2015; 135:1240–1248.

60. Chin SJ, Vickery BP, Kulis MD, et al. Sublingual versus oral immunotherapy for peanut-allergic children: a retrospective comparison. *J Allergy Clin Immunol*. 2013;132: 476–478.

61. Kim EH, Bird JA, Kulis M, et al. Sublingual immunotherapy for peanut allergy: clinical and immunologic evidence of desensitization. *J Allergy Clin Immunol*. 2011;127: 640–646.

62. de Boissieu D, Dupont C. Sublingual immunotherapy for cow's milk protein allergy: a preliminary report. *Allergy*. 2006;61:1238–1239.

63. Dioszeghy V, Mondoulet L, Dhelft V, et al. The regulatory T cells induction by epicutaneous immunotherapy is sustained and mediates long-term protection from eosinophilic disorders in peanut-sensitized mice. *Clin Exp Allergy*. 2014;44:867–881.

64. Dupont C, Kalach N, Soulaines P, Legoue-Morillon S, Piloquet H, Benhamou PH. Cow's milk epicutaneous immunotherapy in children: a pilot trial of safety, acceptability, and impact on allergic reactivity. *J Allergy Clin Immunol*. 2010;125:1165–1167.

65. Jones SM, Sicherer SH, Burks AW, et al. Epicutaneous immunotherapy for the treatment of peanut allergy in children and young adults. *J Allergy Clin Immunol*. 2017;139: 1242–1252.

66. Sampson HA, Shreffler WG, Yang WH, et al. Effect of varying doses of epicutaneous immunotherapy vs placebo on reaction to peanut protein exposure among patients with peanut sensitivity: a randomized clinical trial. *JAMA*. 2017;318:1798–1809.

67. Fleischer DM, Sussman GL, Begin P, et al. Effect of epicutaneous immunotherapy on inducing peanut desentisation in peanut-allergic children: Topline peanut epicutaneous immunotherapy efficacy and safety (PEPITES) randomized clinical trial results. *J Allergy Clin Immunol*. 2018;141:AB410.

68. Jones SM, Agbotounou WK, Fleischer DM, et al. Safety of epicutaneous immunotherapy for the treatment of peanut allergy: a phase 1 study using the Viaskin patch. *J Allergy Clin Immunol*. 2016;137:1258–1261.

69. Srivastava KD, Siefert A, Fahmy T, Caplan MJ, Li XM, Sampson HA. Investigation of peanut oral immunotherapy with CpG/peanut nanoparticles in a murine model of peanut allergy. *J Allergy Clin Immunol*. 2016;138:536–543.

70. Roy K, Mao HQ, Huang SK, Leong KW. Oral gene delivery with chitosan — DNA nanoparticles generates immunologic protection in a murine model of peanut allergy. *Nat Med*. 1999;5:387–391.

71. Wood RA, Sicherer SH, Burks AW, et al. A phase 1 study of heat/phenol-killed, E. coli-encapsulated, recombinant modified peanut proteins Ara h 1, Ara h 2, and Ara h 3 (EMP-123) for the treatment of peanut allergy. *Allergy.* 2013;68:803–808.

72. Yang M, Yang C, Mine Y. Multiple T cell epitope peptides suppress allergic responses in an egg allergy mouse model by the elicitation of forkhead box transcription factor 3- and transforming growth factor-beta-associated mechanisms. *Clin Exp Allergy.* 2010;40: 668–678.

73. Swoboda I, Balic N, Klug C, et al. A general strategy for the generation of hypoallergenic molecules for the immunotherapy of fish allergy. *J Allergy Clin Immunol.* 2013;132: 979–981.

74. Wang J, Patil SP, Yang N, et al. Safety, tolerability, and immunologic effects of a food allergy herbal formula in food allergic individuals: a randomized, double-blind, placebo-controlled, dose escalation, phase 1 study. *Ann Allergy Asthma Immnol.* 2010; 105:75–84.

75. Wang J, Jones SM, Pongracic JA, et al. Safety, clinical, and immunologic efficacy of a Chinese herbal medicine (Food allergy herbal formula-2) for food allergy. *J Allergy Clin Immunol.* 2015;136:962–970.

76. Li XM, Srivastava K, Grishin A, et al. Persistent protective effect of heat-killed *Escherichia coli* producing "engineered," recombinant peanut proteins in a murine model of peanut allergy. *J Allergy Clin Immunol.* 2003;112:159–167.

77. Srivastava KD, Kattan JD, Zou ZM, et al. The Chinese herbal medicine formula FAHF-2 completely blocks anaphylactic reactions in a murine model of peanut allergy. *J Allergy Clin Immunol.* 2005;115:171–178.

Adherence and pharmacoeconomics

Drew Murphy, MD

Chief Medical Officer, Allergy, Asthma Allergy and Sinus Center, West Chester, PA, United States

Allergic rhinitis (AR) is one of the most common diseases in the United States, affecting approximately 1 in 5 persons, and is associated with significant clinical and economic burden.[1] Globally, estimates suggest that AR may affect as many as 500 million people.[2] In the United States, the prevalence of AR is about 15% based upon physician diagnosis and 30% based on patient-reported symptoms.[3] In Europe, the prevalence of AR is about 23%.[4] AR tends to be underdiagnosed by healthcare professionals and its impact, underappreciated by patients. Typically patients have longstanding symptoms before proper diagnosis is made[4-7] Poorly controlled AR can be associated with a number of comorbid conditions, e.g., asthma, recurrent otitis media, and recurrent sinusitis. It can also be associated with a number of symptoms that can greatly impact the patient's quality of life, e.g., impaired sleep with resultant poor school/work performance (aka presentism), decreased energy, depressed mood, and low frustration tolerance These symptoms can result in millions of lost work and school days annually, which adds to healthcare cost burden of poorly controlled asthma.[3,4,8,9] Thus, poorly controlled AR can be associated with considerable direct and indirect costs to the patient, the payer, and the national healthcare system.

In 2005, estimated total direct US costs of AR exceeded $11 billion ($14 billion in 2011), with 60% of expenditures for prescription medications. AR is often associated with additional comorbid disease, including asthma sinus and otitis media for which additional billions of dollars are reportedly spent to treat these conditions.[10,11]

Standard medical treatment for AR includes identification and avoidance of known allergens and pharmacotherapy. Pharmacotherapy includes use of nonsedating oral antihistamines, topical nasal antihistamines, and topical nasal steroids.[1,3,12] These medications can be used regularly to prevent the development of AR symptoms or as needed with the onset of symptoms. Even with use of these medications patients still will not have optional control of their symptoms—up to 33% of children and ~60% of adults will have suboptimal control of their AR symptoms with pharmacotherapy alone.[8,13]

For patients with more severe AR, who have not responding to pharmacotherapy, or are having troublesome medication side effects of treatment, or just simply want to reduce the use of medication, allergen immunotherapy (AIT) should be considered.[1,14] AIT is different from avoidance and pharmacotherapy in that it is a disease-modifying treatment. AIT has been reported to mitigate the development of asthma,[15–18] the development of new allergen sensitivities,[19–25] and has been shown to maintain efficacy after discontinuation of treatment.[19,25–32]

Currently two forms of AIT are available: subcutaneous immunotherapy (SCIT) and sublingual immunotherapy (SLIT) each with its advantages and disadvantages. SCIT is effective for seasonal allergens as well as perennial disease in dust mite allergy patients.[33,34] SCIT, however, does have the disadvantage in that it needs be administered in a physician's office with appropriate emergency equipment present. SLIT had emerged as an alternative form of AIT from SCIT[35] and had shown to be an effective form of AIT[36]

Healthcare has become increasingly costly to patients and society. With the emergence of new forms of AIT, it is appropriate to consider the cost-effectiveness of these new AIT medicines as well as to undertake a pharmacoeconomic analysis to understand the role SLIT and SCIT plays in the medical management of patient with allergic diseases, particularly AR. In this chapter we will review the healthcare economic data for SCIT, SLIT, and SCIT versus SLIT primarily in patients with allergic disease.

SCIT studies

Ariano and colleagues[37] examined the pharmacoeconomics of SCIT and drug therapy compared to drug therapy alone in 30 patients with a 2-year history of *Parietaria*-induced AR and asthma. The patients were treated with SCIT and drug therapy or drug therapy alone for 3 years and had 3 years of follow-up. Symptoms score and drug use improved significantly in the SCIT group starting in year 1 and maintained this effect through the 3 years posttreatment follow-up. Within the second year of treatment SCIT offered ~15% savings that increased to 48% in year 3. This significant savings continued through the follow-up years and at year 6 (3 years post SCIT treatment) there was an 80% cost reduction in favor of SCIT treatment. The net savings for each patient at the final evaluation was $830/year. The authors concluded that this economic savings have significant individual and societal benefits.

An examination of the cost savings utilizing ragweed SCIT was evaluated in a randomized double-blind placebo-controlled trial[38] of 77 adolescents and adults with ragweed-induced asthma. Patients received ragweed SCIT or placebo over a 2-year period and the cost-efficacy of ragweed SCIT in patients with asthma was examined. Cost of asthma medication used and cost of allergen extracts used were evaluated over the two-year period. Over the course of the study, asthma medication costs in the SCIT group were ~30% less ($840 vs. $1,194, combined cost for 2 years) than in the placebo group. However, there was a 2-year cost of immunotherapy supplies and administration $527 for the SCIT group that offset the cost savings.

A 2005 Danish study[39] looked at direct and indirect cost of AIT in patients with seasonal grass pollen allergy and perennial mite allergic patients. This study revealed significant direct and indirect cost savings for patients undergoing AIT.

Prior to starting immunotherapy direct costs were Danish Krone (DKK) 2580 per patient per year and in the years post AIT the cost was DKK 1072 per patient per year. This represents an almost 60% reduction in direct cost per patient per year. When looking at direct and indirect cost combined, preimmunotherapy cost was DKK 16,285 per patient per year and postimmunotherapy cost was reduced 78% to DKK 3570 per patient per year. This study provides further support that SCIT for grass and dust mite allergic patients is cost-effective.

In 2007, Keiding and colleagues[40] evaluated the cost-effectiveness of SCIT versus drug therapy in adult patients with seasonal AR caused by grass pollen not controlled by oral antihistamines, topical steroids, or sodium cromoglycate in Austria, Denmark, Finland, Germany, the Netherlands, and Sweden. This analysis was based upon the UK Immunotherapy Study Group (UKIS) 1-year randomized multi-European center randomized placebo-controlled parallel group trial.[41] This was a one-year trial, and the economic analysis extended to three total years of SCIT and 6 years of follow-up. From the healthcare system perspective, the use of SCIT versus symptomatic treatment was cost-effective with estimates of cost-effectiveness of €10 000–€25 000 per quality-adjusted life year. From a societal and patient perspective when indirect costs were included, that is, less days lost from work and thus increased productivity and wages, SCIT was found to be even more cost-effective.

A 2008 study based upon the German healthcare system[42] performed economic analysis evaluating the cost-effectiveness of SCIT and standard treatment versus standard treatment alone for AR and allergic asthma. After 15 years of treatment there were more symptomatic patients in the SCIT group versus the standard treatment group and the symptomatically treated group was more likely to develop asthma of various severities. The total cost per patient was approximately €2100 higher for the symptomatically treated group versus the SCIT group (€26,100 vs. €24,000 symptomatic group vs. SCIT group, respectively), and this was equivalent to about €140/year cost savings per patient in the SCIT treated group. From a societal point of view, the SCIT reached an ICER of €−19,787 per additional QALY which implies that SCIT and standard treatment were more effective and less costly that symptomatic treatment alone. There was variation in the ICER with adults being the largest beneficiary most likely reflecting a more significant reduction in indirect costs.

Hankin and colleagues in a 2008 study evaluated the cost-effectiveness of SCIT in a Florida medicaid population.[43] In this study the authors examined the Medicaid claims of children newly diagnosed with AR and compared healthcare utilization and costs in the 6 month prior to initiating SCIT to the 6 months after initiating SCIT. In the posttreatment time period, SCIT significantly improved health services utilization. Pharmacy claims, outpatient visit, and hospitalizations were all decreased significantly in the post 6-month treatment period versus the 6 months prior to SCIT initiation. This decreased utilization was associated with significantly decreased costs associated with each of these three categories. Overall healthcare costs decreased from $185° to $1635 ($P < .001$) from the pre-SCIT period to the post-SCIT period.

In an extension of the above data, Hankin et al.[44] utilized a retrospective matched cohort design to determine whether children with newly diagnosed AR who received SCIT incurred less healthcare utilization and fewer costs during an 18-month follow-up period compared to a matched group of children with AR who did not receive SCIT. Children treated with SCIT incurred significantly lower 18-month median per patient total healthcare costs ($3247 vs. $4872), outpatient costs exclusive of immunotherapy-related care ($1107 vs. $2626), and pharmacy costs ($1108 vs. $1316) compared with the matched controls ($P < .001$ for all). Consistent with the previous study, the difference in total healthcare costs was evident within the first few months of initiating immunotherapy. This current study demonstrated these early savings in healthcare costs persisted and, importantly, increased through the 18 months of the study.

Evaluating comparable data in the adult population revealed similar findings.[45] A retrospective claims data analysis of mean 18-month healthcare cost of adult and pediatric patients newly diagnosed with AR and started in SCIT revealed significant savings. Overall SCIT-treated patients had a 38% lower 18 month mean healthcare cost ($6637 vs. $10,644, $P < 0.0001$). Specifically, SCIT treatment in adults results in a 30% reduction in costs ($10,457 SCIT vs. $14,854 controls, $P < 0.0001$) and in children treated with SCIT the reductions was 42% ($5253 AIT vs. $9118 controls, $P < 0.0001$). This reduction in costs was evident within the first 3 months and continued through the 18 months of treatment. Together these three studies demonstrate quite clearly that initiating SCIT treatment for AR in pediatric and adult Florida Medicaid patients is cost-effective.

A German study in 2000[42] compared the cost-effectiveness of SCIT in addition to standard versus the use of SCIT alone. The combination of SCIT and standard therapy was associated with a cost savings of €140 per patient. From a society perspective, SCIT reaches an overall ICER of € 19,787 per additional QALY. That means SCIT and ST were both more effective and less costly compared with symptomatic treatment only. In European countries, even an ICER up to €50,000 per QALY will be rated as cost-effective. Against this background, the SCIT was demonstrated to be a cost-effective treatment.

A study published in 2013[46] evaluated the economic impact of a previous pediatric allergic asthma study. In this study dust mite allergic asthma patients were treated with SCIT to dust mites, for 3 years, and standard therapy versus standard therapy alone. The study investigated the cost and cost-effectiveness of SCIT to dust mites on total medication costs and incremental medication cost. The study was not able to evaluate the effect of SCIT on outpatient visit costs or hospitalizations. In the first year of treatment, there was no difference between the two groups in medication cost. In year 3, there were significant reductions in total medications costs in the SCIT versus standard treatment group (€ 193 vs. € 498, $P < .001$) as well as a reduction in allergy drug costs (€168 vs. € 453, $P < .002$). This cost-effectiveness analysis suggested that while SCIT was associated with additional cost savings over the course of treatment, this is likely due to SCIT's "disease modifying" effect.

Pharmacoeconomic data on sublingual immunotherapy

One of the initial studies analyzing the cost-effectiveness of SLIT[47] was an Italian study. In this retrospective study, 135 pediatric patients with seasonal and perennial AR and/or asthma, data were analyzed comparing the 1 year prior to SLIT and the 3 years of data on SLIT. Outcome measures evaluated included number of exacerbations, visits, absence form nursery or school, direct cost consisting of euros spent on drugs, specialists' visit, and SLIT and indirect cost including costs associated with lost time at school and parental lost time from work. Across the board, treatment with SLIT resulted in lowered number of exacerbations, medical visits, and lost days from school and work. Direct cost decreased 56% from € 506 to € 224 and indirect costs decreased 81% from €2166 to €406 from the pre-SLIT period to treatment with SLIT. Overall cost decreased 76% from € 2672 pre-SLIT to €629 during SLIT treatment. This reduced healthcare cost for patients with seasonal or perennial AR and if they had asthma as well. These data suggest that SLIT could significantly lower overall healthcare costs for the treatment of AR and asthma.

Several studies evaluated the healthcare economics of a randomized trial of grass allergen tablet in adult patients with allergic rhinoconjunctivitis.[48] These studies took a societal perspective, and the analysis had a nine-year horizon. In the northern European cohort[49] of this SLIT study, there was a significant improvement in the QALY in the SLIT group (0.976 vs. 0.947, $P < .001$). In order to be considered cost-effective it was calculated that a drug must generate one QALY for less than € 29,200. In this analysis the SLIT tablet was cost-effective for all the northern European countries studies for annual treatment cost below € 2200. Similarly in the Southern European cohort[49] SLIT was cost-effective at an annual cost in the range of €1500−€ 1900. And finally, analysis of the study data from the United Kingdom, the cost of QALY gained was €6380,[50] again suggesting that SLIT treatment provided a pharmacoeconomic benefit.

The Sublingual Immunotherapy Pollen Allergy Italy (SPAI) study evaluated the costs of using SLIT in association with standard therapy compared to standard treatment alone in 2200 adults with pollen-induced AR and asthma.[50] This study demonstrated that SLIT treatment resulted in a 20.6% reduction in direct costs (- € 626) and 43.7% reduction in indirect cost (- €1487). This resulted in a combined 32.8% reduction in direct and indirect costs with the use of SLIT in this population.

The Sublingual Immunotherapy in Allergic Patients (SIMAP) study[51] was a 1-year observational evaluation of efficacy, safety, and cost in 102 Italian children and adults with grass pollen−induced AR who had received SLIT or standard drug treatment. Mean annual cost of treatment was higher in the SLIT versus SDT group (€311 vs. €180, $P < .0001$). The difference in total costs was mainly because of costs of SLIT. Patients with AR and asthma generated more cost than those with AR alone in both groups.

Ruggeri and colleagues evaluated the cost-effectiveness of a 5-grass pollen tablet in adult patients with grass pollen−induced AR.[52] In this study cost-effectiveness was stratified by low, medium, and high burden of disease based upon average adjusted symptom score (AAdSS). This analysis demonstrates that low AAdSS patients did not benefit from use of a 5-grass pollen SLIT. However, patients with medium to high AAdSS did benefit. The 5-grass pollen SLIT was found to cost € 1, 024/QALY for patients with medium AAdSS and € 1035/QALY for patients with high AAdSS. These numbers were below the "critical" threshold €30,000/QALY, indicating that for patients with medium to high AAdSS, SLIT was a cost-effective treatment. It is important to note that in patients with low AAdSS, SLIT was not cost-effective and the use of SLIT simply added to the cost of treatment, thus illustrating the importance of proper patient selection for treatment.

Ronaldson and colleagues[53] performed a cost—utility analysis in a model that follows two hypothetical cohorts of 1000 children with grass pollen allergic rhinoconjunctivitis, with or without asthma, who are treated with SLIT and symptomatic medications or symptomatic medication only. The results of this analysis demonstrated that the SLIT-treated group will obtain an incremental effectiveness of 0.10 QALYs per patient. The cost of SLIT treatment was € 1202 higher than the standard drug treatment (SDT) group. However, the ICER for the SLIT treated group was €12, 168/QALY, and this is below the threshold of €20,000—€30,000/QALY that is used in the United Kingdom. The interpretation of these data is that grass AIT is cost-effective.

A 2016 study by Pederson et al.[54] evaluated the cost-effectiveness of SLIT dust mite tablet in adult patients with asthma. This was a cost—utility analysis based upon a phase III randomized controlled trial comparing the efficacy of ACARIZAX (SLIT dust mite tablet) with placebo in adult patient with dust mite allergic asthma. Both groups were allowed to continue conventional pharmacotherapy for their asthma. The SLIT-treated group led to an additional 0.66 QALY at an incremental cost of € 2673. This equates to an ICER of € 4041 which is below the threshold of €40,000, thus suggesting that use of dust mite in this adult allergic asthma population was cost-effective.

A similar study performed a pharmacoeconomic analysis[55] of house dust mite SLIT plus pharmacotherapy versus SDT alone in patients with AR. This study examined nine-year time horizons, demonstrating that SLIT resulted in an additional QALY of 0.31 at an incremental cost of € 2276. This resulted in an ICER of € 7,516, indicating that SLIT with house dust mite in addition to pharmacotherapy is cost-effective compared to pharmacotherapy alone in German patients with moderate to severe house dust mite—induced AR.

Cost-effectiveness of SCIT versus SLIT

Pokladnikova and colleagues[56] performed an economic evaluation of SCIT versus SLIT in adults with rhinoconjuctivitis to grass. They evaluated the effect from the point of view of third-party payers, the patients and society. After 3 years of treatment SLIT and SCIT were comparable in their clinical outcomes, with each producing a significant reduction in symptoms scores and drug intake. However, they did note that SCIT demonstrated a slightly better improvement in the visual analog scale and use of antihistamines versus SLIT in the third year of study. From an economic point of view, SLIT proved to be generally less expensive; however, from a patient perspective SCIT was financially preferable to SLIT particularly in the patient population that did not have any loss of income or travel expenses to receive SCIT. From the third-party payer perspective, the three-year direct medical costs were €416 versus €482 for SLIT and SCIT groups, respectively. When consider both direct and indirect cost, 3 years treatment with €684 versus €1004 (p, 0.001)in the SLIT versus SCIT group respectively. If, however, the patients in the SCIT group had no loss of income or productivity from receiving SCIT in the office setting, then SCIT was financially preferable to SLIT.

A Danish study[57] evaluated the budget impact of grass pollen—induced rhinoconjunctivitis comparing SQ-standardized grass AIT (Grazax; *Phleum pratense*, 75,000 SQ-T/2800 BAU; ALK, Denmark) with SCIT (Alutard; *P. pratense*, 100,000 SQ-U/mL; ALK, Denmark). Their analysis revealed the total direct and indirect costs using SLIT with Grazax€3789. This would be €3460 cheaper than using SCIT with Alutard. The authors suggest that this savings could be utilized to treat an additional 600 patients with SLIT at no additional cost to the healthcare system.

In a German 2012 study, Westerhout and colleagues[58] evaluated the cost-effectiveness of grass pollen AIT (Oralair, Grazax, and Alk Depot SQ) in grass pollen allergic rhinoconjunctivitis versus SDT. Patients were treated for 3 years and assessed for a period of 9 years using a Markov model. The cost—utility ratio of Oralair versus symptomatic treatment of €14,728 per QALY. Oralair was the dominant strategy compared to Grazax and Alk Depot SQ, with estimated incremental costs of -€1142 (95%CI: €1255; -€1038) and -€54 (95%CI: €188; €85) and incremental QALYs of 0.015 (95%CI: 0.025; 0.056) and 0.027 (95%CI: 0.022; 0.075), respectively.

In 2014 Dranitsaris and Ellis[59] performed an indirect comparison of double-blind placebo-controlled trials on efficacy, safety, and cost between Oralair, Grazax, and SCIT for the prevention of AR. Twenty trials met the inclusion criteria for their study. The results suggested that use of Oralair was cheaper than Grazax or SCIT. In the first year of treatment Oralair use resulted in a cost savings of $948 versus seasonal SCIT, $1168 versus Grazax, and $2471 versus year round SCIT. The majority of the increase cost associated with SCIT were related to indirect cost (lost productivity and travel cost to clinic) and cost associated with administration of SCIT in the office. In evaluating the cost of years two and three combined, a similar pattern emerged with Oralair offering a cost savings of $868 versus SCIT year round, $1883 versus SCIT seasonal, and $2344 versus Grazax. This model assumes that administration of SCIT would result in decreased productivity (lost hours from work for administration of SCIT). Interestingly if one were to make SCIT administration available such that there was no lost time from work, then the total cost for SCIT year round would be $1721 versus $1889.6, making Oralair approximately 9% more expensive, suggesting that the cost difference between SLIT and SCIT could be drastically impacted depending upon the availability of physician office hours to administer SCIT.

Verheggen and colleagues[60] using a Markov model and a 9-year time horizon, evaluated the cost-effectiveness of Oralair (5-grass tablet) versus subcutaneous allergoid component for the treatment of grass pollen—induced allergic rhinoconjunctivitis. SLIT using Oralair was associated with higher overall costs at €458/patient over the study period, and it was shown to be superior in terms of effectiveness compared with SCIT. Their results showed that for the single allergen grass class, SLIT resulted in an increase of QALYs of 0.036 and ICER of € 12,593 versus the allergoid SCIT for grass. They predicted the probability of SLIT tablet to be the most cost-effective treatment option at 76%.

In a 2017 study by Rheinhold and Bruggenjurgen[61] they compared the cost-effectiveness of SCIT with Allergovit and SLIT with Oralair. They used a Markov model with a time frame of 9 years. This study selected one SCIT preparation as the comparator as opposed to the Verheggen study (Verheggen BG, Westerhout K, Schreder C, and Augustin M Health economic comparison of SLIT allergen and SCIT allergic immunotherapy in patients with seasonal grass allergic rhinoconjunctivitis in Germany. Clinical and Translational Alergy 2015; 5: 1—10) which used a variety of SCIT preparations which may have complicated the interpretation of their results. In the current study, over the 9-year treatment period the total per person cost was approximately 14% more for SLIT versus SCIT (€1159 for Allergovit vs. € 1322 for Oralair). In addition, SCIT treatment resulted in 7.122 QALYs with cost per QALY gained at €11,000 versus €41,405 cost fot QALY gain with SLIT. As a reference, cost-effective therapy should be less that €40,000—€50,000 per QALY gained. In this study, SCIT was more cost-effective than SLIT for treatment of grass pollen—induced rhinoconjunctivitis.

Conclusions

The preponderance of the data suggests that AIT, either with SLIT or SCIT, is a cost-effective treatment option for patients with AR or asthma. The limitations of most of these studies are that they were single or at most dual allergen studies, and the majority of the studies were performed in European centers so the applicability to US patients may be limited. This is particularly relevant in the SCIT versus SLIT comparison. Typical AIT in the United States is multiallergen versus single allergen treatment. SCIT in the United State is reimbursed by the number of doses or in the case of Medicare, and some commercial carriers, "one dose is one cc". This reimbursement is irrespective of the number of allergens that may be present in a particular SCIT treatment bottle(s) such that a single vial of SCIT will be reimbursed the same if there is one allergen or if there are numerous allergens present. Contrasting this with SLIT tablet AIT, one tablet will contain one allergen, e.g., grass and

Table 15.1 Economic studies of SCIT.

Reference	Country	Type	Sample	Comparators	Perspective	Data sources	Time horizon	Results
SCIT versus SDT								
Schadlich, 2000[62]	Germany	CEA	Adults with AR due to pollen or HDM	SCIT for 3 years plus SDT as needed; SDT	Society, healthcare system, third-party payer	Clinical trials, observational studies, epidemiological studies, survey, expert opinion, literature	10 years	SCIT < SDT over time breakeven point of cumulative reached in the 7th year
Petersen, 2005[39]	Denmark	CEA	Adolescents and adults with grass pollen and HDM allergy who received SCIT	SCIT for 3–5 years plus SDT as needed; SDT	Society	National health service records, patient questionnaire	9 years	SCIT > SDT four years of SCIT were associated with additional direct costs of 13,676 DKK (€1841) per patient
Ariano, 2006[37]	Italy	CCA	Adults with SAR and asthma caused by sensitization to *Parietaria* pollen	SCIT for 3 years plus SDT as needed; SDT	Healthcare system, society	RCT, patient records, literature	6 years	SCIT < SDT SCIT reduced cost of about 15% at year 2%, 48% at year 3, 80% reduction found 3 years after stopping SCIT
Keiding, 2007[40]	Austria, Denmark, Finland, Germany, Netherlands, Sweden	CEA CUA	Adults with grass pollen –induced ARC who did not respond adequately to SDT	SCIT for 3 years plus SDT as needed; SDT	Healthcare system, society	RCT, patient diaries, RQLQ, literature	9 years	From societal perspective SCIT was more effective and less expensive versus SDT in the range of €10,000 –25,000 per QALY per the healthcare system

Continued

Table 15.1 Economic studies of SCIT.—*cont'd*

Reference	Country	Type	Sample	Comparators	Perspective	Data sources	Time horizon	Results
Omnes, 2007[63]	France	CEA	Adults and adolescents with HDM and pollen AR with or without allergic asthma	SCIT four 3 years for adults and 4 years for adolescents plus SDT as needed; SDT	Society	Literature, expert opinion	6 years for adults and 7 years for adolescents	The ICER per additional improved patient ranged from €349 (in adolescents with HDM allergy) to €722 (in adults with pollen allergy
Bruggenjurgen, 2008[42]	Germany	CUA	Children and adults with AR and/or asthma	SCIT for 3 years plus SDT as needed; SDT	Third-party payer, society	Literature, expert opinion	15 years	Breakeven point = 10 years. After 15 years, patients who received SCIT plus SDT were more likely to have no symptoms, less likely to develop. Total societal cost after 15 years—annual cost savings of €140 per SCIT-treated patient.
Hankin, 2008[43]	U.S.	CCA	Children with AR who received SCIT	Before and after SCIT	Healthcare system	Retrospective claims data (medicaid)	1 year	Mean (SD) total healthcare costs 6 months before SCIT: $1850 ($2354) 6 months after SCIT: $1635 ($3525) $P < .0001$ Weighted mean 6-month savings/patient: $401
Hankin, 2010[64]	U.S.	CCA	Children with AR who received SCIT and matched controls who did not receive SCIT	SCIT for 18 months plus SDT as needed; SDT as needed for 18 months	Healthcare system	Retrospective claims data (medicaid)	18 months	Median 18-month total healthcare costs SCIT: $3247 SDT: $4872 $P < .001$

Study	Country	Type	Population	Intervention	Perspective	Data source	Time horizon	Findings
Reinhold, 2012[65]	Germany	BIA	Children and adults with AR were allergic asthma who did or did not receive SCIT	SCIT for 1 year; SDT as needed	Healthcare system	Literature, expert opinion	Annually from 2011 to 2050	The cost of offering SCIT to a larger number of patients in earlier stages of disease would result in additional costs of €300–€350 per additionally healed patient.
Hankin 2013[45]	U.S.	CCA	Adults and children with AR who received SCIT and matched controls who did not receive SCIT	SCIT plus SDT as needed for 18 months; SDT as needed for 18 months	Healthcare system	Retrospective claims data (medicaid)	18 months	Mean (SD) 18-month per patient total healthcare costs SCIT versus SDT: Children 42% reduction Adults: 30% reduction $P < .0001$

SCIT versus SDT subset analysis

Study	Country	Type	Population	Intervention	Perspective	Data source	Time horizon	Findings
Creticos, 1996[38]	United States	CCA	Adolescents and adults with at least 1 year of asthma exacerbated by seasonal ragweed exposure	SCIT for 2 years plus SDT as needed; SDT	Healthcare system	RCT, patient diaries, literature, authors' assumptions	2 years	Compared costs of asthma medications: Reduced medication costs were counterbalanced by AIT costs.
Donahue, 1999[66]	United States	CCA	Children and adults with AR who received SCIT	SCIT for 3.5 years plus SDT as needed; SCIT for <3.5 years with SDT as needed	Healthcare system	Retrospective claims data (HMO)	3.5 years	Overall cost of SCIT completers was nearly 3-fold greater than the group that discontinued SCIT. Total cost of SCIT + other healthcare costs SCIT completers = $1206 SCIT noncompleters = $668 Note: AR and asthma

Continued

Table 15.1 Economic studies of SCIT.—cont'd

Reference	Country	Type	Sample	Comparators	Perspective	Data sources	Time horizon	Results
								costs before SCIT were 30% higher in the SCIT completed group, suggesting a greater disease burden than the group that discontinued SCIT
Accelerated versus conventional SCIT								
Mauro, 2006[67]	Italy	CEA	Adults with persistent AR due to HDM	Accelerated buildup schedule of SCIT lasting 3 weeks; traditional buildup schedule of SCIT lasting 13 weeks	Society	RCT, physician records, literature, authors' assumptions	1 year	Higher costs total cost per patient in the buildup phase with conventional buildup
SLIT versus SDT								
Berto, 2005[47]	Italy	CEA	Children and adolescents with AR and/or allergic asthma	1 year of SDT before SLIT and SLIT for 3 years	Healthcare system, society	A retrospective before-and-after study, patient records, literature	4 years	MCD = year before SLIT versus year after SLIT MCD (direct): $481 versus $213 MCD (indirect): $2538 versus$598
Berto, 2006[50]	Italy	CCA	Adolescents and adults with pollen-induced AR with or without asthma	SLIT for 3 years plus SDT as needed; SDT	Healthcare system, society	Retrospective cohort study, patient records, literature, authors' assumptions	6 years	SLIT was dominant over SDT from both a payer and societal perspective. 6-year mean savings per patient who received SLIT versus SDT:

Study	Country		Population	Comparison	Perspective	Data sources	Time horizon	Results
Bachert, 2007[68]	Denmark, Finland, Germany, The Netherlands, Norway, Sweden, United Kingdom	CUA	Adults with grass pollen–induced ARC	SLIT for 3 years plus SDT as needed; SDT	Society	RCT, patient diaries, literature, EQ-5D, authors' extrapolations	9 years	$639 (payer perspective) $2662 (societal perspective) From a payer perspective, assuming an annual cost of AIT of $1,860, cost per QALY ranged from $16,033 to $22,646 y
Beriot-mathiot, 2007[69]	Sweden	CUA	Adults with grass pollen ARC	SLIT for 3 years (continuous/preventive) plus SDT as needed; SLIT for 3 years (seasonal) plus SDT as needed; SDT	Societal	RCT, patient diaries, literature, EQ-5D, authors' extrapolations	1, 5, 9, 12, and 15 years	SLIT was cost-effective if sustained effect after treatment is ≥ 2 years based on a threshold of €29,000 per QALY, whereas seasonal SLIT pattern was cost-effective regardless of time horizon with ICER of €21,829.
Canonica[62]	Italy, France, Spain, Austria	CUA	Adults with grass pollen–induced ARC	SLIT for 3 years plus SDT as needed; SDT	Society	RCT, patient diaries, literature, EQ-5D, patient questionnaire, authors' assumptions	9 years	Based on an annual cost of €1200 for SLIT, the cost per QALY gained ranged from €13,870 to €21,659. SLIT was cost-effective at a cost of <€1900
Berto, 2008[51]	Italy	CCA	Children and adults with grass pollen–induced AR	SLIT for 1 year; SDT for 1 year	Third-party payer	Observational study	1 year	Mean annual direct costs for SLIT and SDT were €311.4 and €179.8, respectively
Nasser, 2008[49]	United Kingdom	CUA	Adults with grass pollen–induced AR and asthma	SLIT for 3 years plus SDT as needed; SDT	Society	RCT, patient diaries, literature	9 years	QALY gained @ 9 years = 0.197 equivalent to an extra 72 days of perfect health for patients

Continued

Table 15.1 Economic studies of SCIT.—cont'd

Reference	Country	Type	Sample	Comparators	Perspective	Data sources	Time horizon	Results
Ariano, 2009[70]	Italy	CCA	Children and adults with allergic asthma sensitized to HDM	SLIT for 3 years plus SDT as needed; SDT	Healthcare system	RCT, patient and physician diaries, literature	5 years	treated with SLIT when compared with those receiving placebo Healthcare costs for those receiving SLIT plus SDT were higher in year 1, the same in years 2 and 3, and significantly lower in years 4 and 5, when compared with patients receiving SDT. For asthmatic patients, annual cost savings at year 5 = 23%.
Ruggeri, 2013[52]	Italy	CEA	Adults with the grass pollen–induced ARC	SLIT for 3 years plus SDT as needed; SDT	Third-party payer, society	2 RCT, retrospective claims data	4 years	ICER for SLIT was <£30,000.
SCIT versus SLIT								
Pokladnikova, 2008[56]	Czech Republic	CEA	Adults with grass pollen–induced ARC	SLIT for 3 years; SCIT for 3 years	Third-party payer, society	RCT; patient records; patient questionnaire; literature	3 years	Payer perspective, the total average direct medical cost per patient of 3-year AIT was: ~ SLIT € 416 versus SCIT € 482 Patient perspective: direct and indirect costs over 3-year SIT costs per patient: SLIT € 684 versus SCIT € 1004
Westerhout, 2012[58]	Germany	CEA CUA	Adults with moderate/ severe seasonal	SLIT (Oralair; OA) for 3 years plus SDT as	Healthcare system	Meta-analysis of RCTs, literature,	9 years	Analysis suggest OA to be cost-effective

						authors' assumptions		
Ronberg, 2012[57]	Denmark	BIA	Adults with grass pollen –induced AR	ARC due to grass pollen	SLIT (Grazax) for 3 years; SCIT (Alutard) for 3–5 years	needed; SLIT (Grazax; GRZ) for 3 years plus SDT as needed; SCIT (Alk Depot SQ; ALD) plus SDT as needed; SDT	Healthcare system	Literature, expert opinion	3–5 years	Direct treatment costs per patient were 28% (€1291) lower with SLIT versus SCIT. Patient direct and indirect costs were 81% (€2169) lower with SLIT versus SCIT total cost savings associated with SLIT versus SCIT were €3460 (48%) per patient.	compared to GRZ and ALD and SDT

ALD, Alk Depot SQ; AR, allergic rhinitis; ARC, allergic rhinoconjuctivitis; BIA, budget impact analysis; CCA, cost–consequence analysis; CEA, cost-effectiveness analysis; CUA, cost –utility analysis; EQ-5D, EuroQol-5D questionnaire; GRZ, Grazax; HDM, house dust mite; HMO, health maintenance organization; ICER, incremental cost-effectiveness ratio; OA, Oralair; QALY, quality-adjusted life year; MCD, mean cost difference; PEFR, pulmonary expiratory flow rate; RQLQ, Rhinoconjuctivitis Quality of Life Questionnaire; SCIT, subcutaneous allergy immunotherapy; SLIT, sublingual allergy immunotherapy; SDT, standard drug treatment.

Adapted with permission from Hankin et al. the global burden of untreated and undertreated allergic rhinitis andsystematic literature review of patterns and outcomes of allergy immuno-therapy for the treatment of patients with allergic rhinitis.2014 manuscript in preparation.

dust mite SLIT. Thus the patient would have to administer two separate tablets. Clearly, multiallergen SCIT would be less expensive than SLIT. Suggest adding Cox Sublingual immunotherapy for aeroallergens: status in the United States 2014 as ref.

One of the arguments for SLIT over SCIT is the limitation of administration of SCIT in a physician's office and the subsequent indirect cost of lost time from work/ productivity. Most, if not all, of the studies on cost-effectiveness assumes that all patients will receive SCIT at a physician's office and this will be during normal business hours. None of the studies collected data directly from patients about the economic impact that SCIT had on them. Furthermore, it needs to be recognized, at least in the United States, if is it possible for patients to receive SCIT treatments outside of standard "business hours" or that in today's electronic world that patients will "do work" during the time they are in the physician's office for SCIT treatment.

Overall, SLIT and SCIT are clinically efficacious and cost-effective treatment options for patients with AR and asthma. Whether SCIT is more cost-effective than SLIT or vice versa remains to be determined and will require more detailed analysis of the cost, both direct and indirect, in patients with multiallergen AIT in the United States Tables 15.1–15.3.

Table 15.2 SLIT-estimated costs based on US-licensed extract manufacturers' list price.

Allergen	Monthly Costs[a]	Average cost/mL Average of two US allergen extract manufacturers' 2013 list price
Cat	$ 82.74 (2000 BAU)	50 mL vial/$13.79 per ml
Dust mite	$ 121.63 (2800 AU DF)	50 mL vial/$14.48 per ml
Standardized grass	$ 7.19 (~2800 BAU)	50 mL vial/$8.56/mL
Ragweed	$ 60.00 (~50mcg)	30 mL vial 1:20 w/v[b]/$6.60/mL
Cat, dust mite, and grass	$ 211.56 month or 2538.72 a year	

DF, *Dermatophagoides farinae*; AU, *allergy units*; BAU, *bioequivalent allergy units*.
[a] *Costs-based average of two US-licensed extract manufacturers' 2013 catalog*

- *Using highest bulk extract available 30 or 50 mL*
- *Estimated dose from clinical trials or Allergen Immunotherapy: A Practice Parameters Third Update*[14]
- *Assumes daily dosing.*

[b] *1/10 w/v = ~150 mcg of Amb a 1 per ml.*

Table 15.3 Allergy immunotherapy Economics and Adherence.

Economics of AIT-see Table 2 for detailed information on the individual studies evaluating cost-effectiveness of AIT versus pharmacotherapy (aka *CER*, comparative effectiveness research)
- Various designs, outcomes, and duration:
  - Designs: budget impact analysis; cost–consequence analysis; cost-effectiveness analysis; cost–utility analysis, and retrospective claims
  - Outcomes: assessed which include ICER, QALY, asthma prevented, and societal, payer, patient, and actual cost
- Ten economic analyses compared SDT versus AIT—only one showed greater costs with AIT versus AIT
- Different CERs and "breakeven time points"—from 3 months to 10 years
  - One 12-year large retrospective claims study ("real-life") involving Florida Medicaid Data which included ∼7.5 million people found 18-month median total cost savings of 30% in adults and 42% in children with new onset AR who received AIT versus matched controls that did not.[45]
- One study compared cluster versus conventional buildup and found cost savings with cluster.[67] Total cost per patient in the buildup phase amounted to €184.40 with accelerated SCIT and €429.35 with traditional SCIT. There was no difference between treatments in occurrence of side effects per patient and per injection
- Both SCIT and SLIT have been shown to be cost-effective compared with SDT for the treatment of AR.
- Whereas the cost of SLIT allergen may be higher than SCIT, SLIT requires fewer physician visits than SCIT, resulting in lower treatment costs and indirect costs (travel, lost working hours).
- Of the 4 economic studies comparing SLIT and SCIT, 3 found SLIT to be a more cost-effective treatment option and 1 found SCIT to be more cost-effective.
- In general, the longer the time horizon, the greater AIT cost-effectiveness compared with SDT

Adherence:
- Studies have reported widely varying rates of premature discontinuation for both SCIT and SLIT.
  - SCIT: rates of SCIT premature discontinuation: ranged from 6% to 84% (15 studies).[43,66,71–82] Seven studies reported discontinuation rates ranging from 6% to 30%,[73–78,83] 5 studies from 31% to 50%,[72,79–82] and 3 studies reported discontinuation rates greater than 50%.[43,66,71]
  - SLIT adherence in short-term studies. Studies that quantitatively measured adherence to SLIT over 1 year or less reported high adherence rates (84%–97%).[84–92]
  - SLIT long-term studies that assessed adherence quantitatively by measuring the amount of SLIT returned during clinical trials reported adherence rates of 72%–91%.[21,93–96]
- RCTs: Rates of adherence to SLIT have been generally good (70%–90%); however, adherence to SLIT is substantially lower when based on physician estimates (29%) and examination of pharmacy SLIT refill data (38%).
- Real-world SLIT adherence
  - The highest rate of SLIT premature discontinuation was reported in a retrospective analysis of pharmacy claims data in the Netherlands.[83] Among 3690 Dutch adults who initiated SLIT, only 7% completed 3 years of treatment.[83]

Continued

Table 15.3 Allergy immunotherapy Economics and Adherence.—*cont'd*

- • A study that examined sales data from 2 large SLIT manufacturers found that less than 20% of SLIT prescriptions were continued after 3 years.[97]
  - • In a study that examined SLIT prescription renewal rates, only 50% of patients who were prescribed SLIT renewed their prescriptions in the 2 subsequent years.[81]
- • SCIT versus SLIT: three of the 4 studies that compared rates of premature discontinuation to both SCIT and SLIT found higher rates of premature discontinuation in patients who received SLIT than in those who received SCIT.
- • Reason for discontinuation: the most common reasons patients cite for discontinuing SCIT are inconvenience, concurrent illness, lack of efficacy, improvement in symptoms, change of residence, and adverse reactions.
- • The most common reasons patients cite for discontinuing SLIT are the inability to take the medication as scheduled/compliance, inconvenience, lack of efficacy, concurrent illness, cost, and adverse effects.
- • Potential interventions to improve adherence
  - • Improve patient education: patients may have poor perception of what to expect from AIT Study surveying AIT patients' knowledge found:[98]
    - • 60% unaware of any treatment duration
    - • 33% did not know about the risk of side effects
    - • 35% considered AIT to be entirely safe
    - • 3% recognize all their allergens without mistakes
- • Increase visit frequency[99]

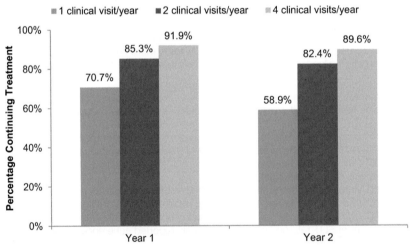

- • Electronic messaging: studies have demonstrated improved medication adherence and disease management with text messages and other forms of electronic reminders significantly increased medication adherence.

AIT Outcomes: Efficacy, Safety, Cost-efficacy, and Adherence
- ■ AIT Outcome: Essentially no "gold standard" for AIT outcome
  - ■ Most "accepted" −20% improvement in CMS score
  - ■ But questions remain: what is clinically meaningful? Are we measuring what matters to the patient?
  - ■ Need a patient-centered Allergy Immunotherapy Outcome Assessment Tool

Table 15.3 Allergy immunotherapy Economics and Adherence.—*cont'd*

- Safety: SLIT better safety profile compared with SCIT but both acceptable safety when administered appropriately (i.e., medically supervised setting)
- Economics: significant cost-savings seen with AIT in various study designs
- Adherence: In RCT, adherence is generally good but problematic with both forms of AIT in real life. Interventions to improve adherence are needed

References

1. Bousquet J, Khaltaev N, Cruz AA, et al. Allergic rhinitis and its impact on asthma (ARIA) 2008 update (in collaboration with the world health organization, GA(2)LEN and AllerGen). *Allergy*. 2008;63(suppl 86):8−160.
2. Ozdoganoglu T, Songu M. The burden of allergic rhinitis and asthma. *Ther Adv Respir Dis*. 2012;6:11−23.
3. Wheatley LM, Togias A. Clinical practice. Allergic rhinitis. *N Engl J Med*. 2015;372:456−463.
4. Bauchau V, Durham SR. Prevalence and rate of diagnosis of allergic rhinitis in Europe. *Eur Respir J*. 2004;24:758−764.
5. Maurer M, Zuberbier T. Undertreatment of rhinitis symptoms in Europe: findings from a cross-sectional questionnaire survey. *Allergy*. 2007;62:1057−1063.
6. Sazonov V, Ambegaonkar BM, Bolge SC, et al. Frequency of diagnosis and treatment of allergic rhinitis among adults with asthma in Germany, France, and the UK: national Health and Wellness Survey. *Curr Med Res Opin*. 2009;25:1721−1726.
7. Nolte H, Nepper-Christensen S, Backer V. Unawareness and under treatment of asthma and allergic rhinitis in a general population. *Respir Med*. 2006;100:354−362.
8. Meltzer EO, Blaiss MS, Derebery MJ, et al. Bur-den of allergic rhinitis: results from the pediatric allergies in America survey. *J Allergy Clin Immunol*. 2009;124(suppl):S43−S70.
9. Long AA. Findings from a 1000-patient internet-based survey assessing the impact of morning symptoms on individuals with allergic rhinitis. *Clin Ther*. 2007;29:342−351.
10. Shaaban R, Zureik M, Soussan D, et al. Rhinitis and onset of asthma: a longitudinal population-based study. *Lancet*. 2008;372:1049−1057.
11. Blaiss MS. Allergic rhinitis: direct and indirect costs. *Allergy Asthma Proc*. 2010;31:375−380.
12. Greiner AN, Hellings PW, Rotiroti G, Scadding GK. Allergic rhinitis. *Lancet*. 2011;378:2112−2122.
13. White P, Smith H, Baker N, Davis W, Frew A. Symptom control in patients with hay fever in UK general practice: how well are we doing and is there a need for allergen immunotherapy? *Clin Exp Allergy*. 1998;28:266−270.
14. Cox L, Nelson H, Lockey R, et al. Allergen immunotherapy: a practice parameter third update. *J Allergy Clin Immunol*. 2011;127(suppl):S1−S55.
15. Moller C, Dreborg S, Ferdousi HA, et al. Pollen immunotherapy reduces the development of asthma in children with seasonal rhinoconjunctivitis (the PAT-study). *J Allergy Clin Immunol*. 2002;109:251−256.

16. Niggemann B, Jacobsen L, Dreborg S, et al. Five- year follow-up on the PAT study: specific immunotherapy and long-term prevention of asthma in children. *Allergy.* 2006;61: 855—859.

17. Jacobsen L, Niggemann B, Dreborg S, et al. Specific immunotherapy has long-term preventive effect of seasonal and perennial asthma: 10-year follow-up on the PAT study. *Allergy.* 2007;62:943—948.

18. Novembre E, Galli E, Landi F, et al. Coseasonal sublingual immunotherapy reduces the development of asthma in children with allergic rhinoconjunctivitis. *J Allergy Clin Immunol.* 2004;114:851—857.

19. Des Roches A, Paradis L, Menardo JL, Bouges S, Daures JP, Bousquet J. Immunotherapy with a standardized dermatophagoides pteronyssinus extract. VI. Specific immunotherapy prevents the onset of new sensitizations in children. *J Allergy Clin Immunol.* 1997;99:450—453.

20. Pajno GB, Barberio G, De Luca F, Morabito L, Parmiani S. Prevention of new sensitizations in asthmatic children monosensitized to house dust mite by specific immunotherapy. A six-year follow-up study. *Clin Exp Allergy.* 2001;31:1392—1397.

21. Marogna M, Spadolini I, Massolo A, Canonica GW, Passalacqua G. Randomized controlled open study of sublingual immunotherapy for respiratory allergy in real-life: clinical efficacy and more. *Allergy.* 2004;59:1205—1210.

22. Purello-D'Ambrosio F, Gangemi S, Merendino RA, et al. Prevention of new sensitizations in monosensitized subjects submitted to specific immunotherapy or not. A retrospective study. *Clin Exp Allergy.* 2001;31:1295—1302.

23. Reha CM, Ebru A. Specific immunotherapy is effective in the prevention of new sensitivities. *Allergol Immunopathol.* 2007;35:44—51.

24. Inal A, Altintas DU, Yilmaz M, Karakoc GB, Kendirli SG, Sertdemir Y. Prevention of new sensitizations by specific immunotherapy in children with rhinitis and/or asthma monosensitized to house dust mite. *J Investig Allergol Clin Immunol.* 2007;17:85—91.

25. Eng PA, Borer-Reinhold M, Heijnen IA, Gnehm HP. Twelve-year follow-up after discontinuation of preseasonal grass pollen immunotherapy in childhood. *Allergy.* 2006;61: 198—201.

26. Mosbech H, Osterballe O. Does the effect of immunotherapy last after termination of treatment? Follow-up study in patients with grass pollen rhinitis. *Allergy.* 1988;43: 523—529.

27. Jacobsen L, Nuchel Petersen B, Wihl JA, Lowenstein H, Ipsen H. Immunotherapy with partially purified and standardized tree pollen extracts. IV. Results from long- term (6-year) follow-up. *Allergy.* 1997;52:914—920.

28. Hedlin G, Heilborn H, Lilja G, et al. Long-term follow-up of patients treated with a three-year course of cat or dog immunotherapy. *J Allergy Clin Immunol.* 1995;96:879—885.

29. Durham SR, Varney VA, Gaga M, et al. Grass pollen immunotherapy decreases the number of mast cells in the skin. *Clin Exp Allergy.* 1999;29:1490—1496.

30. Di Rienzo V, Marcucci F, Puccinelli P, et al. Long-last- ing effect of sublingual immunotherapy in children with asthma due to house dust mite: a 10-year prospective study. *Clin Exp Allergy.* 2003;33:206—210.

31. Marogna M, Bruno M, Massolo A, Falagiani P. Long-lasting effects of sublingual immunotherapy for house dust mites in allergic rhinitis with bronchial hyperreactivity: a long-term (13-year) retrospective study in real life. *Int Arch Allergy Immunol.* 2007;142: 70—78.

32. Ariano R, Kroon AM, Augeri G, Canonica GW, Passalacqua G. Long-term treatment with allergoid immunotherapy with Parietaria. Clinical and immunologic effects in a randomized, controlled trial. *Allergy.* 1999;54:313–319.

33. Calderon MA, Alves B, Jacobson M, Hurwitz B, Sheikh A, Durham S. Allergen injection immunotherapy for seasonal allergic rhinitis. *Cochrane Database Syst Rev.* 2007;1: CD001936.

34. Calderon MA, Penagos M, Lagos M, et al. Allergen injection immunotherapy for perennial allergic rhinitis. *Cochrane Database Syst Rev.* 2016;(2) (in press).

35. Canonica GW, Cox L, Pawankar R, et al. Sublingual immunotherapy: world Allergy organization position paper 2013 update. *World Allergy Organ J.* 2014;7:6.

36. Durham S, Penagos M. *J Allergy Clin Immunol.* 2016;137:339–349.

37. Ariano R, Berto P, Tracci D, Incorvaia C, Frati F. Pharmacoeconomics of allergen immunotherapy compared with symptomatic drug treatment in patients with allergic rhinitis and asthma. *Allergy Asthma Proc.* 2006;27:159–163.

38. Creticos PS, Reed CE, Norman PS, et al. Ragweed immunotherapy in adult asthma. *N Engl J Med.* 1996;334:501–506.

39. Petersen KD, Gyrd-Hansen D, Dahl R. Health-economic analyses of sub- cutaneous specific immunotherapy for grass pollen and mite allergy. *Allergol Immunopathol.* 2005;33: 296–302.

40. Keiding H, Jorgensen KP. A cost-effectiveness analysis of immunotherapy with SQ allergen extract for patients with seasonal allergic rhinoconjunctivitis in selected European countries. *Curr Med Res Opin.* 2007;23:1113–1120.

41. Frew AJ, Powell RJ, Corrigan CJ, Durham SR. Efficacy and safety of specific immunotherapy with SQ allergen extract in treatment-resistant seasonal allergic rhinoconjunctivitis. *J Allergy Clin Immunol.* 2006;117:319–325.

42. Bruggenjurgen B, Reinhold T, Brehler R, et al. Cost-effectiveness of specific subcutaneous immunotherapy in patients with allergic rhinitis and allergic asthma. *Ann Allergy Asthma Immunol.* 2008;101:316–324.

43. Hankin CS, Cox L, Lang D, et al. Allergy immunotherapy among Medicaid- enrolled children with allergic rhinitis: patterns of care, resource use, and costs. *J Allergy Clin Immunol.* 2008;121:227–232.

44. Hankin CS, Cox L, Lang D, et al. Allergy immunotherapy among medicaid- benefits for children with allergic rhinitis: a large-scale, retrospective, matched cohort study. *Ann Allergy Asthma Immunol.* 2010;104:79–85.

45. Hankin CS, Cox L, Bronstone A, Wang Z. Allergy immunotherapy: reduced healthcare costs in adults and children with allergic rhinitis. *J Allergy Clin Immunol.* 2013;131: 1084–1091.

46. Rienhold T, Osterman J, THum-Oltmer S, Bruggenjurgen B. Influence of subcutaneous specific immunotherapy on drug costs in children suffering from allergic asthma. *Clin Transl Allergy.* 2013;3:30–38.

47. Berto P, Bassi M, Incorvaia C, et al. Cost effectiveness of sublingual immunotherapy in children with allergic rhinitis and asthma. *Eur Ann Allergy Clin Immunol.* 2005;37: 303–308.

48. Dahl R, Kapp A, Colombo G, et al. Efficacy and safety of sublingual immunotherapy with grass allergen tablet for seasonal allergic rhinoconjunctivitis. *J Allergy Clin Immunol.* 2006;118:434–440.

49. Nasser S, Vestenbaek U, Beriot-Mathiot A, Poulsen PB. Cost-effectiveness of specific immunotherapy with Grazax in allergic rhinitis co-existing with asthma. *Allergy.* 2008;63:1624—1629.

50. Berto P, Passalacqua G, Crimi N, et al. Economic evaluation of sublingual immunotherapy vs symptomatic treatment in adults with pollen-induced respiratory allergy: the sublingual immunotherapy pollen allergy italy (SPAI) study. *Ann Allergy Asthma Immunol.* 2006;97:615—621.

51. Berto P, Frati F, Incorvaia C, et al. Comparison of costs of sublingual immunotherapy and drug treatment in grass-pollen induced allergy: results from the SIMAP database study. *Curr Med Res Opin.* 2008;24:261—266.

52. Ruggeri M, Oradei M, Frati F, et al. Economic evaluation of 5-grass pollen && tablets versus placebo in the treatment of allergic rhinitis in adults. *Clin Drug Investig.* 2013;33:343—349.

53. Ronaldson S, Taylor M, Bech R, et al. Economic evaluation of SQ-standardized grass allergy immunotherapy tablet (Grazax ®) in children. *Clin Outcomes Res.* 2014;6, 197—196.

54. Hahn-Peterson J, Worm M, Andreasen JN, Taylor M. Cost utility analysis if the SQ HDM SLIT-tablet in house list mite allergic asthma patients in a German setting. *Clin Transl Allergy.* 2016;6:35—42.

55. Green W, Klein-Tebbe J, Klimek L, Hahn-Pederson J, Andreasen J and Tylor M Cost effectiveness of SQ HDM SLIT tablet in addition to pharmacotherapy for the treament of house dust mite allergic rhinitis in Germany

56. Pokladnikova J, Krcmova I, Vlcek J. Economic evaluation of sublingual vs subcutaneous allergen immunotherapy. *Ann Allergy Asthma Immunol.* 2008;100:482—489.

57. Ronborg SM, Svendsen UG, Micheelsen JS, Ytte L, Andreasen JN, Ehlers L. Budget impact analysis of two immunotherapy products for treatment of grass pollen-induced allergic rhinoconjunctivitis. *Clin Outcomes Res.* 2012;4:253—260.

58. Westerhout KY, Verheggen BG, Schreder CH, Augustin M. Cost effective- ness analysis of immunotherapy in patients with grass pollen allergic rhino- conjunctivitis in Germany. *J Med Econ.* 2012;15:906—917.

59. Dranitsaris G, Ellis AK. Sublingual or subcutaneous immunotherapy for seasonal allergic rhinitis: an indirect analysis of efficacy, safety and cost. *J Eval Clin Pract.* 2014;20:225—238.

60. Verheggen BG, Westerhout K, Schreder C, Augustin M. Health economic comparison of SLIT allergen and SCIT allergic immunotherapy in patients with seasonal grass - allergic rhino conjunctivitis in Germany. *Clin Transl Allergy.* 2015;5:1—10.

61. Reinhold T, Bruggenjurden. Cost-Effectiveness of grass pollen SCIT compared with SLIT and symptomatic treatment. *Allergo J Int.* 2017;26:7—15.

62. Schadlich PK, Brecht JG. Economic evaluation of specific immunotherapy versus symptomatic treatment of allergic rhinitis in Germany. *Pharmacoeconomics.* 2000;17:37—52.

63. Omnes LF, Bousquet J, Scheinmann P, et al. Pharmacoeconomic assessment of specific immunotherapy versus current symptomatic treatment for allergic rhinitis and asthma in France. *Allerg Immunol.* 2007;39:148—156.

64. Hankin CS, Cox L, Lang D, et al. Allergen immunotherapy and health care cost benefits for children with allergic rhinitis: a large-scale, retrospective, matched cohort study. *Ann Allergy Asthma Immunol.* 2010;104:79—85.

65. Reinhold M, Willich S, Brüggenjürgen B. Subcutaneous specific immunotherapy: economic implications from the perspective of statutory health insurance — a population based cost-effectiveness estimation. *Allergologie*. 2012;35:539—550.

66. Donahue JG, Greineder DK, Connor-Lacke L, Canning CF, Platt R. Utilization and cost of immunotherapy for allergic asthma and rhinitis. *Ann Allergy Asthma Immunol*. 1999; 82:339—347.

67. Mauro M, Russello M, Alesina R, et al. Safety and pharmacoeconomics of a cluster administration of mite immunotherapy compared to the traditional one. *Eur Ann Allergy Clin Immunol*. 2006;38:31—34.

68. Bachert C, Vestenbaek U, Christensen J, Griffiths UK, Poulsen PB. Cost-effectiveness of grass allergen tablet (GRAZAX(R)) for the prevention of seasonal grass pollen induced rhinoconjunctivitis — a Northern European perspective. *Clin Exp Allergy*. 2007;37: 772—779.

69. Beriot-Mathiot A, Vestenbaek U, Bo Poulsen P. Influence of time horizon and treatment patterns on cost-effectiveness measures: the case of allergen-specific immunotherapy with Grazax. *J Med Econ*. 2007;10:215—228.

70. Ariano R, Berto P, Incorvaia C, et al. Economic evaluation of sublingual immunotherapy vs. symptomatic treatment in allergic asthma. *Ann Allergy Asthma Immunol*. 2009;103: 254—259.

71. Mabry RL. Desensitization versus intraturbinal injection of corticosteroid for nasal allergy: indications, effectiveness, and patient acceptance. *South Med J*. 1982;75: 423—425.

72. Cohn JR, Pizzi A. Determinants of patient compliance with allergen immunotherapy. *J Allergy Clin Immunol*. 1993;91:734—737.

73. Lower T, Henry J, Mandik L, Janosky J, Friday Jr GA. Compliance with allergen immunotherapy. *Ann Allergy*. 1993;70:480—482.

74. Rhodes BJ. Patient dropouts before completion of optimal dose, multiple allergen immunotherapy. *Ann Allergy Asthma Immunol*. 1999;82:281—286.

75. More DR, Hagan LL. Factors affecting compliance with allergen immunotherapy at a military medical center. *Ann Allergy Asthma Immunol*. 2002;88:391—394.

76. Dam Petersen K, Gyrd-Hansen D, Kjaergaard S, Dahl R. Clinical and patient based evaluation of immunotherapy for grass pollen and mite allergy. *Allergol Immunopathol*. 2005;33:264—269.

77. Tinkelman D, Smith F, Cole 3rd WQ, Silk HJ. Compliance with an allergen immunotherapy regime. *Ann Allergy Asthma Immunol*. 1995;74:241—246.

78. Pajno GB, Vita D, Caminiti L, et al. Children's compliance with allergen immunotherapy according to administration routes. *J Allergy Clin Immunol*. 2005;116:1380—1381.

79. Mahesh PA, Vedanthan PK, Amrutha DH, Giridhar BH, Prabhakar AK. Factors associated with non-adherence to specific allergen immunotherapy in management of respiratory allergy. *Indian J Chest Dis Allied Sci*. 2010;52:91—95.

80. Hsu NM, Reisacher WR. A comparison of attrition rates in patients undergoing sublingual immunotherapy vs subcutaneous immunotherapy. *Int Forum Allergy Rhinol*. 2012; 2:280—284.

81. Sieber J, De Geest S, Shah-Hosseini K, Mosges R. Medication persistence with long-term, specific grass pollen immunotherapy measured by prescription renewal rates. *Curr Med Res Opin*. 2011;27:855—861.

82. Ruiz FJ, Jimenez A, Cocoletzi J, Duran E. Compliance with and abandonment of immunotherapy. *Rev Alerg Mex*. 1997;44:42—44.

83. Kiel MA, Roder E, Gerth van Wijk R, Al MJ, Hop WC, Rutten-van Molken MP. Real-life compliance and persistence among users of subcutaneous and sublingual allergen immunotherapy. *J Allergy Clin Immunol.* 2013;132(2):353−360.

84. Jansen A, Andersen KF, Bruning H. Evaluation of a compliance device in a subgroup of adult patients receiving specific immunotherapy with grass allergen tablets (GRAZAX) in a randomized, open-label, controlled study: an a priori subgroup analysis. *Clin Ther.* 2009;31:321−327.

85. Durham SR, Yang WH, Pedersen MR, Johansen N, Rak S. Sublingual immunotherapy with once-daily grass allergen tablets: a randomized controlled trial in seasonal allergic rhinoconjunctivitis. *J Allergy Clin Immunol.* 2006;117:802−809.

86. Passalacqua G, Musarra A, Pecora S, et al. Quantitative assessment of the compliance with a once-daily sublingual immunotherapy regimen in real life (EASY project: evaluation of A novel SLIT formulation during a Year). *J Allergy Clin Immunol.* 2006;117: 946−948.

87. Passalacqua G, Musarra A, Pecora S, et al. Quantitative assessment of the compliance with once-daily sublingual immunotherapy in children (EASY project: evaluation of a novel SLIT formulation during a year). *Pediatr Allergy Immunol.* 2007;18:58−62.

88. Halken S, Agertoft L, Seidenberg J, et al. Five-grass pollen 300IR SLIT tablets: efficacy and safety in children and adolescents. *Pediatr Allergy Immunol.* 2010;21:970−976.

89. Bufe A, Eberle P, Franke-Beckmann E, et al. Safety and efficacy in children of an SQ-standardized grass allergen tablet for sublingual immunotherapy. *J Allergy Clin Immunol.* 2009;123:167−173 e7.

90. Lombardi C, Gani F, Landi M, et al. Quantitative assessment of the adherence to sublingual immunotherapy. *J Allergy Clin Immunol.* 2004;113:1219−1220.

91. Wahn U, Tabar A, Kuna P, et al. Efficacy and safety of 5-grass-pollen sublingual immunotherapy tablets in pediatric allergic rhinoconjunctivitis. *J Allergy Clin Immunol.* 2009; 123:160−166 e3.

92. Shaikh WA, Shaikh SW. Allergies in India: a study on medication compliance. *J Indian Med Assoc.* 2009;107:462−463.

93. Ott H, Sieber J, Brehler R, et al. Efficacy of grass pollen sublingual immunotherapy for three consecutive seasons and after cessation of treatment: the ECRIT study. *Allergy.* 2009;64:179−186.

94. Marogna M, Tomassetti D, Bernasconi A, et al. Preventive effects of sublingual immunotherapy in childhood: an open randomized controlled study. *Ann Allergy Asthma Immunol.* 2008;101:206−211.

95. Roder E, Berger MY, de Groot H, Gerth van Wijk R. Sublingual immunotherapy in youngsters: adherence in a randomized clinical trial. *Clin Exp Allergy.* 2008;38: 1659−1667.

96. Pajno GB, Caminiti L, Crisafulli G, et al. Adherence to sublingual immunotherapy in preschool children. *Pediatr Allergy Immunol.* 2012;23:688−689.

97. Senna G, Lombardi C, Canonica GW, Passalacqua G. How adherent to sublingual immunotherapy prescriptions are patients? The manufacturers' viewpoint. *J Allergy Clin Immunol.* 2010;126:668−669.

98. Sade K, Berkun Y, Dolev Z, Shalit M, Kivity S. Knowledge and expectations of patients receiving aeroallergen immunotherapy. *Ann Allergy Asthma Immunol.* 2003;91:444−448.

99. Vita D, Caminiti L, Ruggeri P, Pajno GB. Sublingual immunotherapy: adherence based on timing and monitoring control visits. *Allergy.* 2010;65:668−669.

AIT and immunomodulatories in investigation

Unconventional but promising routes for allergen immunotherapy: an update on intralymphatic and epicutaneous immunotherapy

Gabriela Senti, MD [1], **Pål Johansen, PhD** [2], **Marta Paulucci, MSc** [2], **Thomas M. Kündig, MD** [2]

[1]*Direction Research and Education University, University Hospital Zurich, Zurich, Switzerland;* [2]*Department of Dermatology, University Hospital Zurich & University of Zurich, Zurich, Switzerland*

Introduction

Respiratory allergies and food allergies are important socioeconomic burden with approximately 6% of the population suffering from food allergies[1] and up to 30% of the population suffering from respiratory allergies.[2] Pharmacotherapy ameliorates IgE-mediated symptoms, but it is only a "symptomatic" treatment that cannot prevent progression of disease, e.g., from rhinoconjunctivitis to asthma and to food allergies. The only disease-modifying treatment that also has a long-term effect is allergen immunotherapy (AIT).[3−10] More than a century ago, Noon[11] introduced subcutaneous immunotherapy (SCIT) for the treatment of hay fever. However, despite its high efficacy, long-lasting symptom amelioration, and high cost-effectiveness,[9,10] less than 5% of allergy patients choose to undergo AIT. Additionally, patient compliance and treatment adherence with AIT are generally poor.[12] This is primarily because the current routes of AIT (SCIT and the more recently introduced sublingual immunotherapy (SLIT)) have major disadvantages. Subcutaneous AIT has the disadvantage that it requires from 12 to 70 visits to a medically supervised clinic and an observation period after administration (Fig. 16.1A). Thus, SCIT requires a fair amount of patient time, which has a cost, i.e., lost time from work, cost related to travel, etc.). In addition, many SCIT patients quit treatment due to lack of efficacy or due to systemic allergic reactions or bothersome large local reactions.[13−17] In Europe, SLIT is being used routinely, and the method is gradually

Immunotherapies for Allergic Disease. https://doi.org/10.1016/B978-0-323-54427-6.00016-X

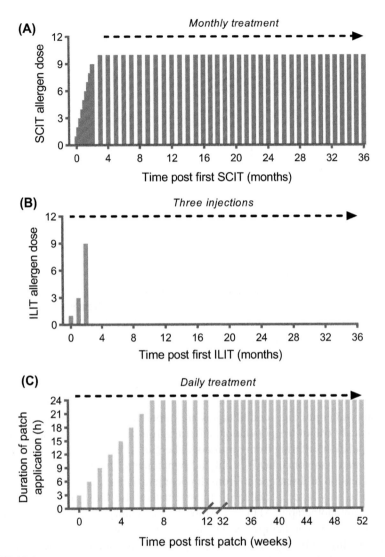

FIGURE 16.1

Illustration of representative dosing schemes of SCIT (A), ILIT (B), and EPIT (C). SCIT is typically administered in weekly to monthly intervals over 3 years, with an initial dose-increasing phase of 4–12 weeks. ILIT is typically administered every 4 weeks, and the number of injections is typically three, with a dose escalation throughout. In EPIT, the allergen-containing patch is applied to the skin and left there for a certain time. The duration of application and the intervals between each patch application have varied, but for the most developed patches, a dose escalation (duration of a single application) period of 12 weeks and daily applications for 1 year have been recommended. SCIT, subcutaneous immunotherapy; ILIT, intralymphatic immunotherapy; EPIT, epicutaneous allergen immunotherapy.

spreading to the United States.[18] The introduction of SLIT could widen the scope of AIT and allow an increased number of patients to receive therapy as the treatment is home-based. Generally, the first SLIT dose is administered in a medically supervised setting. If well tolerated, SLIT is subsequently self-administered at home. Despite daily treatment for 3 years, adherence to SCIT appears to be better than to SLIT,[23] and for SLIT, the cost seems to be the main factor for discontinuation.[13,19−22] While both SCIT and SLIT are efficacious, when appropriately used, adherence to both AIT types is similar concerning patients remaining on therapy. In one study, the percentages of patients who prematurely discontinued treatment were 11%−77% for SCIT, while 22%−93% for SLIT.[23] Hence, it is important to involve the patient in the decision to use AIT and which form of therapy to be utilized.

While AIT is considered both efficacious and safe,[7,24−27] there remains room for improvement. This review therefore discusses alternative routes to the regulatory authority approved SCIT and SCIT, with a special focus on how the route can improve efficacy, safety, and patient compliance. These are dependent variables, as improved efficacy will allow reducing the number of allergen administrations, or treatment duration, or allergen dose, which by consequence should improve patient compliance and safety. Both intralymphatic immunotherapy (ILIT) and epicutaneous immunotherapy (EPIT) (Fig. 16.1B−C) have potential to become alternative routes of AIT with better or comparable treatment adherence and efficacy. Fig. 16.1 illustrates representative dosing schemes of SCIT, ILIT, and EPIT. SCIT is typically administered in weekly to monthly intervals over 3 years, with an initial dose-increasing phase of 4−12 weeks (Fig. 16.1A). Phase I/II clinical trials with ILIT have typically been performed by intralymphatic administrations of allergen every 4 weeks, and the number of injections are typically three (Fig. 16.1B). Typically, the dose has been increased from the first to the last ILIT injection. In some trials, shorter intervals and more injections have been applied. In EPIT trials, the allergen-containing patch is applied to the skin and left there for a certain period of time. The duration of application and the intervals between each patch application have varied in different trials, but for the most developed patches, a dose escalation (duration of a single application) period of 12 weeks and daily applications for 1 year have been recommended (Fig. 16.1C).

Fig. 16.2 illustrates the routes of AIT by means of SCIT and ILIT (Fig. 16.2A) and EPIT (Fig. 16.2B). It shows that all routes aim at delivering AIT allergen to draining lymph nodes. In SCIT, the allergen is administered to the subcutaneous tissue that often contains much fatty tissue and low concentrations of professional antigen-presenting cells (APCs) such as dendritic cells (DCs). In EPIT, the allergen has to penetrate the epidermal barrier of the skin, upon which it can encounter epidermal DCs or Langerhans cells (LCs), which again can carry allergens through lymphatic vessels to the draining lymph node. In ILIT, the lymph node is located by means of ultrasound and the allergen is directly injected into the lymph node that contains large number of DCs, but also other APCs such as macrophages and B cells. In the following, we especially review the recent developments of ILIT and EPIT.

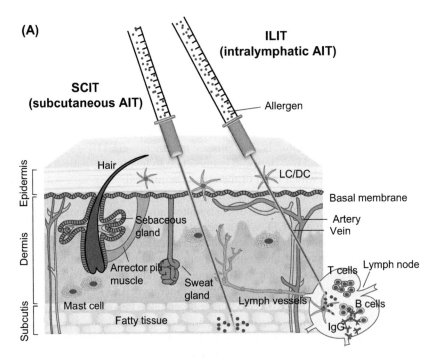

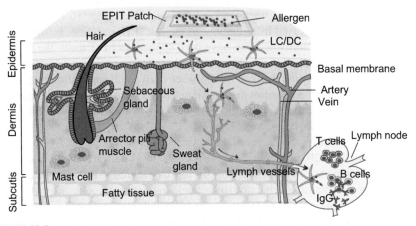

FIGURE 16.2

Illustration of the routes of AIT by means of SCIT and ILIT (A) and by means of EPIT (B). All routes aim at delivering AIT allergen to draining lymph nodes. In SCIT, the allergen is administered to the subcutaneous tissue that often contains much fatty tissue and low concentrations of professional antigen-presenting cells such as dendritic cells (DCs). In ILIT, the lymph node is located by means of ultrasound and the allergen is directly injected

Measures to enhance AIT efficacy

To reduce the number of allergen administrations and thus to shorten the duration of AIT, immunogenicity of the administered allergen has to be enhanced. A straightforward approach would simply be to increase the allergen dose. AIT has a clear dose-dependent effect,[28] but the dose-dependent allergic side effects limit the dose that can be given. Rendering allergens hypoallergenic by chemical modification to allergoids,[29–31] by recombinant modification,[31–34] or by using non-IgE-binding[35–38] or immunoregulatory[39,40] peptides may also permit increased allergen doses, but the modifications often negatively affect allergen immunogenicity. A reduction of injection numbers may also be achieved by replacing the classically used aluminum salts with a more T helper (Th) 1 promoting adjuvant, such as the Toll-like receptor (TLR) ligands CpG oligodeoxynucleotide,[41] monophosphoryl lipid A,[42–45] or microcrystalline tyrosine.[46]

The number of injections may also be reduced by changing to a more efficient route of allergen delivery. Ideally, this route would be characterized by a high density of APCs. The latter are present at highest density in secondary lymphatic organs, such as lymph nodes. Indeed, when allergen was administered directly into lymph nodes, the number of injections could be reduced to only three.[47–49] This so-called ILIT is discussed in more details below.

Measures to improve AIT safety

To improve safety of AIT, inadvertent allergen delivery to the blood vasculature must be avoided, ideally by delivery of the allergen to nonvascularized tissue. SLIT fulfills this criterion because allergen is delivered to the oral mucosa, which is covered by a multilayered epithelium. However, the allergen diffuses down into deeper mast cell—containing layers, and this diffusion is responsible for the frequently observed oral side effects.[50–52] The tissue below the epithelium also contains a high density of blood vessels. However, without microtrauma to this vasculature, it rarely happens that significant amounts of allergen reach the

---

into the lymph node that contains large number of DCs, but also other APCs such as macrophages and B cells. These cells can take up AIT allergen and present this to lymphocytes for induction of allergen-specific antibody and T-cell responses, including tolerance-mediating CD4 Tregs. The annotated doses for SCIT and ILIT are arbitrary. In EPIT, the allergen penetrates the epidermal barrier of the skin, upon which it encounters epidermal DCs or LCs. The LCs, in part activated by keratinocytes, migrate to dermis and subsequently via lymphatic vessels to a subcutaneous draining lymph for stimulation of allergen-specific B and T cell responses, including allergen-neutralizing IgG antibodies and Tregs. SCIT, subcutaneous immunotherapy; ILIT, intralymphatic immunotherapy; EPIT, epicutaneous allergen immunotherapy.

circulation, for which reason SLIT has proved safe in terms of systemic allergic side effects.[50,51] The same should hold true for EPIT, where allergen is administered to the nonvascularized epidermis. An advantage of EPIT over SLIT is that keratinocytes can additionally be activated by physical irritation, such as abrasion or adhesive tape stripping, or also by adding adjuvants.[53] Such epithelial irritation increases the expression of proinflammatory cytokines, such as IL-1α and TNF-α, which skew the immune response toward Th1.[54] These effects can activate LCs to leave the epidermis and migrate into draining lymph nodes for activation of T and B cells. Therefore, EPIT may reduce side effects by minimizing the risk of allergen inadvertently reaching the blood vasculature, but also shorten treatment duration by increasing immunogenicity. We have also observed that epicutaneously administered allergen rapidly and efficiently diffuses down into the dermis.[55]

Intralymphatic allergen immunotherapy

The concept that antigen localization is a key parameter that determines the strength of the immune response was pioneered in Zurich by the work of Rolf Zinkernagel, Nobel laureate in Medicine. Because an immune response requires the interaction of three important immune cells (APCs, T cells, and B cells), a reaction is more likely to happen at a site where these three cell types are present in high numbers. This premise holds for antigens targeted to lymphoid organs, in particular lymph nodes, whereas antigens outside such organs are largely ignored by the immune system.[56] A great number of preclinical and clinical studies have demonstrated the potency of intralymphatic administration of peptides, proteins, DNA, RNA, bacteria, viruses, or DCs, as comprehensively reviewed.[57] In mice, ILIT with bee venom allergens; food allergens; and allergen extracts from grass pollen, birch pollen, and cat dander stimulated robust antiallergic and protective B- and T-cell immune responses.[58-61] Compared with SCIT, ILIT enhanced efficiency of immunization, inducing allergen-specific IgG2a antibody responses 10 to 20 times higher with only 0.1% of the allergen dose.[62] Moreover, ILIT enhanced IL-2, IFN-γ, IL-4, and IL-10 secretion from lymphocytes when compared with SCIT, suggesting that ILIT did not polarize the response toward Th1, Th2, or Th17, but generated overall stronger responses.[62] The mechanism by which ILIT works is not necessarily different from that of conventional SCIT. However, ILIT facilitates the delivery of more allergen to lymph nodes than SCIT or any other route, as demonstrated in biodistribution studies in mice[62,63] and humans.[63] Hence, the immune responses and, consequentially, the therapeutic efficacy of ILIT are potentially stronger than of SCIT. Moreover, because ILIT allows for administration of lower allergen doses, it would be expected to have a lower incidence of unwanted allergic side effects because allergic adverse events are proportional to the administered allergen dose.

ILIT using allergen extracts

In a Swiss trial, 165 patients with seasonal rhinoconjunctivitis due to grass pollen sensitization were randomized to receive either 54 SCIT injections with pollen extract over 3 years (cumulative allergen dose: 4,031,540 units) or three ILIT injections over 2 months (3000 units).[47] Both for ILIT and SCIT, 25-gauge needles were used, and ILIT was not associated with more injection-associated pain.[47] Patients who received ILIT experienced increased tolerance to nasal allergen provocation within 4 months of treatment. The tolerance was long lasting and comparable to the tolerance achieved after 3 years of SCIT. Grass pollen ILIT caused symptom amelioration, reduced skin prick test reactivity, decreased specific serum IgE, and it was associated with fewer allergic adverse events than SCIT. As compared to SCIT patients, ILIT patients showed enhanced compliance, mostly likely because of they only had to comply with getting three injections. Out of 66 patients allocated to receive ILIT, 58 (88%) started and completed the treatment. In contrast, only 54 out of 99 (55%) patients allocated to receive SCIT completed their therapy.

In the described study, ILIT was not compared with placebo but with perennial SCIT with grass pollen extract. However, an independent Swedish study confirmed the results of ILIT in a double-blind placebo-controlled trial,[49] and another placebo-controlled trial by the same group conformed their previous findings in polysensitized patients who received ILIT for both grass and birch allergy, by split injections into their left and right inguinal lymph nodes.[64] The latter trial found that ILIT induced effector memory T cells and CCR5+ TH1-type central memory cells,[64] as well as regulatory T cells (Tregs), both biomarkers that have been reported to correlate with successful AIT.[65] A further Scandinavian open label 3-year clinical study in 10 patients with grass and birch pollen allergy revealed statistically significant clinical efficacy and the induction of both grass pollen− and birch pollen−specific Tregs,[66] and ILIT were also shown to induce allergen-specific non-IgE producing plasmablasts and increased cutaneous tolerance.[67]

In an open-label South Korean study in 11 patients with sensitization to house dust mite, cat, or dog allergens, ILIT was found to improve rhinitis symptoms and to improve quality of life for at least 1 year.[68] As compared to pretreatment levels, ILIT was found to reduce the use of rescue medication and to alleviate allergic symptoms during allergen exposure in daily life. However, the study also reported two cases of grade 3 (Mueller classification) allergic adverse events in highly sensitized patients receiving combined *Der f* and *Der p* ILIT.[68] One patient reacted with anaphylaxis to the first ILIT with 30 μg allergen. A second patient did not react to the first ILIT with 30 μg allergen, but showed symptoms of anaphylaxis after ILIT with 100 μg allergen 4 weeks later. Despite the severe reactions, the patients choose to undergo further ILIT with reduced allergen doses. The two patients did not experience further adverse allergic reactions. Interestingly, when questioned about the personal cost contribution to AIT, the ILIT patients reported increased willingness to pay for treatment.[69]

A pediatric allergology group performed a double-blind placebo-controlled clinical trial in 15 adolescent patients with grass pollen allergy, and the study showed excellent safety and a strong treatment effect after three injections during 8 weeks.[70] Again, ILIT compliance was excellent as all patients completed the trial.

ILIT using recombinant and modified allergens

In a randomized placebo-controlled double-blind trial, we investigated the efficacy of ILIT with a recombinant cat dander allergen that was also modified to target major histocompatibility complex class II (MAT-Fel d 1).[48] Three MAT-Fel d 1 ILIT injections with 1 month interval improved nasal allergen tolerance and stimulated antigen-specific Treg responses and IgG4 without any significant allergic adverse events. Interestingly, MAT-Fel d 1 ILIT was found to induce IgG4 but no IgG1 antibody production,[71] likely also because of the immunomodulatory properties of the MAT component of the allergen.[72]

Time interval between injections in ILIT

In a double-blind placebo-controlled clinical trial in patients with seasonal allergic rhinitis due to grass pollen sensitization, Witten and colleagues[73] found that three or six ILIT sessions induced some desired immunological changes, such as Treg responses and elevated IgG4. However, the authors reported no improvement of clinical parameters, such as symptom amelioration or reduced need to take other antiallergic medication. If anything, symptoms tended to worsen. The authors concluded that their data were conflicting by us[47,48] and Hylander and colleagues.[49] However, Witten and colleagues[73] used a different protocol. While we and Hylander,[49] as well as Patterson in the ILIT report in adolescents,[70] used a 4-week time interval between injections, Witten and colleagues[73] used only 2-week intervals. It is well known from vaccine immunology that shortening the time interval from four to 2 weeks interferes with memory B cell formation and affinity maturation, which both require phases where only small amounts of antigen are present in lymph follicles. Small amounts enable competition for the antigen, which again positively selects for high-affinity memory B cells. Similar effects are postulated for affinity and functionality of the T cell response.[74] For example, Patel and colleagues[75] observed that four peptide injections (Cat-PAD) with 4-week intervals improved allergen tolerance in patients at 1-year follow-up, whereas the same total AIT peptide dose given through eight injections with 2-week intervals did not produce significant tolerance in the rhinoconjunctival provocation using environmental exposure chambers. Of note, interim analysis in the same study at 18−22 weeks revealed improved tolerance in both treatment groups as compared with placebo. Furthermore, shortening the time interval between injections is known to shift the immune response toward Th2,[76] which may explain why Witten and colleagues[73] observed symptoms to worsen. We evaluated the question of ILIT time intervals in a murine allergy model and found that the ILIT-mediated induction of IgG1 and IgG2a was independent of the dosing interval, but that the IgG2s response had higher affinity when prolonging the time interval between dosing.[77] In conclusion, ILIT directly into a subcutaneous lymph node is (1) readily feasible, (2) practically painless, (3) reduces the required allergen dose, (4) reduces the number of required AIT sessions to three, (5) reduces the treatment duration from 3 years to 2 months, (6) enhances safety, and (7) enhances patient compliance.

Outlook for ILIT

The organ with the highest density of immune cells certainly is the lymph node. Upon uptake of antigen or AIT allergen, skin-resident APCs migrate to the draining lymph nodes, as this is the only place where a sufficient number of T cells are present.[56,57] The same is true for the subsequent cognate interaction between antigen-specific T cells and B cells. As there is also a high density of immature DCs present in lymph nodes, direct administration of a vaccine or allergen into a lymph node should certainly be the most efficient route for immunization. As discussed above, this method has also been used since the 1950s in various animal models and using various vaccines. It is therefore not surprising that there are now several clinical trials in allergy demonstrating high clinical efficacy after only three injections. Due to the high efficacy of the route, not only the number of injections can be reduced, but also the allergen dose, rendering this route safer than conventional SCIT.

Good-quality ILIT requires ultrasound and is certainly more cumbersome than EPIT or SCIT, but with only three injections, ILIT leads to a high treatment adherence, and the high clinical efficacy should also lead to high treatment satisfaction. One technical concern of ILIT that may be raised is the location of lymph nodes in obese persons, which may represent more than 50% of the patients.[78] However, lymphadenectomy is a normal procedure in radiology and oncology, and obesity does not affect the number of retrieved lymph nodes and the rate of intraoperative complications in gynecologic cancers.[79] Especially, the accessibility of inguinal lymph nodes, as utilized in ILIT, should not be particularly impaired in obese patients, as the groin area is not particularly prone to obesity, and the abdominal skin folds can be "lifted off" the groin area for ultrasound-guided injections.

Epicutaneous allergen immunotherapy

In the vaccine field, the delivery of antigen across the skin is referred to as "transcutaneous" vaccination.[80] We believe that in the context of AIT, in order to be in line with the terms SCIT and SLIT, this route should be called epicutaneous immunotherapy,[81] and we introduced the acronym EPIT for this route.[82] The nomenclature "subcutaneous" and "sublingual" immunotherapy both refer to the site of allergen administration, i.e., the "subcutaneous tissue" or the "sublingual" space, and not to the further penetration or further immunological transport of the allergen.

The epicutaneous route of vaccination is by no means new. This is actually the original route, used in ancient times in India, Tibet, and other parts of Asia, from where it arrived in England in the early 18th century.[83] There, Edward Jenner applied cowpox virus to scarified human skin. After the world became free of pox, this route of vaccination was somewhat forgotten, but at the beginning of the 21st century, epicutaneous vaccination had a revival, driven by the increasing interest in novel needle-free vaccination routes. Epicutaneous vaccination against *Escherichia coli*–induced traveler's diarrhea made the first step.[84] Soon after, animal models showed success in transcutaneous/epicutaneous vaccination against *Helicobacter pylori*,[85] influenza virus,[86] and diphtheria toxin.[87] The protective mechanism in all of these applications relies on induction of humoral immunity dominated by IgG1 and IgA. Studies testing epicutaneous vaccination against human immunodeficiency virus also found induction of mucosal cytotoxic T cells together with secretion of mucosal antibodies.[88]

One major advantage of EPIT is that the skin contains several types of immune cells, DCs, LCs, T cells, NK cells, macrophages.[89] Especially DCs and LCs are good in priming T cells, for which reason epicutaneous vaccination has also been tested for cancer immunotherapy. Indeed, promising results was achieved for the induction of CD8+ T cell responses,[90,91] and EPIT was successfully applied to induce suppressive T cell responses in experimental allergic encephalomyelitis.[91,92] At current, several vaccines for transcutaneous or epicutaneous vaccination are undergoing clinical testing, as reviewed in Ref. 93.

History of EPIT in allergy

We have discussed the fascinating and mostly forgotten history of EPIT as an allergy treatment in previous reviews.[81,94] Allergen EPIT was introduced already in 1917. Besredka showed that EPIT induced specific antibodies.[95] Five years later, in 1921, Vallery-Radot and Hangenau reported the first case study on successful EPIT in human.[96] In patients with allergy to horse dander, they found that allergen administration onto scarified skin ameliorated systemic allergic symptoms. A decade later, when SCIT, introduced by Noon and Freeman in 1911,[11] was being more widely used, also the risks of subcutaneous pollen extract injection became apparent. At the time, suffering from a "pollen shock" during SCIT was recognized as a considerable danger of subcutaneous allergen administration in highly sensitized patients. Therefore, a method called intradermal allergen-specific immunotherapy was developed.[97,98] This idea was based on an observation by Phillips,[98] that hay fever patients often reported symptom amelioration after intradermal pollen tests. Philipps therefore started treating highly sensitive patients by intradermal administration of pollen extract. Interestingly, intradermal AIT was found to be both safe and efficacious. Symptom relief was reported already after administration of three doses.[98] Similarly, Ramirez treated grass pollen–allergic patients by so-called "cuti-vaccination," the administration of pollen extract onto scarified skin.[99] Therefore, already in the 1930s it was suggested that the subcutaneous route might not be optimal for AIT.[97]

In the 1950s and 1960s, EPIT was revisited by French allergologists.[99,100] Pautrizel[100] administered allergen extract onto only rubbed, not scarified, epidermis. Results were reported to be excellent, but a large number of applications were required to reach symptom relief. Blamoutier[95,99] applied allergen extract onto scarified skin: "On the proximal volar aspect of the lower arm, in a square area of 4 × 4 cm, chessboard-like horizontal and vertical scratches are made with a needle [...] These scratches should be superficial and not cause bleeding."[101] Allergic side effects of the epicutaneous method were rare and considered milder than after conventional SCIT.[98–100] Therefore, the method became used all over Europe.[101–103] Symptom relief reported to be rapid, and the relative safety of the method allowed performing coseasonal treatment. Also, the reported clinical efficacy seemed to surpass SCIT.[101] Despite better safety and better clinical efficacy than SCIT, and despite reproducibility of the method across Europe, this route, in France called "méthode de quadrillage cutané," was then forgotten, and in the second half of the last century SCIT became the gold standard.

EPIT with aeroallergens

While the scientific and historical evidence for EPIT in allergy is strong, there existed no double-blind placebo-controlled clinical trials. This led us revisit EPIT with the aim of offering more convenience for patients, i.e., a safe route that would allow for self-administration at home. This should be goal achievable with EPIT. Moreover, a needle-free method would be important especially for children. We performed three clinical trials testing efficacy and safety of EPIT. In order to keep epithelial barrier disruption minimal, we replaced skin scarification by adhesive tape stripping.[104,105] A normal, self-adhesive tape (e.g., Scotch tape) was stuck to the skin and lifted off, repeated 6 times with a new part of tape. Such tape stripping represents a barrier disruption which is likely somewhere in between rubbing the skin performed by Pautrizel[100] and scarification with a needle performed by Blamoutier.[95] Besides enhancing the penetration of allergens by removing or at least damaging the *stratum corneum*,[105] tape stripping also activates of keratinocytes to express and secrete a number of proinflammatory cytokines (IL-1, IL-6, IL-8, TNFα, and IFNγ). The latter induce maturation of LCs and their emigration to draining lymph nodes.[106,107] In a first double-blind placebo-controlled trial, we found that application of 12 patches containing grass pollen extract significantly ameliorated symptoms in hay fever patients. We could also confirm the abovementioned historic studies reporting excellent safety, as we observed no systemic allergic side effects. Adverse events were limited to mild local eczematous reactions under the skin patch.[104] Over the entire trial with 12 patch applications per patient, mild eczema was seen in 15 out of the 21 patients receiving allergen EPIT, and only in 5 out of the 15 placebo patients. When looking at a single patch application, eczema under the patch was observed in roughly half of the allergen EPIT patients. This eczema had a severity score between 3 and 6 on a scale from 0 to 18. It was concluded that patch-associated eczema correlated with symptom amelioration.

In a second dose escalation trial, we included 132 patients with grass pollen allergy. The aim of this trial was to find the optimal treatment dose for EPIT. Patients in this trial received six patches during the pollen season. There was a clear positive correlation between the allergen dose in the patch and the clinical effect,[108] and also the local adverse effects were clearly dose dependent. The most frequently reported local adverse event was pruritus under the patch, followed by eczema observed after patch removal. Interestingly, with every subsequent patch application, we observed a reduction of local adverse events. After the sixth and last patch application, approximately half as many local adverse events were reported. This reduction could not be explained by local degranulation of mast cells or depletion of immune cells, as the protocol asked to apply each of the six patches to a different area of the arm. Apparently, the reduction of local adverse events was explained by induction of immunological tolerance. In a third clinical trial, the immunological changes induced during EPIT were investigated. EPIT induced allergen-specific IgG4.[109] The clinical efficacy observed in our three double-blind placebo-controlled trials have been independently confirmed by Agostinis et al., demonstrating safety and efficacy of EPIT in children with grass pollen allergy. Symptoms of hay fever and use of rescue medication were significantly reduced in patients receiving allergen EPIT.[110]

There are no head-to-head clinical comparisons of EPIT to other routes AIT, but such appraisals have been done in murine models. In the mouse, EPIT with Phl p 5 was equivalent or better than SLIT.[111] Although IgG2a titers induced by EPIT and SLIT were comparable and although reduction of IgE levels was similar, in the asthma model, only EPIT could significantly reduce eosinophil numbers in the bronchoalveolar lavage. Our own comparison of SCIT with EPIT using ovalbumin in a murine model also found that EPIT and SCIT were comparably efficient.[53]

When comparing the three double-blind placebo-controlled clinical trials we performed, we could see a clear linear dependence on the total allergen dose administered.[109] A strategy to improve EPIT should therefore be to deliver higher allergen doses. Thus, in our last clinical trial, we changed from tape stripping to abrasion of the skin using a conventional nail file. While abrasion was mild and did not cause any visible alteration or damage to the skin, we were surprised by a number of systemic allergic reactions.[109] The systemic side effects correlated with the degree of *stratum corneum* disruption with six grade 3 systemic allergic reactions after skin preparation by abrasion (n = 26, 23%) and only one grade 3 reaction after tape stripping (n = 239, 0.4%). The latter number was not different from that observed after placebo EPIT (n = 277, 0.4%). Obviously, due to the tight barrier function of the *stratum corneum*, a relatively high dose of allergen must be used in EPIT. Controlling skin penetration by preparing the skin therefore becomes a highly critical parameter for the safety of EPIT.

Epicutaneous immunotherapy with food allergens

A clinical trial using the Viaskin EDS (DBV Technologies, Bagneux, France) tested efficacy and safety of EPIT in children with cow's milk allergy. There was a tendency toward increased cumulative tolerance doses after a 3-month treatment period.[112] Treatment was well tolerated and no systemic allergic reactions occurred. The only reported side effects were local eczematous skin reactions. Good safety is pivotal for considering EPIT as a treatment option for food allergies, where conventional SCIT has a high rate of anaphylactic reactions.[113]

In a phase I study, peanut EPIT with the Viaskin patch showed good safety and tolerability during a 2-week treatment period.[114] This phase I study was followed by a phase II study in 74 peanut-allergic patients of 4–25 years of age. In this double-blind placebo-controlled multicenter clinical trial, the participants were treated either with placebo EPIT or peanut EPIT at two doses.[115] After 52 weeks, treatment showed success in 12% of the placebo patients, in 46% of patients treated with the 100 µg dose, and in 48% of patients treated with the 250 µg dose, respectively. The changes in successfully consumed peanut doses were 43 mg in the 100 µg group, and 130 mg of protein in the 250 µg group, while no improvement was observed after placebo EPIT; one peanut contains approximately 240 mg peanut proteins. Treatment success was found to be better in younger children, but safe with predominantly mild local reactions at the patch site. Peanut EPIT increased peanut-specific IgG4 levels and the IgG4 to IgE ratio, and decreased basophil activation and peanut-specific Th2 cytokines. While statistically significant, the authors concluded that treatment response was "modest."[115] In another phase IIb dose-ranging trial in peanut-allergic patients with a median age of 11 years, administration of Viaskin patches with 250 µg peanut extract over 12 months resulted in a significant response versus placebo,[116] and the serum titers allergen-specific Igg4 was increased.[117] The following phase III trial with 356 peanut-allergic children found a significant difference in treatment response after 12 months when compared with placebo, but failed to meet another prespecified criterion, i.e., ≥15% lower bound of the confidence interval; the latter was 12.4%.[118] While this is only an arbitrary criterion, the overall clinical efficacy of 35.3% versus 13.6% in the placebo group was rather modest. Adverse events were common but mostly local skin reactions to the patch. Treatment adherence was very high with 98.5%, despite daily patch applications, and the patients participating in a further peanut EPIT trial was rather satisfied with the treatment.[119] It is yet unclear whether the data out of the clinical trial program, especially the data from the phase III trial, will give peanut EPIT an advantage over oral peanut immunotherapy.[120,121] While there can be not much doubt that EPIT works, it is yet unclear when the first EPIT therapies will enter the market.

Based on the encouraging data of EPIT on eosinophilic gastrointestinal disease in mice[111] and piglets,[122] Spergel et al. performed a randomized placebo-controlled study to assess safety and efficacy of cow milk EPIT with a Viaskin patch in children with milk-induced eosinophilic esophagitis.[123] While the intent to treat population showed no significant improvement, the per-protocol population, albeit only seven allergen versus two placebo-treated patients, showed significantly reduced eosinophil counts.

Methods to improve EPIT

Enhancing penetration into the skin

As known for classical SCIT,[28] also in EPIT there is a dose-response relation-ship.[109,115,116] Increasing the dose reaching the skin should therefore improve EPIT, and a well-known practice in dermatology to enhance penetration of active compounds into the skin is occlusion. This is the method typically used in the above-described EPIT trials. All these trials have used a patch that was worn for several hours. Occlusion enhances penetration into the skin by hydration of the *stratum corneum*, which generates water channels and facilitates diffusion of hydrophilic molecules, such as allergens. Any form of occlusion, such as the allergen patches used by us[104,108,109] and others,[110] hydrates the skin by accumulation of sweat.[111,112,124,125] The Viaskin EPIT system is using an occlusion system initially developed for diagnostic purposes as an alternative system to the conventional Finn chamber used in atopy patch test.[125] Briefly, sweat dissolves the allergens, which then have been demonstrated to accumulate in the *stratum corneum*, where they efficiently target immune cells of the superficial skin layer[126] that rapidly migrate to the draining lymph nodes.[111] We had chosen to apply the grass pollen extract onto the skin in a patch where the allergens were mixed into petrolatum/Vaseline. The reason for this choice was that hydrophilic proteins poorly dissolve in petrolatum, so that the allergens would diffuse from a supersaturated phase into the hydrated *stratum corneum*. Skin penetration may additionally be enhanced by adding so-called penetration enhancers, such as salicylic acid,[110] or by packing the antigen into lipid-based colloidal systems.[127,128] Finally, skin penetration can be enhanced by microporation, using a microneedle patch[86,129] or a laser.[130,131]

A simple way to deliver more EPIT allergen is to increase the area of the patch. Assuming that only a small fraction of the loaded allergen diffuses into the skin, a larger patch should be assumed to deliver more allergen. In our clinical trials, the patch size was 15 sq cm.[84,132,133] The Viaskin patch is considerably approximately 1/10 of that size.[84,132,133] However, while these two trial series cannot be compared due to the use of different allergens, lack of skin preparation before application of the Viaksin patch, and different allergen doses in the patches, it can only be speculated that the patch size matters.

While all above methods enhance penetration into the skin, the remaining question is to which degree these different methods activate keratinocytes, as discussed below. The activation of keratinocytes may be important for activation of LCs. It could be speculated that the different outcomes of these methods, such as the relative inefficacy of the Viaskin EDS chamber, may well be explained by the assumption that hydration alone does not activate keratinocytes to the same extent as tape stripping or abrasion. In fact, a heavily disrupted skin barrier has been observed to polarize the immune response toward Th1, whereas slight skin barrier disruption rather induces Th2- and Treg-dominated responses.[54] The evidence in this area is conflicting. In mouse models of peanut allergy, intact skin and not stripped skin were found to be crucial for efficacy and safety of immunotherapy.[134] In a mouse model with ovalbumin, no therapeutic effect was observed if the skin was not tape stripped before allergen application.[53]

We have also tested microneedle patches and laser microporation of the *stratum corneum* to enhance allergen penetration into the epidermis.[53] In these clinical trials, we found that once the allergen had passed across the *stratum corneum* and therefore penetrated into the live layers of the epidermis, the basal membrane represented no barrier to diffusion into the dermis. Even when only perforating the upper 10 μm of the epidermis, i.e., only the *stratum corneum*, we could observe formation of hives only minutes after application of allergens.

Adjuvants for epicutaneous use

Adjuvants in EPIT represent another strategy to enhance efficacy. Aluminum salts, today still the adjuvant used in most marketed vaccines,[135] is not suitable for epicutaneous administration.[136] Thus far, cholera toxin and heat-labile enterotoxin have been successfully used as adjuvants in epicutaneous vaccination against infectious diseases of mice and humans.[84,132,133] However, imidazoquinolines (TLR7 or TLR8 ligands) and CpG (TLR9 ligand) are currently being tested as adjuvants for epicutaneous vaccination against cancer.[90,137] Our group recently tested the immune-enhancing and immune-modulatory potential of diphenylcyclopropenone when used as adjuvant in EPIT.[53] More recently, Cabauatan et al.[138,139] described birch pollen—specific AIT in a guinea pig model, using the patch delivery system mentioned above that had been originally developed for epicutaneous vaccination against traveler's diarrhea.[84] Recombinant Bet v 1 was administered in a skin patch that also contained heat-labile *E. coli* toxin (LT) as an adjuvant. Patch vaccination induced IgG responses that are comparable to subcutaneous vaccination with rBet v 1 adjuvanted with alum, but only when the patch contained LT.

Keratinocytes can also be activated by physical measures, such as tape striping. Complete removal of the SC required at least 30 consecutive tapes.[140] Tape striping has been found to upregulate TLR9,[141] and consequently adding CpG to tape-stripped skin strongly modulated the immune response to EPIT CpG modulation of immune response in mice.[142] In our mouse models with ovalbumin, EPIT showed no therapeutic effect if the skin was not tape stripped before allergen application.[53] In contrast, in a mouse model of peanut allergy, intact skin and not stripped skin was found to be crucial for efficacy and safety of immunotherapy.[134] The data in this area are therefore conflicting.

The above discussion circles around which adjuvant would best induce a Th1 response, i.e., interpreting AIT as classical vaccination. However, which adjuvants could be used to enhance regulatory T cells? EPIT has been demonstrated to induce Foxp3+ Treg cells that suppressing both local and systemic allergen-driven immune responses[143−145] and can prevent new sensitizations to other allergens.[145] This effect was mediated by CD4+CD25 + T cells, as shown by adoptive transfer experiments. In one study, we therefore modified EPIT by adding retinoids and vitamin D3 as adjuvants, both known to enhance induction of Treg cells, but at least in mice, we could not observe further immunological improvement of EPIT.[53] Both retinoids and vitamin D3 are highly lipophilic, low molecular weight, and can penetrate the skin. However, this negative result could still just be due to technical and dosing problems.

Outlook for EPIT

The discussed historic as well as preclinical and clinical data in grass pollen and peanut allergy leave no doubt that EPIT works and could be a good alternative route for AIT. However, there is room for improvements and optimization. EPIT in the mouse model shows similar clinical efficacy to SCIT. While there are no head-to-head comparisons in human clinical trials, it looks like our grass pollen studies may have clinical efficacy that is comparable to SCIT, but only when high doses of allergen were used. Mouse models suggest that tape stripping of the skin before patch application is necessary for the clinical effect, but also, EPIT using the Viaskin peanut patch seems to work, although with modest efficacy. There are several differences between our patch and the Viaskin trials. In our grass pollen trials, the skin was prepared by tape stripping, the allergen was administered to the skin in petrolatum Vaseline, where the allergen was only poorly solvable, and the patch was approximately 10 times larger in terms of area. It is likely that more allergen was delivered in these grass pollen EPIT trials. However, grass pollen extract and peanut extract EPIT cannot simply be compared as there are more serious safety concerns around peanut AIT. Thus, one has to be more careful when trying to increase the allergen EPIT dose and when using methods to prepare the skin to enhance penetration. Another concern, which EPIT in peanut allergy is the risk of sensitization via the skin.[146–148] The difference between "sensitization" and "desensitization," apart from allergen dosage, most likely lies in the immune environment present at the time of application, such as presence of atopic dermatitis and preparation of the skin.

Thus, while the skin is a highly interesting "immune organ" for administration of AIT, one main problem is that the skin also is an organ that protects the human body from the environment. This protection includes a highly impermeable *stratum corneum* that represents the main obstacle for allergen delivery into the live skin. Although we prepared the skin by tape stripping to remove part of the *stratum corneum*, we came to a practical limit in terms of the dose that could be administered. We used 30 µg of major grass pollen allergen Phl p 1 per patch, corresponding to 1 mL of the 10-fold concentration that is used for the skin prick solution. A higher concentration would not only generate considerable material costs, but the application to any accidently impaired skin barrier would represent a considerate risk for systemic allergic effects. Future research should therefore focus on enhancing penetration of the *stratum corneum* into the viable layers of the skin where LCs reside, and on adjuvants suitable for epicutaneous administration.

Acknowledgments

T. Kündig and P. Johansen received financial support from Swiss National Science Foundation (Berne, Switzerland), *Stiftung für wissenschaftliche Forschung*, University of Zurich (Zurich, Switzerland), *Innosuisse*, and *Truus und Gerrit van Riemsdijk Stiftung* (Vaduz, Lichtenstein).

References

1. Lyons SA, Burney PGJ, Ballmer-Weber BK, et al. Food allergy in adults: substantial variation in prevalence and causative foods across Europe. *J Allergy Clin Immunol Pract*. 2019;7:1920−1928.
2. Pawankar R, Canonica GW, Holgate ST, Lockey RF. Allergic diseases and asthma: a major global health concern. *Curr Opin Allergy Clin Immunol*. 2012;12:39−41.
3. Zielen S, Devillier P, Heinrich J, Richter H, Wahn U. Sublingual immunotherapy provides long-term relief in allergic rhinitis and reduces the risk of asthma: a retrospective, real-world database analysis. *Allergy*. 2018;73:165−177.
4. Cardona V, Luengo O, Labrador-Horrillo M. Immunotherapy in allergic rhinitis and lower airway outcomes. *Allergy*. 2017;72:35−42.
5. Hoffmann HJ, Valovirta E, Pfaar O, et al. Novel approaches and perspectives in allergen immunotherapy. *Allergy*. 2017;72:1022−1034.
6. Schmitt J, Schwarz K, Stadler E, Wustenberg EG. Allergy immunotherapy for allergic rhinitis effectively prevents asthma: results from a large retrospective cohort study. *J Allergy Clin Immunol*. 2015;136:1511−1516.
7. Jutel M, Agache I, Bonini S, et al. International consensus on allergy immunotherapy. *J Allergy Clin Immunol*. 2015;136:556−568.
8. Demoly P, Kleine-Tebbe J, Rehm D. Clinical benefits of treatment with SQ house dust mite sublingual tablet in house dust mite allergic rhinitis. *Allergy*. 2017;72:1576−1578.
9. Roberts G, Pfaar O, Akdis CA, et al. EAACI guidelines on allergen immunotherapy: allergic rhinoconjunctivitis. *Allergy*. 2018;73:765−798.
10. Asaria M, Dhami S, van Ree R, et al. Health economic analysis of allergen immunotherapy for the management of allergic rhinitis, asthma, food allergy and venom allergy: a systematic overview. *Allergy*. 2018;73:269−283.
11. Noon L. Prophylactic inoculation against hay fever. *Lancet*. 1911;177:1572−1573.
12. Incorvaia C, Mauro M, Ridolo E, et al. Patient's compliance with allergen immunotherapy. *Patient Prefer Adherence*. 2008;2:247−251.
13. Pajno GB, Vita D, Caminiti L, et al. Children's compliance with allergen immunotherapy according to administration routes. *J Allergy Clin Immunol*. 2005;116: 1380−1381.
14. Cohn JR, Pizzi A. Determinants of patient compliance with allergen immunotherapy. *J Allergy Clin Immunol*. 1993;91:734−737.
15. Lower T, Henry J, Mandik L, Janosky J, Friday Jr GA. Compliance with allergen immunotherapy. *Ann Allergy*. 1993;70:480−482.
16. Tinkelman D, Smith F, Cole 3rd WQ, Silk HJ. Compliance with an allergen immunotherapy regime. *Ann Allergy Asthma Immunol*. 1995;74:241−246.
17. Rhodes BJ. Patient dropouts before completion of optimal dose, multiple allergen immunotherapy. *Ann Allergy Asthma Immunol*. 1999;82:281−286.

18. Tsabouri S, Mavroudi A, Feketea G, Guibas GV. Subcutaneous and sublingual immunotherapy in allergic asthma in children. *Front Pediatr.* 2017;5:82.

19. Marogna M, Spadolini I, Massolo A, Canonica GW, Passalacqua G. Randomized controlled open study of sublingual immunotherapy for respiratory allergy in real-life: clinical efficacy and more. *Allergy.* 2004;59:1205—1210.

20. Lombardi C, Gani F, Landi M, et al. Quantitative assessment of the adherence to sublingual immunotherapy. *J Allergy Clin Immunol.* 2004;113:1219—1220.

21. Passalacqua G, Musarra A, Pecora S, et al. Quantitative assessment of the compliance with a once-daily sublingual immunotherapy regimen in real life (EASY Project: evaluation of a novel SLIT formulation during a year). *J Allergy Clin Immunol.* 2006;117:946—948.

22. Senna G, Ridolo E, Calderon M, Lombardi C, Canonica GW, Passalacqua G. Evidence of adherence to allergen-specific immunotherapy. *Curr Opin Allergy Clin Immunol.* 2009;9:544—548.

23. Cox LS, Hankin C, Lockey R. Allergy immunotherapy adherence and delivery route: location does not matter. *J Allergy Clin Immunol Pract.* 2014;2:156—160.

24. Cox L, Calderon MA. Subcutaneous specific immunotherapy for seasonal allergic rhinitis: a review of treatment practices in the US and Europe. *Curr Med Res Opin.* 2010;26:2723—2733.

25. Cox L, Nelson H, Lockey R, et al. Allergen immunotherapy: a practice parameter third update. *J Allergy Clin Immunol.* 2011;127:S1—S55.

26. Bousquet J, Lockey R, Malling HJ. Allergen immunotherapy: therapeutic vaccines for allergic diseases. A WHO position paper. *J Allergy Clin Immunol.* 1998;102:558—562.

27. Pitsios C, Demoly P, Bilo MB, et al. Clinical contraindications to allergen immunotherapy: an EAACI position paper. *Allergy.* 2015;70:897—909.

28. Frew AJ, Powell RJ, Corrigan CJ, Durham SR, Group UKIS. Efficacy and safety of specific immunotherapy with SQ allergen extract in treatment-resistant seasonal allergic rhinoconjunctivitis. *J Allergy Clin Immunol.* 2006;117:319—325.

29. Henmar H, Lund G, Lund L, Petersen A, Wurtzen PA. Allergenicity, immunogenicity and dose-relationship of three intact allergen vaccines and four allergoid vaccines for subcutaneous grass pollen immunotherapy. *Clin Exp Immunol.* 2008;153:316—323.

30. Burks AW, Calderon MA, Casale T, et al. Update on allergy immunotherapy: American academy of allergy, asthma & immunology/European academy of allergy and clinical immunology/PRACTALL consensus report. *J Allergy Clin Immunol.* 2013;131:1288—1296.

31. Benito-Villalvilla C, Soria I, Subiza JL, Palomares O. Novel vaccines targeting dendritic cells by coupling allergoids to mannan. *Allergo J Int.* 2018;27:256—262.

32. Valenta R, Niespodziana K, Focke-Tejkl M, et al. Recombinant allergens: what does the future hold? *J Allergy Clin Immunol.* 2011;127:860—864.

33. Campana R, Huang HJ, Freidl R, et al. Recombinant allergen and peptide-based approaches for allergy prevention by oral tolerance. *Semin Immunol.* 2017;30:67—80.

34. Valenta R, Campana R, Niederberger V. Recombinant allergy vaccines based on allergen-derived B cell epitopes. *Immunol Lett.* 2017;189:19—26.

35. Muller U, Akdis CA, Fricker M, et al. Successful immunotherapy with T-cell epitope peptides of bee venom phospholipase A2 induces specific T-cell anergy in patients allergic to bee venom. *J Allergy Clin Immunol.* 1998;101:747—754.

36. Worm M, Lee HH, Kleine-Tebbe J, et al. Development and preliminary clinical evaluation of a peptide immunotherapy vaccine for cat allergy. *J Allergy Clin Immunol.* 2011;127:89—97.

37. Worm M, Patel D, Creticos PS. Cat peptide antigen desensitisation for treating cat allergic rhinoconjunctivitis. *Expert Opin Investig Drugs*. 2013;22:1347−1357.

38. Pellaton C, Perrin Y, Boudousquie C, et al. Novel birch pollen specific immunotherapy formulation based on contiguous overlapping peptides. *Clin Transl Allergy*. 2013;3:17.

39. Creticos PS. Advances in synthetic peptide immuno-regulatory epitopes. *World Allergy Organ J*. 2014;7:30.

40. Couroux P, Patel D, Armstrong K, Larche M, Hafner RP. Fel d 1-derived synthetic peptide immuno-regulatory epitopes show a long-term treatment effect in cat allergic subjects. *Clin Exp Allergy*. 2015;45:974−981.

41. Creticos PS, Schroeder JT, Hamilton RG, et al. Immunotherapy with a ragweed-toll-like receptor 9 agonist vaccine for allergic rhinitis. *N Engl J Med*. 2006;355:1445−1455.

42. Dubuske LM, Frew AJ, Horak F, et al. Ultrashort-specific immunotherapy successfully treats seasonal allergic rhinoconjunctivitis to grass pollen. *Allergy Asthma Proc*. 2011; 32:239−247.

43. Mothes N, Heinzkill M, Drachenberg KJ, et al. Allergen-specific immunotherapy with a monophosphoryl lipid A-adjuvanted vaccine: reduced seasonally boosted immunoglobulin E production and inhibition of basophil histamine release by therapy-induced blocking antibodies. *Clin Exp Allergy*. 2003;33:1198−1208.

44. Drachenberg KJ, Wheeler AW, Stuebner P, Horak F. A well-tolerated grass pollen-specific allergy vaccine containing a novel adjuvant, monophosphoryl lipid A, reduces allergic symptoms after only four preseasonal injections. *Allergy*. 2001;56:498−505.

45. Zielen S, Gabrielpillai J, Herrmann E, Schulze J, Schubert R, Rosewich M. Long-term effect of monophosphoryl lipid A adjuvanted specific immunotherapy in patients with grass pollen allergy. *Immunotherapy*. 2018;10:529−536.

46. Leuthard DS, Duda A, Freiberger SN, et al. Microcrystalline tyrosine and aluminum as adjuvants in allergen-specific immunotherapy protect from IgE-mediated reactivity in mouse models and act independently of inflammasome and TLR signaling. *J Immunol*. 2018;200:3151−3159.

47. Senti G, Prinz Vavricka BM, Erdmann I, et al. Intralymphatic allergen administration renders specific immunotherapy faster and safer: a randomized controlled trial. *Proc Natl Acad Sci USA*. 2008;105:17908−17912.

48. Senti G, Crameri R, Kuster D, et al. Intralymphatic immunotherapy for cat allergy induces tolerance after only 3 injections. *J Allergy Clin Immunol*. 2012;129:1290−1296.

49. Hylander T, Latif L, Petersson-Westin U, Cardell LO. Intralymphatic allergen-specific immunotherapy: an effective and safe alternative treatment route for pollen-induced allergic rhinitis. *J Allergy Clin Immunol*. 2013;131:412−420.

50. Cox LS, Larenas Linnemann D, Nolte H, Weldon D, Finegold I, Nelson HS. Sublingual immunotherapy: a comprehensive review. *J Allergy Clin Immunol*. 2006;117: 1021−1035.

51. Canonica GW, Bousquet J, Casale T, et al. Sub-lingual immunotherapy: world allergy organization position paper 2009. *Allergy*. 2009;64(Suppl 91):1−59.

52. Canonica GW, Cox L, Pawankar R, et al. Sublingual immunotherapy: world allergy organization position paper 2013 update. *World Allergy Organ J*. 2014;7:6.

53. von Moos S, Johansen P, Waeckerle-Men Y, et al. The contact sensitizer diphenylcyclopropenone has adjuvant properties in mice and potential application in epicutaneous immunotherapy. *Allergy*. 2012;67:638−646.

54. Swamy M, Jamora C, Havran W, Hayday A. Epithelial decision makers: in search of the 'epimmunome'. *Nat Immunol*. 2010;11:656−665.

55. Spina L, Weisskopf M, von Moos S, Graf N, Kundig TM, Senti G. Comparison of microneedles and adhesive-tape stripping in skin preparation for epicutaneous allergen delivery. *Int Arch Allergy Immunol.* 2015;167:103−109.

56. Zinkernagel RM, Ehl S, Aichele P, Oehen S, Kundig T, Hengartner H. Antigen localisation regulates immune responses in a dose- and time-dependent fashion: a geographical view of immune reactivity. *Immunol Rev.* 1997;156:199−209.

57. Johansen P, Mohanan D, Martinez-Gomez JM, Kundig TM, Gander B. Lympho-geographical concepts in vaccine delivery. *J Control Release.* 2010;148:56−62.

58. Johansen P, Senti G, Martinez Gomez JM, et al. Toll-like receptor ligands as adjuvants in allergen-specific immunotherapy. *Clin Exp Allergy.* 2005;35:1591−1598.

59. Johansen P, Senti G, Martinez Gomez JM, Wuthrich B, Bot A, Kundig TM. Heat denaturation, a simple method to improve the immunotherapeutic potential of allergens. *Eur J Immunol.* 2005;35:3591−3598.

60. Martinez-Gomez JM, Johansen P, Rose H, et al. Targeting the MHC class II pathway of antigen presentation enhances immunogenicity and safety of allergen immunotherapy. *Allergy.* 2009;64:172−178.

61. Mohanan D, Slutter B, Henriksen-Lacey M, et al. Administration routes affect the quality of immune responses: a cross-sectional evaluation of particulate antigen-delivery systems. *J Control Release.* 2010;147:342−349.

62. Martinez-Gomez JM, Johansen P, Erdmann I, Senti G, Crameri R, Kundig TM. Intra-lymphatic injections as a new administration route for allergen-specific immunotherapy. *Int Arch Allergy Immunol.* 2009;150:59−65.

63. Senti G, Freiburghaus AU, Kundig TM. Epicutaneous/transcutaneous allergen-specific immunotherapy: rationale and clinical trials. *Curr Opin Allergy Clin Immunol.* 2010;10:582−586.

64. Hellkvist L, Hjalmarsson E, Kumlien Georen S, et al. Intralymphatic immunotherapy with 2 concomitant allergens, birch and grass: a randomized, double-blind, placebo-controlled trial. *J Allergy Clin Immunol.* 2018;142:1338−1341.

65. Jutel M, Agache I, Bonini S, et al. International consensus on allergen immunotherapy II: mechanisms, standardization, and pharmacoeconomics. *J Allergy Clin Immunol.* 2016;137:358−368.

66. Ahlbeck L, Ahlberg E, Nystrom U, Bjorkander J, Jenmalm MC. Intralymphatic allergen immunotherapy against pollen allergy: a 3-year open follow-up study of 10 patients. *Ann Allergy Asthma Immunol.* 2018;121:626−627.

67. Schmid JM, Nezam H, Madsen HH, Schmitz A, Hoffmann HJ. Intralymphatic immunotherapy induces allergen specific plasmablasts and increases tolerance to skin prick testing in a pilot study. *Clin Transl Allergy.* 2016;6:19.

68. Lee SP, Choi SJ, Joe E, et al. A pilot study of intralymphatic immunotherapy for house dust mite, cat, and dog allergies. *Allergy Asthma Immunol Res.* 2017;9:272−277.

69. Lee SP, Jung JH, Lee SM, et al. Intralymphatic immunotherapy alleviates allergic symptoms during allergen exposure in daily life. *Allergy Asthma Immunol Res.* 2018;10:180−181.

70. Patterson AM, Bonny AE, Shiels WE, Erwin EA. Three-injection intralymphatic immunotherapy in adolescents and young adults with grass pollen rhinoconjunctivitis. *Ann Allergy Asthma Immunol.* 2015;116:168−170.

71. Freiberger SN, Zehnder M, Gafvelin G, Gronlund H, Kundig TM, Johansen P. IgG4 but no IgG1 antibody production after intralymphatic immunotherapy with recombinant MAT-Feld1 in human. *Allergy.* 2016;71:1366−1370.

72. Zaleska A, Eiwegger T, Soyer O, et al. Immune regulation by intralymphatic immunotherapy with modular allergen translocation MAT vaccine. *Allergy*. 2014;69:1162–1170.

73. Witten M, Malling HJ, Blom L, Poulsen BC, Poulsen LK. Is intralymphatic immunotherapy ready for clinical use in patients with grass pollen allergy? *J Allergy Clin Immunol*. 2013;132:1248–1252.

74. Kedl RM, Kappler JW, Marrack P. Epitope dominance, competition and T cell affinity maturation. *Curr Opin Immunol*. 2003;15:120–127.

75. Patel D, Couroux P, Hickey P, et al. Fel d 1-derived peptide antigen desensitization shows a persistent treatment effect 1 year after the start of dosing: a randomized, placebo-controlled study. *J Allergy Clin Immunol*. 2013;131:103–109.

76. Guery JC, Galbiati F, Smiroldo S, Adorini L. Selective development of T helper (Th)2 cells induced by continuous administration of low dose soluble proteins to normal and beta(2)-microglobulin-deficient BALB/c mice. *J Exp Med*. 1996;183:485–497.

77. Hjalmsdottir A, Wackerle-Men Y, Duda A, Kundig TM, Johansen P. Dosing intervals in intralymphatic immunotherapy. *Clin Exp Allergy*. 2016;46:504–507.

78. Hales CM, Carroll MD, Fryar CD, Ogden CL. *Obesity Among Adults and Youth: United States, 2015–2016*. Hyattsville, MD: National Center for Health Statistics; 2017.

79. Salman MC, Usubutun A, Ozlu T, Boynukalin K, Yuce K. Obesity does not affect the number of retrieved lymph nodes and the rate of intraoperative complications in gynecologic cancers. *J Gynecol Oncol*. 2010;21:24–28.

80. Matsuo K, Hirobe S, Okada N, Nakagawa S. Frontiers of transcutaneous vaccination systems: novel technologies and devices for vaccine delivery. *Vaccine*. 2013;31:2403–2415.

81. Senti G, von Moos S, Kundig TM. Epicutaneous allergen administration: is this the future of allergen-specific immunotherapy? *Allergy*. 2011;66:798–809.

82. Senti G, Johansen P, von Moos S, Kundig TM. A bizarre attack on the freedom of scientific expression. *Allergy*. 2015;70:1037–1038.

83. Dinc G, Ulman YI. The introduction of variolation 'A La Turca' to the West by Lady Mary Montagu and Turkey's contribution to this. *Vaccine*. 2007;25:4261–4265.

84. Frech SA, Dupont HL, Bourgeois AL, et al. Use of a patch containing heat-labile toxin from *Escherichia coli* against travellers' diarrhoea: a phase II, randomised, double-blind, placebo-controlled field trial. *Lancet*. 2008;371:2019–2025.

85. Hickey DK, Aldwell FE, Tan ZY, Bao S, Beagley KW. Transcutaneous immunization with novel lipid-based adjuvants induces protection against gastric *Helicobacter pylori* infection. *Vaccine*. 2009;27:6983–6990.

86. Sullivan SP, Koutsonanos DG, Del Pilar Martin M, et al. Dissolving polymer microneedle patches for influenza vaccination. *Nat Med*. 2010;16:915–920.

87. Ding Z, Verbaan FJ, Bivas-Benita M, et al. Microneedle arrays for the transcutaneous immunization of diphtheria and influenza in BALB/c mice. *J Control Release*. 2009;136:71–78.

88. Belyakov IM, Hammond SA, Ahlers JD, Glenn GM, Berzofsky JA. Transcutaneous immunization induces mucosal CTLs and protective immunity by migration of primed skin dendritic cells. *J Clin Investig*. 2004;113:998–1007.

89. Richmond JM, Harris JE. Immunology and skin in health and disease. *Cold Spring Harb Perspect Med*. 2014;4:a015339.

90. Rechtsteiner G, Warger T, Osterloh P, Schild H, Radsak MP. Cutting edge: priming of CTL by transcutaneous peptide immunization with imiquimod. *J Immunol*. 2005;174:2476–2480.

91. Bynoe MS, Evans JT, Viret C, Janeway Jr CA. Epicutaneous immunization with auto-antigenic peptides induces T suppressor cells that prevent experimental allergic encephalomyelitis. *Immunity.* 2003;19:317—328.

92. Bynoe MS, Viret C. Antigen-induced suppressor T cells from the skin point of view: suppressor T cells induced through epicutaneous immunization. *J Neuroimmunol.* 2005;167:4—12.

93. Zheng Z, Diaz-Arevalo D, Guan H, Zeng M. Noninvasive vaccination against infectious diseases. *Hum Vaccines Immunother.* 2018;14:1717—1733.

94. Senti G, Kundig TM. Novel delivery routes for allergy immunotherapy: intralymphatic, epicutaneous, and intradermal. *Immunol Allergy Clin N Am.* 2016;36:25—37.

95. Blamoutier P, Blamoutier J, Guibert L. Treatment of pollinosis with pollen extracts by the method of cutaneous quadrille ruling. *Presse Med.* 1959;67:2299—2301.

96. Vallery-Radot P, Hangenau J. Asthme d'origine équine. Essai de désensibilisation par des cutiréactions répétées. *Bull Soc Méd Hôp Paris.* 1921;45.

97. Hurwitz SH. Medicine: seasonal hay fever-some problems in treatment. *Cal West Med.* 1930;33:520—521.

98. Phillips EW. Relief of hay-fever by intradermal injections of pollen extract. *JAMA.* 1926;86:182—184.

99. Blamoutier P, Blamoutier J, Guibert L. Traitement co-saisonnier de la pollinose par l'application d'extraits de pollens sur des quadrillages cutanés: Résultats obtenus en 1959 et 1960. *Rev Fr Allerg.* 1961;1:112—120.

100. Pautrizel R, Cabanieu G, Bricaud H, Broustet P. Allergenic group specificity & therapeutic consequences in asthma; specific desensitization method by epicutaneous route. *Sem Hop.* 1957;33:1394—1403.

101. Eichenberger H, Storck H. Co-seasonal desensitization of pollinosis with the scarification-method of Blamoutier. *Acta Allergol.* 1966;21:261—267.

102. Martin-DuPan RBF, Neyroud M. Treatment of pollen allergy using the cutaneous checker square method of Blamoutier and Guilbert. *Schweiz Rundsch Med Prax.* 1971;60:1469—1472.

103. Palma-Carlos AG. Traitement co-saisonnier des pollinoses au Portugal par la méthode des quadrillages cutanés. *Rev Fr Allerg.* 1967;7:92—95.

104. Senti G, Graf N, Haug S, et al. Epicutaneous allergen administration as a novel method of allergen-specific immunotherapy. *J Allergy Clin Immunol.* 2009;124:997—1002.

105. Dickel H, Goulioumis A, Gambichler T, et al. Standardized tape stripping: a practical and reproducible protocol to uniformly reduce the stratum corneum. *Skin Pharmacol Physiol.* 2010;23:259—265.

106. Nickoloff BJ, Naidu Y. Perturbation of epidermal barrier function correlates with initiation of cytokine cascade in human skin. *J Am Acad Dermatol.* 1994;30:535—546.

107. Dickel H, Gambichler T, Kamphowe J, Altmeyer P, Skrygan M. Standardized tape stripping prior to patch testing induces upregulation of Hsp90, Hsp70, IL-33, TNF-alpha and IL-8/CXCL8 mRNA: new insights into the involvement of 'alarmins'. *Contact Dermatitis.* 2010;63:215—222.

108. Senti G, von Moos S, Tay F, et al. Epicutaneous allergen-specific immunotherapy ameliorates grass pollen-induced rhinoconjunctivitis: a double-blind, placebo-controlled dose escalation study. *J Allergy Clin Immunol.* 2012;129:128—135.

109. Senti G, von Moos S, Tay F, Graf N, Johansen P, Kundig TM. Determinants of efficacy and safety in epicutaneous allergen immunotherapy: summary of three clinical trials. *Allergy.* 2015;70:707—710.

110. Agostinis F, Forti S, Di Berardino F. Grass transcutaneous immunotherapy in children with seasonal rhinoconjunctivitis. *Allergy*. 2010;65:410−411.

111. Mondoulet L, Dioszeghy V, Larcher T, et al. Epicutaneous immunotherapy (EPIT) blocks the allergic esophago-gastro-enteropathy induced by sustained oral exposure to peanuts in sensitized mice. *PLoS One*. 2012;7:e31967.

112. Dupont C, Kalach N, Soulaines P, Legoue-Morillon S, Piloquet H, Benhamou PH. Cow's milk epicutaneous immunotherapy in children: a pilot trial of safety, acceptability, and impact on allergic reactivity. *J Allergy Clin Immunol*. 2010;125:1165−1167.

113. Scurlock AM, Jones SM. An update on immunotherapy for food allergy. *Curr Opin Allergy Clin Immunol*. 2010;10:587−593.

114. Jones SM, Agbotounou WK, Fleischer DM, et al. Safety of epicutaneous immunotherapy for the treatment of peanut allergy: a phase 1 study using the Viaskin patch. *J Allergy Clin Immunol*. 2016;137:1258−1261.

115. Jones SM, Sicherer SH, Burks AW, et al. Epicutaneous immunotherapy for the treatment of peanut allergy in children and young adults. *J Allergy Clin Immunol*. 2017;139, 1242-12452 e9.

116. Sampson HA, Shreffler WG, Yang WH, et al. Effect of varying doses of epicutaneous immunotherapy vs placebo on reaction to peanut protein exposure among patients with peanut sensitivity: a randomized clinical trial. *JAMA*. 2017;318:1798−1809.

117. Koppelman SJ, Peillon A, Agbotounou W, Sampson HA, Martin L. Epicutaneous immunotherapy for peanut allergy modifies IgG4 responses to major peanut allergens. *J Allergy Clin Immunol*. 2019;143:1218−1221.

118. Fleischer DM, Greenhawt M, Sussman G, et al. Effect of epicutaneous immunotherapy vs placebo on reaction to peanut protein ingestion among children with peanut allergy: the PEPITES randomized clinical trial. *JAMA*. 2019;321:946−955.

119. Lewis MO, Brown-Whitehorn TF, Cianferoni A, Rooney C, Spergel JM. Peanut-allergic patient experiences after epicutaneous immunotherapy: peanut consumption and impact on QoL. *Ann Allergy Asthma Immunol*. 2019;123:101−103.

120. Zylke JW. Epicutaneous immunotherapy vs placebo for peanut protein ingestion among peanut-allergic children. *JAMA*. 2019;321:956.

121. Matthews JG, Zawadzki R, Haselkorn T, Rosen K. Clarification of epicutaneous immunotherapy trial phase 3 results and methods for qualitative survey design. *Ann Allergy Asthma Immunol*. 2018;121:641−642.

122. Mondoulet L, Kalach N, Dhelft V, et al. Treatment of gastric eosinophilia by epicutaneous immunotherapy in piglets sensitized to peanuts. *Clin Exp Allergy*. 2017;47:1640−1647.

123. Spergel JM, Elci OU, Muir AB, et al. Efficacy of epicutaneous immunotherapy in children with milk-induced eosinophilic esophagitis. *Clin Gastroenterol Hepatol*. 2019. https://doi.org/10.1016/j.cgh.2019.05.014 (in press).

124. Mondoulet L, Dioszeghy V, Vanoirbeek JA, Nemery B, Dupont C, Benhamou PH. Epicutaneous immunotherapy using a new epicutaneous delivery system in mice sensitized to peanuts. *Int Arch Allergy Immunol*. 2010;154:299−309.

125. Kalach N, Soulaines P, de Boissieu D, Dupont C. A pilot study of the usefulness and safety of a ready-to-use atopy patch test (Diallertest) versus a comparator (Finn Chamber) during cow's milk allergy in children. *J Allergy Clin Immunol*. 2005;116:1321−1326.

126. Soury D, Barratt G, Ah-Leung S, Legrand P, Chacun H, Ponchel G. Skin localization of cow's milk proteins delivered by a new ready-to-use atopy patch test. *Pharm Res.* 2005; 22:1530−1536.

127. Rattanapak T, Birchall J, Young K, et al. Transcutaneous immunization using microneedles and cubosomes: mechanistic investigations using optical coherence tomography and two-photon microscopy. *J Control Release.* 2013;172:894−903.

128. Rattanapak T, Young K, Rades T, Hook S. Comparative study of liposomes, transfersomes, ethosomes and cubosomes for transcutaneous immunisation: characterisation and in vitro skin penetration. *J Pharm Pharmacol.* 2012;64:1560−1569.

129. Bal SM, Ding Z, van Riet E, Jiskoot W, Bouwstra JA. Advances in transcutaneous vaccine delivery: do all ways lead to Rome? *J Control Release.* 2010;148:266−282.

130. Weiss R, Hessenberger M, Kitzmuller S, et al. Transcutaneous vaccination via laser microporation. *J Control Release.* 2012;162:391−399.

131. Scheiblhofer S, Thalhamer J, Weiss R. Laser microporation of the skin: prospects for painless application of protective and therapeutic vaccines. *Expert Opin Drug Deliv.* 2013;10:761−773.

132. Yu XL, Cheng YM, Shi BS, et al. Measles virus infection in adults induces production of IL-10 and is associated with increased CD4+ CD25+ regulatory T cells. *J Immunol.* 2008;181:7356−7366.

133. Glenn GM, Rao M, Matyas GR, Alving CR. Skin immunization made possible by cholera toxin. *Nature.* 1998;391:851.

134. Mondoulet L, Dioszeghy V, Puteaux E, et al. Intact skin and not stripped skin is crucial for the safety and efficacy of peanut epicutaneous immunotherapy (EPIT) in mice. *Clin Transl Allergy.* 2012;2:22.

135. Marrack P, McKee AS, Munks MW. Towards an understanding of the adjuvant action of aluminium. *Nat Rev Immunol.* 2009;9:287−293.

136. Scharton-Kersten T, Yu J, Vassell R, O'Hagan D, Alving CR, Glenn GM. Transcutaneous immunization with bacterial ADP-ribosylating exotoxins, subunits, and unrelated adjuvants. *Infect Immun.* 2000;68:5306−5313.

137. Stoitzner P, Sparber F, Tripp CH. Langerhans cells as targets for immunotherapy against skin cancer. *Immunol Cell Biol.* 2010;88:431−437.

138. Cabauatan CR, Campana R, Niespodziana K, et al. Heat-labile *Escherichia coli* toxin enhances the induction of allergen-specific IgG antibodies in epicutaneous patch vaccination. *Allergy.* 2017;72:164−168.

139. Killingbeck SS, Ge MQ, Haczku A. Patching it together: epicutaneous vaccination with heat-labile *Escherichia coli* toxin against birch pollen allergy. *Allergy.* 2017;72:5−8.

140. Solberg J, Ulrich NH, Krustrup D, et al. Skin tape stripping: which layers of the epidermis are removed? *Contact Dermatitis.* 2019;80:319−321.

141. Inoue J, Aramaki Y. Toll-like receptor-9 expression induced by tape-stripping triggers on effective immune response with CpG-oligodeoxynucleotides. *Vaccine.* 2007;25: 1007−1013.

142. Inoue J, Yotsumoto S, Sakamoto T, Tsuchiya S, Aramaki Y. Changes in immune responses to antigen applied to tape-stripped skin with CpG-oligodeoxynucleotide in mice. *J Control Release.* 2005;108:294−305.

143. Dioszeghy V, Mondoulet L, Dhelft V, et al. Epicutaneous immunotherapy results in rapid allergen uptake by dendritic cells through intact skin and downregulates the allergen-specific response in sensitized mice. *J Immunol.* 2011;186:5629−5637.

144. Dioszeghy V, Mondoulet L, Puteaux E, et al. Differences in phenotype, homing properties and suppressive activities of regulatory T cells induced by epicutaneous, oral or sublingual immunotherapy in mice sensitized to peanut. *Cell Mol Immunol*. 2017;14: 770–782.

145. Mondoulet L, Dioszeghy V, Puteaux E, et al. Specific epicutaneous immunotherapy prevents sensitization to new allergens in a murine model. *J Allergy Clin Immunol*. 2015;135:1546–1557.

146. Tordesillas L, Goswami R, Benede S, et al. Skin exposure promotes a Th2-dependent sensitization to peanut allergens. *J Clin Investig*. 2014;124:4965–4975.

147. Hourihane JO, Dean TP, Warner JO. Peanut allergy in relation to heredity, maternal diet, and other atopic diseases: results of a questionnaire survey, skin prick testing, and food challenges. *BMJ*. 1996;313:518–521.

148. Lack G, Fox D, Northstone K, Golding J, Avon Longitudinal Study of Parents and Children Study Team. Factors associated with the development of peanut allergy in childhood. *N Engl J Med*. 2003;348:977–985.

Modified allergens: peptides, fragments, and recombinant allergens

17

Mark W. Tenn, BHSc [1,2], **Anne K. Ellis, MD, MSc, FRCPC** [1,2]

[1]*Departments of Medicine and Biomedical & Molecular Sciences, Queen's University, Kingston, ON, Canada;* [2]*Allergy Research Unit, Kingston General Health Research Institute, Kingston, ON, Canada*

Introduction

Allergen immunotherapy (AIT) is the only disease-modifying treatment available for allergic diseases. Following the first reported use of AIT to treat grass pollen allergy by Leonard Noon,[1] many clinical trials have demonstrated the clinical benefit of AIT for allergic rhinitis (AR) and allergic asthma. In two comprehensive systematic reviews with metaanalyses, use of AIT reduced both symptom scores and use of rescue medication in patients with AR or allergic asthma.[2,3] However, both analyses reported an increase in local and systemic adverse reactions in patients treated with AIT compared with placebo.

Traditional AIT uses whole allergen extracts prepared from natural sources such as animal dander, house dust mite (HDM), and various types of pollen.[4] During the manufacturing process, the 3D structure of major protein allergens is preserved. Thus, extract-based therapies are often accompanied by a relatively high frequency of immediate or late-phase reactions in treated patients.[5,6] These reactions are likely mediated by the cross-linking of IgE by native allergen and activation of allergen-specific T cells, respectively. Both the immunogenicity and potency of commercialized extracts also depend on the quality of the source material. The allergen concentrations in extracts are difficult to alter and are often predetermined by the starting material used. Extracts may also be contaminated with bacteria or nonallergenic compounds during purification.[4] Although natural allergen extracts have been proven effective in desensitizing patients to common environmental allergens in the clinic, the risk of adverse reactions and anaphylaxis due to retained IgE or T cell reactivity represents a major concern for both patients and allergists alike.

Over the last 20 years, significant advances have been made in recombinant technologies and the use of modified allergens as an extract alternative with improved safety profiles and lower side effects.[7] Recombinant allergens can be produced with high purity, precise concentrations of allergen, and with defined immunologic characteristics comparable with their native allergen counterparts. Recombinant technologies have also been used to synthesize "hypoallergenic" derivatives that

Immunotherapies for Allergic Disease. https://doi.org/10.1016/B978-0-323-54427-6.00017-1

exhibit reduced IgE and/or T cell reactivity while maintaining their immunogenic properties. These include hypoallergenic fragments, hybrid allergen proteins, and short synthetic T or B cell epitope—derived peptides.

This chapter will provide an overview of the different types of modified allergens, and the methods and rationale for their design. This chapter will also discuss and summarize recent clinical trials reporting the efficacy, safety, and tolerability of modified allergens as an alternative immunotherapy treatment approach for allergic diseases.

Disadvantages of natural allergen extracts

Both local (i.e., near the site of treatment administration) and systemic adverse reactions related to the use of natural allergen extracts during AIT are well documented. In patients receiving sublingual immunotherapy (SLIT), 70%—75% experience local adverse reactions (LARs) confined to the oral mucosa.[5,8] SLIT-LARs often occur during the build-up phase prior to reaching the maintenance dose and commonly include oral and oropharyngeal pruritus, swelling of the lips and tongue, and throat irritation.[5,9] In contrast, up to 82% of patients receiving subcutaneous immunotherapy (SCIT) experience LARs which include pain, erythema, and swelling near the injection site.[6] Severe adverse reactions (SARs) can include life-threatening anaphylaxis, rhinitis and asthma exacerbations, urticaria, chest discomfort/tightness, and other gastrointestinal or neurological symptoms. In a comprehensive review of 66 SLIT studies, SARs were reported in 0.056% of SLIT doses administered.[10] Using 5 years of surveillance data collected between 2008 and 2013 from clinical practices in the United States, Puerto Rico, and Canada, SARs were reported in approximately 1.9% of patients receiving SCIT and in 0.1% of injection visits.[11] Two recent surveys conducted "real-life" clinical assessments on SARs due to AIT (SLIT or SCIT) in European clinical practices (France, Spain, and Germany).[12,13] Both studies reported a higher case prevalence of SARs in SCIT-treated patients compared with patients receiving SLIT (sublingual drops or tablets) in pediatric and adult populations. Moreover, the risk of experiencing SARs was significantly higher in patients treated with natural extract—based SLIT products compared with SLIT products containing allergoids, chemically modified allergens exhibiting reduced IgE reactivity.[12,13] Together, these observations from real-life settings highlight the safety benefit of modified allergens over traditional natural extracts.

Due to their dependency on the raw materials used for extraction, natural allergen extracts are heterogeneous mixtures of relevant allergens and other nonallergenic compounds such as bacterial endotoxin.[14] Having precise control over the concentrations of individual allergens is near impossible as the raw materials dictate the amount of allergen extracted into the final product.[4] This leads to allergen extracts with variable potencies, in vivo biological activity, and even the absence of relevant allergens. For example, when comparing commercialized allergen extracts from different manufacturers, several studies reported large differences in the concentrations of both total protein and of individual major allergens. This was observed for extracts from dog, several mold species, birch, timothy grass, and HDM (*Dermatophagoides fairinae* and *Dermatophagoides pteronyssinus*).[15−21] Large variations in major allergen content were also reported for market-approved extract-based SLIT products for birch pollen, HDM, and timothy grass pollen. A greater than 10-fold difference in the concentration of Bet v 1 was observed in six birch-SLIT products.[22] For five HDM-SLIT products, the concentrations of Der p 1 and Der f 1 ranged from 0.6 to 14.5 µg/mL and 0.2−12.4 µg/mL, respectively.[23] At maintenance dose, the total protein content of Phl p 5 varied greatly across 10 grass-SLIT products ranging from 0.2 to 21.6 µg.[18] The large variability in major allergen content and even the lack of important allergens all together may explain why some AIT products require longer dosing regimens and provide only partial protection. Martin Chapman did a nice study years ago comparing commericial extracts of Alternaria and Aspergillious -in two years and it was frightening how low the content was. Bob Esch did a nice study comparing Alternaria major allergen content years ago with gel blots and demonstrated differences within a company if in normal saline or glycerine/hsa.

Types of recombinant allergens and hypoallergenic derivatives

With the high frequency of adverse reactions related to natural allergen extracts, there is a growing need for safer alternatives that exhibit reduced allergenicity, but maintain immunogenicity comparable with their extract counterparts. Natural extracts contain a variety of conformational IgE-binding epitopes. These epitopes can activate mast cells and basophils, leading to the release of histamine and possibly life-threatening anaphylaxis.[24] Early attempts were made to modify natural allergen extracts using chemicals to alter or destroy conformational IgE-binding epitopes while maintaining immunogenicity (i.e., preservation of linear T cell epitopes); later labeled as allergoids. With the advent of recombinant technologies, cDNA encoding the major protein responsible for allergic symptoms can be isolated and used to produce highly purified recombinant protein free of contamination and nonallergenic material.[7] Moreover, the amino acid sequence can be modified to further reduce allergenicity. The subsequent sections elaborate on key recombinant allergen derivatives and their efficacy as demonstrated in recent AIT clinical trials (see Tables 17.1−17.3).

Allergoids

Allergoids are chemically modified derivatives of whole allergens that demonstrate reduced allergenicity while preserving the ability to elicit tolerogenic immune responses. The reduced allergenic potential stems from the decrease in conformational

Table 17.1 Summary of clinical trials using allergoids and recombinant allergen derivatives.

Allergen	Molecule	Study	Treatment schedule	Safety
Allergoids				
Ragweed	Short ragweed allergoid adsorbed to L-tyrosine and monophosphoryl lipid A	Phase IIb[26]	4 subcutaneous weekly build-up injections	TEAEs reported in 94.7% and 67.7% of allergoid and placebo groups. Primarily consisted of local injection site reactions (pruritus, swelling, pain, warmth).
HDM	Monomeric allergoid containing 1:1 mix of carbamylated Der p and Der f allergoids	Phase II[29]	Once daily sublingual tablets for 12 weeks (total of 84 tablets)	3.4% and up to 7.7% of patients experienced ≥ 1 local treatment-related AE in placebo and active treatment groups.
Grass	Timothy grass pollen allergoid	Phase II[27]	7 preseasonal weekly subcutaneous build-up injections followed by 2 biweekly maintenance dose injections.	65.0% and 50.0%–68.4% of placebo and active treatment group experienced ≥1 TEAE with most being swelling/pruritus at injection site.
	Mixed grass pollen allergoid (Pollinex®)	Prospective, controlled, noninterventional study[28]	4 preseasonal weekly subcutaneous build-up injections	28.6% of patients receiving injections reported local AE (itching and swelling).
Recombinant wild-type allergens				
Grass	Equimolar mixture of rPhl p 1, rPhl p 2, rPhl p 5a, rPhl p 5b, rPhl p 6	DBPC-RCT[31]	10 weekly subcutaneous build-up injections followed by maintenance dose injections with dosing reduced by 50% during the pollen seasons	AEs reported in 5.9% and 10.7% of placebo and active treatment injections, respectively. > 90% of AEs were transient erythema and local swelling. Systemic AEs occurred in 0.96% of active treatment injections.
		Phase II[32]	Total of 13 subcutaneous injections every 4–14 days starting 5 months before the grass pollen season	16% of active treatment groups reported grades I or II systemic AEs. Grades III or IV systemic AEs were not reported.

Allergen	Product	Study	Protocol	Adverse events
Birch	rBet v 1	DBPC-RCT[33]	12 weekly preseasonal subcutaneous build-up injections followed by monthly maintenance dose injections for 2 years	Frequency of local and systemic AEs comparable across all groups. 60.8% of reported TEAEs in rBet v 1 group were immediate local reactions compared to 15.2% in placebo.
		Phase II[34]	Once daily sublingual tablets starting 4 months prior to the birch pollen season and continuing for 1 week after the season	86.0% and 90.2%–96.7% of placebo and active treatment groups reported ≥1 TEAE, respectively (most local reactions). 23 withdrew due to AEs.
Birch and apple	rBet v 1 and rMal d 1	Phase II[35]	Once daily sublingual drop (kept under tongue for 1–2 minutes) for 16 weeks	55% and 95% of placebo and both rBet v 1 and rMal d 1 groups, respectively, experienced ≥ 1 AE after first sublingual administration with most affecting the mouth, ears, and throat,
Cat	rFel d 1 fusion protein	Phase I/IIa[36]	3 intralymphatic build-up injections into the superficial inguinal lymph node 28 days apart	Comparable occurrence of AEs across placebo and active treatment groups (most being local lymph node swelling)

Fragments and recombinant hypoallergenic derivatives

Allergen	Product	Study	Protocol	Adverse events
Birch	2 rBet v 1 fragments (aa 1–73 and aa 74–159) and 1 rBet v 1 trimer	DBPC-RCT[37,40]	8 preseasonal subcutaneous build-up injections every 1–2 weeks followed by maintenance dose injections every 4 weeks until the flowering season	Higher frequency of local swelling and grades I/II systemic AEs in fragment/trimer groups compared with placebo. Common systemic AEs were conjunctivitis, rhinitis, and cough.
Birch	Folding variant of rBet v 1 (rBet v 1-FV)	Phase II[52]	10 weekly subcutaneous injections 8 weekly preseasonal subcutaneous build-up injections with weekly maintenance dose injections continuing until the start of birch pollen season	Drug-related TEAEs reported in 42.9% and 37.5%–87.5% of placebo and active treatment groups with majority as local injection site reactions.
		Phase II[53] DBPC-RCT[54]	8 weekly preseasonal subcutaneous build-up injections followed by maintenance dose injections every 7–28 days with 50% dose reduction during birch pollen season	91.7% and 85.2% of rBet v 1-FV and birch extract group experienced ≥ 1 AE possibly related to study drug. Systemic AEs occurred in 42% of rBet v 1-FV and 41% of birch extract group. 60% of active treatment and 53% of placebo groups experienced injection-related AEs mostly mild in severity and over half as injection site reactions.

TEAEs, Treatment-emergent adverse events; AE, adverse event.

Table 17.2 Summary of clinical trials using synthetic peptides.

Allergen	Molecule	Study	Treatment schedule	Safety
T Cell Epitope-Derived Peptides				
Cat	Equimolar mixture of 7 Fel d 1-derived peptides	Phase IIa(59)	Single-dose intradermal or subcutaneous injection	Transient and self-limiting erythema occurred within 15 minutes and accompanied all intradermal injections. Few local reactions reported for subcutaneous injections
		Phase II(61), 2-yr follow up study(62), phase III(63)	4 intradermal injections every 4 weeks (4x6) or 8 intradermal injections every 2 weeks (8x3)	Drug-related TEAEs reported in 18.8%, 26.9%, and 21.2% of placebo, 8x3, and 4x6 groups respectively with most mild in severity. Drug-related AEs were not reported during 2-yr follow up
		Single-blind, placebo run-in study(60)	2 biweekly intradermal placebo injections followed by 8 weekly intradermal treatment injections	Injection site AEs were not reported
HDM	Mixture of 7 Der p-derived peptides	PC-RCT(64)	Successive cohorts received 4 intradermal injections of 0.03, 0.3, 1, 3, and 12 nmol every 4 weeks	Common TEAEs included nausea, influenza, gastroenteritis, and nasopharyngitis
		DBPC-RCT(65), 2-yr follow up study(66)	12-week treatment period of 4 intradermal injections of 12 nmol or 11 intradermal injections of 12 nmol	Safety information not published
		Phase IIb(68)	12-week treatment period of 4 intradermal injections of 12 nmol, 20 nmol, or 8 intradermal injections of 12 nmol	Safety information not published
Ragweed	Mixture of Amb a 1-derived peptides	PC-RCT(69)	Dosing regimens not published	Safety information not published
Grass	Mixture of 7 peptides derived from Cyn d 1, Lol p 5, Dac g 5, Hol l 5, and Phl p 5	Phase II(70), 1 yr-follow up(71), 2-yr follow up(72)	14-week treatment period of 8 intradermal injections every 2 weeks (8x6Q2W), 4 intradermal injections every 4 weeks (4x12Q4W), or 8 intradermal injections every 2 weeks (8x12Q2W)	20.0% of placebo and 29.6-37.1% of active treatment groups reported ≥ 1 drug-related TEAE. > 30% of all groups reported severe TEAEs (noted as AEs causing interference with daily living)

Contiguous Overlapping Peptides

Bee Venom	3 long synthetic peptides derived from phospholipase A2 (aa 1-60, aa 47-99, aa 90-134)	Phase I(78)	7 subcutaneous build-up injections every 30 minutes followed by 5 maintenance dose injections at days 4, 7, 14, 42, and 70	No local/systemic AEs reported during the build-up phase with late-phase local erythema occurring in 2 patients during maintenance dose injections
Birch	Equimolar mixture of three overlapping peptides derived from Bet v 1 (aa 2-50, aa 48-118, aa 106-160) (named AllerT)	Phase I(79)	Skin testing with AllerT	Positive skin reactions were not reported for AllerT
		Phase I/IIa(80)	5 subcutaneous build-up injections 15 minutes apart on day 1 followed by 4 maintenance dose injections delivered on days 7, 14, 21, and 51	Occurrence of local AEs were comparable between placebo and AllerT groups and included pain, erythema, and induration
		Phase IIb(81)	2-month treatment period of 5 preseasonal subcutaneous injections with half dose delivered on day 1	63.3% and 53.7-59.0% of placebo and AllerT groups respectively reported injection-site reactions (most involving pain and erythema). 26.6% and 64.1-70.7% of placebo and AllerT groups respectively reported systemic AEs

B Cell Epitope-Derived Peptides

Grass	Equimolar mixture of 4 recombinant grass pollen fusion proteins (rPhl p 1, rPhl p 2, rPhl p 5, rPhl p 6) fused to the PreS domain of human hepatitis B virus (named BM32)	Phase I(92)	Skin and patch testing	Immediate and late-phase skin reactions were not reported
		Phase IIa(93)	3 subcutaneous injections administered 3 to 4 weeks apart	94.4% and 94.4-100% of placebo and BM32 groups respectively reported local injection site reactions (most being late-phase). Only BM32 groups reported grade 1 systemic late-phase treatment-associated AEs (primarily allergic rhinitis)
		Phase IIb(95)	3 preseasonal subcutaneous injections, a booster injection, and another 3 preseasonal subcutaneous injections	Year 1: 73.6% and 86.7-88.7% of placebo and BM32 groups reported late-phase local reactions with a higher percentage also reporting late-phase systemic AEs (mostly grade I) compared to placebo. Year 2: Frequencies of local and systemic AEs comparable between BM32 and placebo

HDM, house dust mite; TEAEs, Treatment-emergent adverse events; AE, adverse event.

Table 17.3 Molecules in preclinical development.

Allergen	Molecule	Current phase of development	Main findings
Mosaic proteins			
Grass	Rearranged hybrid proteins derived from Phl p 1, Phl p 2, Phl p 5, and Phl p 6[44]	*In vitro* and in vivo animal work	Reduced binding to allergic patients' IgE.
Birch	Rearranged proteins derived from Bet v 1[41]	*In vitro* and in vivo animal work	Reduced allergen-induced basophil activation and histamine release.
HDM	Rearranged hybrid proteins derived from Der p 1 and Der p 2[43]	*In vitro* and in vivo animal work	Induced allergen-specific blocking IgG antibodies following animal vaccination.
Cat	Rearranged proteins derived from Fel d 1[42]	*In vitro* and in vivo animal work	
Recombinant mutants			
Parietaria pollen	Fusion protein of Par j 1 and Par j 2 containing mutated IgE epitopes[49]	*In vitro* and in vivo animal work	Reduced IgE reactivity, basophil activation, and induced allergen-specific blocking antibodies following vaccination of mice.
	Fusion protein of Par j 1 and Par j 2 containing mutated cysteine residues[50]	*In vitro* and in vivo animal work	Induced T cell proliferation comparable to wild-type allergen, and vaccination reduced allergen-specific IgE and increased allergen-specific IgG1 and IgG2a in sensitized mice.
Carp	Cyp c 1 with mutated calcium-binding domains[45–48]	*In vitro* and in vivo animal and human skin testing	Reduced binding to patients' IgE and basophil activation/histamine release. Cyp c 1 mutant–induced antibodies reduced allergic symptoms in fish allergy mouse model. Yielded smaller skin prick test wheals compared to wild-type Cyp c 1 in fish-allergic patients.

T cell epitope–derived peptides

Peanut	Synthetic peptides derived from Ara h 1[73–75]	In vitro and in vivo animal work	7 synthetic Ara h 1–derived peptides exhibited reduced peanut-allergic basophil activation and induced peanut-specific T cell proliferation. Protected against peanut-induced anaphylaxis in two peanut allergy mouse models

B cell epitope–derived peptides

Birch	Bet v 1–derived peptides fused to KLH[86] Bet v 1–derived peptides fused to the PreS domain[89]	In vitro and in vivo animal and human skin testing (Bet v 1-KLH only)	Reduced binding to allergic patients' IgE. Reduced allergen-induced basophil activation and histamine release. Induced allergen-specific blocking IgG antibodies following animal vaccination. Bet v 1–derived peptides did not elicit positive skin prick test reactions in birch-allergic patients[86]
HDM	Der p 2–derived peptides fused to KLH[87] Der p 23–derived peptides fused to the PreS domain[90]	In vitro and in vivo animal work	
Cat	Fel d 1–derived peptides fused to the PreS domain[88]	In vitro and in vivo animal work	

HDM, house dust mite.

IgE-binding epitopes following modification. Both IgG and linear T cell epitopes are preserved, rendering allergoids a suitable candidate for use in AIT trials. There are many methods for producing allergoids, which have been summarized in a recent review.[25] These include thermal and chemical denaturation, enzymatic and chemical polymerization, carbohydrate conjugation (i.e., addition of sugars), and carbamylation (i.e., treatment with potassium cyanate), which produces monomeric allergoids. Due to the large variety of production methods, not all allergoids are created equal. Some allergoids demonstrate strong immunogenicity while others require an adjuvant (e.g., a carrier protein) to elicit immune responses.[25] Recent research has focused on the evaluation of allergoids for ragweed, timothy grass, and HDM produced using chemical polymerization (i.e., treatment with formaldehyde or glutaraldehyde) and the aforementioned carbamylation.

Polymerized allergoids for ragweed and timothy grass have been recently developed for patients with AR. In a phase IIb trial, the clinical efficacy of ragweed MATA MPL (short ragweed pollen allergoid adsorbed to both L-tyrosine and monophosphoryl lipid A (MPL)) was evaluated using an ultrashort course regimen comprised of only four weekly subcutaneous injections at increasing doses of 300, 700, 2000, and 6000 standardized units/mL.[26] Adsorption to L-tyrosine and MPL served to slow the release of the drug and enhance immunogenicity.[25] After randomization to active treatment or placebo, ragweed-allergic patients underwent a baseline ragweed pollen challenge conducted over 4 days in an environmental challenge chamber (EEC), 4 weeks of treatment, and a final pollen challenges 3 weeks after treatment. Ragweed MATA MPL led to a significant improvement in total symptom scores (48% over placebo) and an increase in ragweed-specific IgG1 and IgG4 compared with placebo.[26] In another recent randomized, double-blind, placebo-controlled, dose-finding study, the efficacy of a new timothy grass pollen allergoid (three doses of 1800, 6000, and 18,000 therapeutic units (TU)/ml) was compared with a market-approved 6-grass pollen allergoid (Allergovit® at 6000 TU/mL) in patients with grass pollen–induced AR.[27] Using a preseasonal treatment regimen of nine subcutaneous injections (seven weekly at increasing dosage and two biweekly at maintenance dose), all three doses of the new timothy grass pollen allergoid significantly reduced late-phase wheal reactions assessed by intracutaneous testing with a 6-grass pollen allergen solution (primary study outcome) and increased *Phleum pratense*–specific IgG4 compared with placebo. These responses were also comparable with those observed in the Allergovit®-treated group.[27] Finally, a prospective, patient-preference, noninterventional study evaluated the use of a market-approved grass pollen allergoid (POLLINEX-G® Quattro Plus 1.0 mL) in an ultrashort course booster treatment regimen in grass-allergic patients exhibiting recurrent AR symptoms after successful completion of any grass AIT prior to enrollment.[28] Patients had a choice between the booster AIT group (four preseasonal weekly subcutaneous injections of 300, 800, and 2000 SU twice) and control group (no injections). Both groups received antiallergic medication upon request throughout the grass pollen season. Compared with the control group, the booster AIT group experienced a 38.4% reduction in combined symptom and medication scores during the peak of grass pollen season. Approximately one-third of patients receiving booster injections also remained medication-free compared with only 2%−4% of the control group.[28] In agreement with safety data concerning SLIT, these studies exhibited comparable frequencies of adverse events (AEs) between allergoid and placebo groups (29%−95% vs. 65% −67%). AEs were primarily local with most being mild injection-site reactions (warmth, pain, swelling, pruritus).

A new monomeric allergoid comprised of a 1:1 mixture of carbamylated *D. pteronyssinus* and *D. farinae* allergoids was evaluated in a recent randomized, double-blind, placebo-controlled, dose-finding study.[29] HDM-allergic patients were randomized to one of four doses of sublingual allergoid-containing tablets (300, 1000, 2000, 3000 standard allergy units (UA)) or placebo taken once daily for 12 weeks. Clinical efficacy was evaluated using conjunctival provocation testing (CPT) with an HDM solution before and after treatment. Compared with placebo, only the 2000 UA dose led to a trending reduction in allergic severity ($P < .1$) and a significantly greater percentage of patients with improved CPT response thresholds ($P = .04$). The monomeric HDM allergoid also demonstrated a favorable safety profile, with up to 7.7% of patients in the 2000 and 3000 UA groups experiencing local treatment−related AEs compared with 3.4% of the placebo group.[29] These included oral discomfort/pruritus, tongue swelling, throat irritation, and oropharyngeal blistering.

Overall, AIT with allergoids can be efficacious in reducing the severity of allergic symptoms compared with placebo. Although the occurrence of local AEs is similar to therapies using natural allergen extracts, SCIT with allergoids often require a shorter treatment regimen to achieve clinical benefit. The superior safety profile of SLIT with allergoids over natural extracts has also been supported in two metaanalyses involving both pediatric and adult patients.[12,13]

Recombinant wild-type allergens

In many native allergens, only a small proportion of protein components are actually responsible for mediating allergic reactivity. Following confirmation of their allergenicity (i.e., binding to IgE from allergic sera),[30] these proteins can be sequenced, and their cDNA transfected into viral vectors and expressed in bacterial cell cultures (e.g., *Escherichia coli* cultures). The final product is a recombinant form of the protein that can be mass produced in a reproducible manner with high purity and consistent structural, molecular, and immunogenic properties. Problems related to quality control, contamination, and variable allergen content inherent in natural extracts can be avoided as the final concentrations of recombinant proteins can be manipulated entirely. The final composition can also contain single or multiple recombinant proteins from the same allergen species.[4] This is advantageous as treatment with recombinant proteins can be tailored to the patient's sensitization profile. For example, approximately, 90% of grass-allergic patients are sensitized to Phl p 1, while only 40%−60% are sensitized to Phl p 2.[31] Recombinant preparations of major allergens from timothy grass, birch, cat, and apple have already been evaluated in AIT studies for the treatment of AR and birch pollen–related oral allergy syndrome (OAS).

One of the earliest AIT studies to use recombinant allergen-based vaccines evaluated the clinical efficacy of a mixture of five recombinant grass pollen allergens for the treatment of grass pollen allergy.[31] In a randomized, double-blind, placebo-controlled trial, grass-allergic patients received either an equimolar mixture of five *P. pratense* allergens (Phl p 1, 2, 5a, 5b, and 6) or placebo. Both were administered using an 18-month treatment regimen spanning two grass pollen seasons; 10 weekly subcutaneous injections at increasing dosage until maintenance, followed by injections 15, 28, and then 42 days apart with dosing reduced by 50% during grass pollen season. The active treatment led to a 38.9% reduction over placebo in combined symptom medication scores during the second pollen season. Increases in both grass-specific IgG1 and IgG4 were seen after only 3–4 months of treatment and persisted throughout the study. Of the 78 treatment-related AEs (10.7% of 731 injections) reported for active treatment, 71 were local (primarily transient erythema and swelling) and seven were systemic (primarily general/localized urticaria), thus demonstrating a favorable safety profile for doses containing up to 40 μg of recombinant protein.[31] In a follow-up dose-finding safety study, up to 120 μg of the same recombinant grass mixture delivered as a single subcutaneous injection was tolerated in grass-allergic patients.[32] Using a modified dosing regimen of 13 subcutaneous injections, 16% of patients on active treatment (2.21% of active treatment injections) experienced mild (grades I or II) systemic AEs, which were well distributed among the four doses evaluated (20, 40, 80, and 120 μg). Mild systemic AEs included mild dyspnea, dizziness and flushing, and urticaria. Severe systemic AEs (grades III or IV) were not reported, supporting the use of SCIT with high doses of recombinant allergens.[32]

Studies comparing the clinical efficacy of recombinant allergens to natural extracts and evaluating their use in SLIT were first conducted with recombinant Bet v 1 (rBet v 1, major birch pollen allergen). In a multicenter, randomized, double-blind, placebo-controlled study, 134 birch-allergic patients received rBet v 1, natural Bet v 1 (nBet v 1, purified from defatted birch pollen), natural birch pollen extract, or placebo.[33] The 2-year treatment period included a preseasonal build-up phase of 12 weekly subcutaneous injections followed by monthly injections of 15 μg Bet v 1 protein (maintenance dose) or placebo for 2 years. During the first birch pollen season, rBet v 1 treatment led to a 49.4% reduction in daily mean total rhinoconjunctivitis symptom scores (TRSS), a 64.2% reduction in daily rescue medication score, and increased levels of Bet v 1–specific IgG antibodies compared with the placebo group. These changes were comparable in magnitude to both nBet v 1 and birch pollen extract, and persisted into the second pollen season. rBet v 1–treated patients experienced a similar rate of systemic reactions (mostly rhinitis and conjunctivitis) but a higher rate of local reactions (primarily local swelling) compared with the other three treatment groups.[33] When rBet v 1 was formulated into a fast-disintegrating sublingual tablet taken daily for 5 months, birch-allergic patients treated with 12.5, 25, or 50 μg doses demonstrated a significant reduction in both average adjusted symptom scores (17.0%−17.7%) and average rescue medication scores (30.3%−33.0%) during the birch pollen season compared with placebo-treated patients.[34] Contrasting historical SLIT safety data, over 90% of the active treatment groups and 86% of the placebo group experienced at least one treatment-related AE. These were predominantly local reactions of throat irritation, oral pruritus, and ear pruritus.[34] More recently, a randomized, double-blind, placebo-controlled study compared the efficacy of rBet v 1 or rMal d 1 (major apple allergen, cross-reactive to Bet v 1) sublingual drops in reducing symptoms of apple OAS in patients with birch pollen−related apple allergy.[35] Sublingual challenge testing with a rMal d 1 challenge solution was done to assess treatment efficacy. After randomization to 300 μL of rBet v 1, rMal d 1, or placebo sublingual drops given once daily for 16 weeks, rMal d 1−induced oral symptoms were significantly reduced in rMal d 1−treated patients compared with placebo with 25% tolerating an additional challenge with 20 g of fresh apple.[35] In contrast, SLIT rBet v 1 treatment had no effect on rMal d 1−induced oral symptoms and decreased the ratio of Mal d 1-specific IgG4/IgE antibodies compared with the increase seen after rMal d 1 treatment. Echoing the safety data from the previous study, 95% and 55% of the active treatment (both rBet v 1 and rMal d 1) and placebo groups, respectively, experienced AEs. Most were local reactions and included oral pruritus, ear pruritus, throat irritation, and oral blisters/edema.[35]

The clinical efficacy of rFel d 1 (major cat dander allergen) was first evaluated using intralymphatic allergen delivery, where allergen is directly injected into the lymph nodes (intralymphatic immunotherapy).[36] Using an increasing dosing regimen of three injections (1, 3, and 10 μg) into a superficial inguinal lymph node, cat-allergic patients were randomized to either a fusion protein preparation of rFel d 1 (MAT-rFel d 1) or placebo. The MAT-rFel d 1 group exhibited a significant increase in both nasal and skin tolerance to cat dander extract, and increased cat dander−specific IgG4 titers 5 weeks after treatment. Additionally, few AEs were reported for up to 88 days after the first injection with most being lymph node swelling and dyspnea, thus demonstrating a favorable safety and efficacy profile with only three intralymphatic injections.[36]

Compared with natural allergen extracts, AIT with recombinant allergens appear to be just as efficacious in reducing allergic symptoms. They are less prone to contamination during production and can be safely administered using subcutaneous, sublingual, and even intralymphatic routes. However, they are still associated with a high frequency of AEs, although most are local reactions and mild in intensity. This is not unexpected as recombinant allergens still contain the same allergenic IgE-binding epitopes found in natural allergen extracts.

Fragments and recombinant hypoallergenic derivatives

The allergenicity of recombinant allergens can be further reduced by directly modifying the protein's DNA sequence. By altering the order of amino acids, the conformation of otherwise reactive IgE-binding epitopes can be disrupted, thus rendering them nonreactive without reducing T cell reactivity.[7] The methods of producing hypoallergenic derivatives from recombinant allergens vary and can include fragmentation, sequence rearrangement, and site-directed mutagenesis. *In vitro* IgE-binding and basophil histamine release assays, as well as in vivo animal immunization experiments are routinely used to assess both allergenicity and immunogenicity of new derivatives.

Using fragmentation, two hypoallergenic derivatives were developed from rBet v 1; two fragments (amino acids 1–73 and 74–159), and one trimer comprising three linked copies of rBet v 1 cDNA.[37] Early studies evaluated the safety and efficacy of these hypoallergenic derivatives in birch-allergic patients using a preseasonal dosing regimen of eight subcutaneous injections followed by maintenance injections (80 μg) every 4 weeks. Treatment with fragments or trimers led to an increase in serum and nasal IgG antibodies against Bet v 1, and a significant reduction in the elevated Bet v 1–specific IgE responses normally seen after the birch pollen season.[37–39] Although trending improvement in nasal symptom scores and patient well-being were also observed, changes in combined symptom medication scores (primary endpoint) during the pollen season were not significant compared with placebo.[40] Moreover, both fragment- and trimer-treated patients experienced a higher frequency of local and systemic AEs compared to the placebo group. Local AEs primarily included swelling at the injection site while systemic AEs included conjunctivitis, rhinitis, cough, and asthmatic exacerbations.[40]

Sequence rearrangement serves as an alternative approach in reducing the IgE reactivity of recombinant allergens. After the characterization of relevant epitopes, the allergen-encoding cDNA is fragmented into smaller parts, which are then recombined in an order differing from the original sequence. This process produces either recombinant mosaic or hybrid mosaic proteins depending on if the parts were derived from a single or two or more allergens.[7] Selective rearrangement disrupts the conformation of IgE epitopes while allowing for the preservation of sequences required for the induction of blocking IgG antibodies and T cell reactivity.

Bet v 1 was reassembled to yield three recombinant mosaic proteins. Using sera from birch-allergic patients, all three mosaic proteins showed a strong reduction in both IgE reactivity and basophil activation compared with rBet v 1. Moreover, IgG blocking antibodies from rabbits immunized with rBet v 1-mosaic proteins strongly inhibited the binding of patients' IgE to rBet v 1 (82%–87% inhibition).[41] Similar findings were observed for recombinant mosaic proteins derived from Fel d 1 and hybrid mosaic proteins derived from two major HDM allergens (Der p 1 and 2), as well as four major allergens from timothy grass pollen (Phl p 1, 2, 5, and 6).[42–44] In addition to reduced IgE and basophil reactivity, immunization of rabbits with grass pollen mosaic proteins induced stronger IgG titers compared with immunization with POLLINEX-G® (registered grass pollen allergoid–based vaccine), and induced IgG antibodies that suppressed airway hyperresponsiveness in a mouse model of grass pollen allergy.[44]

Another approach to constructing recombinant hypoallergenic derivatives is the mutation of specific amino acids on allergen-encoding cDNA. By using site-directed mutagenesis, sequences contributing to IgE binding can be modified without the need of fragmenting the entire cDNA molecule. Using this approach, a hypoallergenic mutant of the major fish allergen paravalbumin was constructed.[45] Based on the observation that calcium depletion significantly reduces the IgE-binding capacity of rCyp c 1, point mutations were introduced into both calcium-binding sites of rCyp c 1 (mCyp c 1). Using sera and peripheral blood mononuclear cells (PBMCs) from fish-allergic patients, mCyp c 1 exhibited a 95% reduction in IgE reactivity, a strong reduction in histamine release from basophils compared with wild-type rCyp c 1, and comparable T cell proliferative responses to that induced by rCyp c 1 and natural Cyp c 1.[45,46] Supporting these findings, skin testing of fish-allergic patients with mCyp c 1 led to a significant reduction in wheal size compared with the wild-type allergen at doses up to 32 µg/mL with no occurrence of late or generalized adverse reactions.[47] Additionally, using a vaccination protocol resembling traditional SCIT regimens, IgG blocking antibodies induced from mCyp c 1—immunized rabbits significantly reduced symptoms of anaphylaxis in a mouse model of fish allergy following an intragastric challenge with carp extract.[48] More recently, two hypoallergenic mutants containing a fusion of rPar j 1 and rPar j 2 (major allergens of *Parietaria* pollen, a common pollen species in Southern Europe) were constructed using different targeting strategies. The first mutant exhibited a 3-amino acid mutation in a region containing an immunodominant IgE epitope on both Par j 1 and Par j 2 (PjEDloop1). Using sera and PBMCs from *Parietaria* pollen-allergic patients, PjEDloop1 demonstrated reduced allergenicity and similar immunogenicity compared with a mix of rPar j 1 and 2, and induced IgG blocking antibodies that strongly inhibited the binding of patients' IgE to rPar j 1 and 2.[49] The second mutant exhibited mutations that disrupted the disulfide bonds on both rPar j 1 and rPar j 2 (PjEDcys). PjEDCys-stimulated PBMCs from *Parietaria* pollen-allergic patients significantly reduced the percentage of Th2 cytokine-secreting cells compared with a mixture of rPar j 1 and 2. Moreover, immunization of *Parietaria* pollen-sensitized mice with three subcutaneous injections of PjEDCys led to a strong reduction in specific IgE and a significant increase in IgG1 and IgG2a antibodies, all against rPar j 1 and 2, compared with control vaccination with phosphate buffered saline.[50]

Akin to the methods used to create allergoids from natural allergen extracts, hypoallergenic structural variants of wild-type recombinant allergens can also be constructed by altering the chemicals used during the purification of said recombinant allergen. Structural variants lose their native 3D conformation, likely reducing the reactivity of conformational-dependent IgE epitopes while preserving both the original cDNA sequence and T cell epitopes. This approach was used to construct a stable monomeric folding variant of rBet v 1 (rBet v 1-FV).[51] In a randomized, double-blind, placebo-controlled, dose-finding study, the efficacy of rBet v 1-FV (four doses of 20, 80, 160, and 320 µg) was evaluated in birch-allergic patients during an 8-hour birch pollen challenge in an EEC.[52] Using a dosing regimen of 10 weekly subcutaneous injections with the last three given as maintenance injections, all four doses led to a significant reduction in total symptom scores (71.9% −81.8%) and an increase in Bet v 1-specific IgG1 titers compared with placebo-treated patients during the 8-hour birch pollen challenge. The frequency of treatment-related AEs ranged from 37.5% to 87.5% with the lowest incidence reported by the 80 μg group (37.5% of patients). This frequency was comparable with the placebo group (42.9% of patients) and primarily included local injection site reactions, thus demonstrating preliminary efficacy and tolerability of an 80 μg dose containing rBet v 1-FV for the treatment of birch pollen allergy.[52] When rBet v 1-FV (80 μg dose) was compared with a standardized birch pollen extract using a shorter preseasonal dosing regimen of eight weekly subcutaneous injections, birch-allergic patients treated with rBet v 1-FV exhibited lower daily combined symptom medication scores during the first birch pollen season compared with the extract-treated group (median 5.86 vs. 12.40).[53] However, the difference between the two active treatments was not significant and equated to the daily use of one antihistamine tablet. Both treatments also led to comparable increases in birch pollen–specific IgG titers. Although the safety profile of rBet v 1-FV was comparable with that of birch pollen extract, a large proportion of both treatment groups experienced at least one possibly treatment-related AE (91.7% and 85.2%, respectively) as well as systemic reactions (42% and 41%, respectively).[53] Finally, a recent randomized, double-blind, placebo-controlled study evaluated the efficacy of rBet v 1-FV in reducing symptoms of birch pollen–related soya allergy in birch-allergic patients with soya allergy.[54] Double-blind, placebo-controlled food challenges with soya protein were used to assess treatment efficacy with the lowest observable AE levels for objective signs and subjective symptoms as primary endpoints. After randomization to eight weekly updosing and then maintenance subcutaneous injections (80 μg) every 7–28 days of rBet v 1-FV or placebo, a trending improvement in the cumulative dose of soya protein required until the first occurrence of objective symptoms was observed in the active group compared with placebo. rBet v 1-FV treatment also led to significant increases in IgG4 antibodies against Bet v 1, and the Bet v 1-homologues Gly m 4 (major soybean allergen) and Cor a 1 (major hazelnut allergen). Injection-related AEs were primarily mild and were reported in 60% and 53% of the active and placebo groups, respectively, with most being local injection site reactions.[54]

Although there are a variety of methods to construct recombinant hypoallergenic derivatives, they all aim to reduce allergenicity and the likelihood of IgE-mediated adverse effects while maintaining immunogenicity comparable with native allergens and natural allergen extracts. These methods allow for greater control in implementing specific modifications into the protein's genetic makeup compared with recombinant wild-type allergens. However, due to the variety of modifications that could be made, many hypoallergenic derivatives of common aeroallergens remain in preclinical as well as preliminary phase I/II stages of development.

Synthetic T cell epitope—derived peptides

Previous iterations of modified allergens (allergoids, recombinant allergens, and hypoallergenic derivatives) are still capable of eliciting IgE-mediated adverse reactions as some IgE epitopes remain unaltered. To address this problem, early studies by Norman et al.[55] and Creticos et al.[56] evaluated synthetic peptides derived from multiple T cell epitopes from Fel d 1 (two 27-amino acid tolerizing peptides) and Amb a 1 (major ragweed allergen, three tolerizing peptides 21—27 amino acids in length) for the treatment of cat and ragweed allergies. When administered subcutaneously, both peptides reduced allergic symptoms. However, they were accompanied by a high rate of late-onset AEs (e.g., asthma) and were discontinued in the late 1990s.[57] Shorter peptides named synthetic peptide immunoregulatory epitopes (SPIREs) were developed soon after. With a length of only 13—17 amino acids, SPIREs are unable to cross-link IgE, strongly reducing the likelihood of serious IgE-mediated AEs such as anaphylaxis. They also contain major T cell epitopes known to bind to major histocompatibility complex (MHC) class II molecules on antigen presenting cells. The binding to MHC class II molecules is thought to induce tolerance and upregulation of allergen-specific regulatory T cells (Tregs).[57,58] To date, SPIREs have been developed for major allergens from cat, HDM, ragweed, grass, and peanut.

SPIREs derived from Fel d 1 were among the first to be developed and extensively tested as a possible treatment for cat allergy. Preliminary MHC class II-binding studies and in vitro proliferation/cytokine secretion assays identified seven short Fel d 1—derived peptides capable of binding to multiple HLA class II molecules. A 7-peptide vaccine was formulated (Cat-PAD, cat-peptide antigen desensitization) and both safety and efficacy were evaluated in a preliminary randomized, double-blind, placebo-controlled, phase IIa study including cat-allergic patients.[59] When Cat-PAD was administered as a single intradermal injection at doses of 0.03, 0.3, 3, and 12 nmol, the 3 nmol dose resulted in the greatest reduction (40%) in late-phase (at 8 hours) skin responses (LPSR) to an intradermal cat allergen challenge compared with placebo 3 weeks after treatment. All four doses were well tolerated with intradermal injections accompanied only by erythema that was transient and self-limiting in nature.[59] A separate placebo run-in pilot study evaluated the safety and efficacy of Cat-PAD in cat-allergic children aged 5—11 years.[60] Using an intradermal dosing regimen of two biweekly placebo injections followed by eight injections of 6 nmol Cat-PAD every 4 weeks, local pain scores at the injection site were low with no local AEs reported. Symptom scores also improved, as assessed by the children's parents and investigator, thus demonstrating tolerability and preliminary efficacy for the use of Cat-PAD in children.[60] Given the favorable safety profile, the efficacy of Cat-PAD was further evaluated in two phase II trials involving a larger cohort of cat-allergic patients.[61,62] Participants were randomized to a dosing regimen of either four intradermal injections of a 6 nmol dose every 4 weeks or eight intradermal injections of a 3 nmol dose every 2 weeks and underwent a 3-hour cat allergen challenge over four consecutive days in an EEC before, 18—22 weeks, and 50—54 weeks (primary endpoint) after the start of treatment.[61] After treatment, only the 6 nmol group exhibited a significant reduction in mean TRSS (primary endpoint) and mean nasal and ocular symptoms (secondary endpoints) compared with placebo at 50—54 weeks. Treatment-emergent AEs (TEAE) considered related to the study drug were reported at similar frequencies across all three groups (18.8%, 21.2%, and 26.9% for the placebo, 6 nmol, and 3 nmol group, respectively) with most being mild in severity.[61] A subsequent randomized, double-blind, placebo-controlled study evaluated the long-term treatment effect of Cat-PAD 2 years after treatment.[62] Following a 3-hour cat allergen challenge over four consecutive days in an EEC, only the 6 nmol group demonstrated a trending reduction in mean TRSS compared with placebo ($P = .13$). Very few AEs were reported with only two cases of bronchospasms unrelated to the study drug in the 6 nmol group.[62] Contrasting both phase II trials, a similar treatment effect was not observed in a recent multicenter, phase III field study of 1245 cat-allergic patients with severe allergy symptoms (mean TRSS $\geq$ 10) and a cat at home. Using two dosing regimens of four intradermal injections of 6 nmol or eight intradermal injections of 6 nmol, the study did not meet its primary endpoint, showing a comparable 58.2%—59.8% improvement in combined scores (sum of TRSS and rescue medication use score) across both treatment and placebo groups 1 year after the start of treatment.[63]

Using a method of in vitro identification and clinical workup similar to Cat-PAD, seven peptides representing immunodominant T cell epitopes from *D. pteronyssinus* were constructed and evaluated as a possible treatment for HDM allergy. Formulated as a 7-peptide vaccine, preliminary safety and efficacy were assessed using an escalating dosing regimen.[64] HDM-allergic patients were randomized to one of five cohorts. The first cohort received four intradermal injections of 0.03 nmol HDM-PAD every 4 weeks. Successive cohorts thereafter received four intradermal injections of 0.3, 1, 3, and 12 nmol, respectively. Two of the 10 participants in each cohort received placebo. Mirroring the Cat-PAD study, the 3 nmol group reported the lowest occurrence of TEAEs, the largest reduction (51.19%) in LPSR, and a significant reduction (36.7%) in CPT score compared with placebo 18—22 weeks after starting treatment.[64] TEAEs primarily included nausea, nasopharyngitis, influenza, and gastroenteritis. The efficacy of HDM-PAD was further evaluated during 4-hour HDM challenges held over three consecutive days in an EEC. When two intradermal 4-weekly dosing regimens of either four injections of 12 nmol (4 × 12 nmol) or 11 injections of 12 nmol (11 × 12 nmol) were compared, only the 4 × 12 nmol group demonstrated a significant reduction in mean TRSS compared with placebo 49—50 weeks after the start of treatment.[65] In the corresponding 2-year follow-up study of HDM-PAD, the 4 × 12 nmol dose regimen exhibited a greater reduction in mean symptom scores during the 4-hour HDM challenges compared with placebo.[66] These reductions were also comparable with those seen in a field setting (22.7% improvement in mean TRSS in the EEC vs. 35.8% improvement in mean TRSS in a field setting).[67] However, similar to Cat-PAD, the treatment effect of HDM-PAD observed at 1 year was not seen in a larger phase IIb field study of 714 HDM-allergic patients with severe allergy symptoms (mean TRSS $\geq$ 12). When three dosing regimens of 4×12 nmol, 4×20 nmol, and 8×12 nmol were compared, all three dosing regimens exhibited a 34.9%—44.3% reduction in combined scores from baseline. However, these differences were not significantly better than that seen with placebo, which resulted in a 39.1% reduction in combined scores.[68]

SPIREs have also been developed for common environmental aeroallergens including ragweed[69] and several grass species. Resembling previous SPIREs for cat and HDM, seven synthetic peptides 10—18 amino acids in length were derived from group 1 (Cyn d 1) and group 5 (Lol p 5, Dac g 5, Hol l 5, and Phl p 5) allergens that are cross-reactive to several grasses including Bermuda, canary, orchard, rye, timothy, velvet, and Kentucky bluegrass. In a recent randomized, double-blind, placebo-controlled study, the safety and efficacy of the seven grass allergen peptides (grass-SPIRE) were evaluated in 282 grass-allergic patients in the environmental exposure unit (EEU).[70] Patients were randomized to one of the three intradermal dosing regimens of eight biweekly injections of 6 nmol (8x6Q2W), eight biweekly injections of 12 nmol (8x12Q2W), or four 4-weekly injections of 12 nmol (4x12Q4W) with treatment ending prior to the start of grass pollen season. After the season (approximately 25 weeks after start of treatment), only the 8x6Q2W group demonstrated a significant improvement in mean TRSS during the posttreatment grass pollen challenges in the EEU (4-day 3-hour challenges) compared with placebo (42% improvement over placebo). The incidence of TEAEs considered related to the study drug was also lower in the 8x6Q2W group compared to the other two doses (29.6% vs. 36.6% and 37.1%) but higher than the placebo group (20.0%).[70] Treatment persistence of grass-SPIRE was further evaluated in two optional follow-up studies taking place after the second (approximately 1 year after treatment) and third (approximately 2 years after treatment) grass pollen season. Following 3-hour grass pollen challenges held over four consecutive days in the EEU, the 8x6Q2W group demonstrated a trending improvement in mean TRSS one ($P = .0535$) and two ($P = .113$) years after the start of treatment compared with placebo-treated patients.[71,72] Thus, a short-course regimen of grass-SPIRE is efficacious in reducing grass-allergic symptoms, with treatment persistence lasting up to 2 years from the first injection.

Only recently has peptide immunotherapy been evaluated as a possible treatment for food allergy. Using a combination of epitope HLA-restriction studies, antigen-specific T cell lines, and in vitro cell proliferation and activation assays, seven short peptides representing major T cell epitopes of Ara h 1 (major peanut allergen) were identified and constructed. Using PBMCs from peanut-allergic patients, these peptides were able to induce T cell proliferation without activating peanut-reactive basophils.[73] Ara h 1 T cell epitope—derived peptides were also evaluated in two separate mouse models of peanut allergy. One mouse model was transgenic for HLA-DRB1*0401. Compared with saline-treated mice, treatment with Ara h 1-derived peptides conferred significant protection against peanut-induced anaphylaxis.[74] The maximum dose of 100 μg of peptide provided the highest protection in a dose-dependent manner.[75] Thus, short synthetic peptides derived from major

T cell epitopes of food allergens represent a possible therapy for the treatment of food allergy. However, this is subjected to further evaluation.

Contiguous overlapping peptides

Contiguous overlapping peptides (COPs) serve as an alternative approach in developing synthetic T cell epitope—based peptides. Several COPs in combination encompass the entire allergen sequence with multiple overlapping regions to ensure the representation of all possible T cell epitopes. Compared to using HLA-restriction studies, COPs overcome the inherent selection bias present when selecting immunodominant T cell epitopes for SPIRE development.[76] They are also more likely to drive IgG antibody production compared with SPIREs.[58,77] Using this approach, COPs have been developed from major allergens of bee venom[78] and birch.

A set of three COPs spanning the entire 159-amino acid sequence of Bet v 1 was constructed.[79] When evaluated individually or in combination as an equimolar 3-peptide vaccine (AllerT), all three COPs exhibited undetectable binding to birch-allergic patients' IgE, a strong reduction in basophil activation, and failed to induce anaphylaxis following an intraperitoneal challenge in Bet v 1—sensitized mice compared with rBet v 1. Moreover, skin testing of birch-allergic patients with AllerT or component COPs did not yield a positive response even at the highest concentration (10 μM). Comparatively, 80% of patients experienced positive skin tests to a 1:10 dilution of rBet v 1 (0.1 μM), thus demonstrating a favorable safety profile.[79] The safety and immunogenicity of AllerT was further evaluated in a randomized, double-blind, placebo-controlled, parallel-group phase I/IIa trial.[80] The trial included 20 birch-allergic patients randomized 3:1 to a preseasonal dosing regimen of five subcutaneous injections delivered 15 minutes apart at increasing doses followed by maintenance dose (95 μg AllerT) injections on days 7, 14, 21, and 51 of AllerT or placebo. After the second birch pollen season (1 year after treatment), a fivefold increase in Bet v 1—specific IgG4 was observed in the AllerT group. This was significantly greater than placebo and persisted into the fourth birch pollen season (3 years after treatment). Changes in Bet v 1—specific IgE were unapparent in both groups throughout the study. The occurrence and severity of local AEs across both groups were comparable, with most being local pain and erythema at the injection site.[80]

Finally, in a subsequent phase IIb study including 239 birch-allergic patients, the efficacy of two doses of AllerT (50 and 100 μg) was evaluated.[81] Using a preseasonal dosing regimen of five subcutaneous injections delivered on days 1 (half-dose), 8, 15, 29, and 57 (all at full dose), the 50 μg group demonstrated a significant reduction in the combined daily rhinoconjunctivitis symptom and medication score (26% over placebo) during the birch pollen season compared with placebo.[81] A nonsignificant reduction was seen in the 100 μg group. After treatment, both doses led to significant increases in Bet v 1—specific IgG4 compared with placebo, which persisted throughout the birch pollen season. TEAEs were reported in 75% of the placebo group and 85%—90% of the AllerT groups with over half of each group reporting local injection site reactions (e.g., local pain, erythema, and swelling). A reduction in $FEV_1 \geq 30\%$ was also reported in 6.5% of AllerT-treated patients, often occurring more than 3 hours after the first or second injection. Only two serious AEs related to AllerT were reported, both resolved with rescue medication (e.g., epinephrine and inhaled β_2-agonists).[81]

Synthetic B cell epitope—derived peptides

The occurrence of late-phase allergic reactions (e.g., asthma) can be common with T cell epitope—based therapies such as SPIREs and COPs.[81,82] Likely due to activated allergen—specific T cells, synthetic peptides derived from B cell epitopes (i.e., IgE binding sites) offers a novel approach to reduce both immediate IgE- and late T cell—mediated AEs.[83] Due to their short length of approximately 20—40 amino acids, B cell epitope—derived peptides lack the proper structural folding required to cross-link IgE antibodies. They also exhibit reduced T cell activation due to the lack of major T cell epitopes. Based on the hapten-carrier principle, these peptides are rendered immunogenic by coupling to a nonallergenic carrier protein capable of providing carrier-specific T cell help and devoid of allergen-specific T cell epitopes.[84,85] Coupling can be achieved through chemical means or through the production of a recombinant fused protein containing both peptide and carrier protein. Tolerance via B cell epitope—derived peptides is thought to arise through the induction of allergen-specific IgG antibodies via carrier-specific T cell help.[83] To date, short B cell epitope—derived peptides have been constructed for major allergens from birch, cat, HDM, and grass.

Similar to recombinant hypoallergenic derivatives, the allergenicity of new B cell epitope—based peptides is often evaluated using in vitro cellular assays (e.g., IgE-binding and basophil activation tests) and in vivo immunization experiments. Six synthetic peptides 25 to 32 amino acids in length were derived from IgE-binding sites of Bet v 1 and chemically conjugated to keyhole limpet hemocyanin (KLH), an immunogenic carrier protein.[86] Using sera and PBMCs from birch-allergic patients, an equimolar mixture of all six peptides showed no IgE reactivity and a substantial reduction in histamine release compared with rBet v 1. Moreover, skin testing of birch-allergic patients with the peptides did not elicit immediate skin reactions at 100 µg/mL, compared with the skin reactions already seen with rBet v 1 at a concentration <0.78 µg/mL. IgG antibodies from peptide-immunized rabbits also blocked the binding of patients' IgE to rBet v 1 and strongly inhibited rBet v 1-induced basophil degranulation.[86] Similar findings were observed for two B cell epitope—based peptides derived from Der p 2 coupled to KLH. Alongside their reduced allergenicity, stimulation of PBMCs from HDM-allergic patients with Der p 2—derived peptides led to lower T cell proliferation compared with stimulation with rDer p 2.[87]

Alongside KLH, the PreS domain derived from hepatitis B virus (HBV) serves as an alternative immunogenic carrier protein. Similar to recombinant wild-type allergens, recombinant fusion proteins consisting of B cell epitope—derived peptides and the PreS domain can be expressed in bacterial cell cultures and purified in a reproducible and homogeneous manner with defined concentrations. This approach has been used to engineer fusion proteins consisting of the PreS domain and B cell epitope—based peptides derived from Fel d 1, Bet v 1, and Der p 23, a new major HDM allergen.[88-90] Similar to KLH-coupled peptides, these fusion proteins demonstrated a substantial reduction in *in vitro* IgE reactivity, basophil activation and histamine release, T cell proliferation, and induced IgG antibodies that inhibited the binding of allergic patients' IgE to sensitized allergens.[88-90]

One of the most extensively studied B cell epitope—based vaccines to date is BM32, a grass pollen allergy vaccine comprising an equimolar mixture of four recombinant fusion proteins. Each fusion protein contains the HBV-derived PreS domain fused to synthetic peptides derived from IgE-binding sites of four major timothy grass pollen allergens (Phl p 1, 2, 5, and 6).[91] During preliminary in vitro and in vivo assessments, BM32 and individual recombinant fusion proteins showed no detectable IgE reactivity, a strong reduction in basophil activation and lymphocyte proliferative responses compared with wild-type grass allergens, and induced anti-BM32 IgG rabbit antibodies that inhibited grass pollen-induced basophil activation from grass-allergic patients.[91] Both skin testing and atopy patch testing (APT) with BM32 did not induce any immediate or late-phase reactions in grass-allergic patients. In comparison, nearly all patients had positive skin testing reactions to grass pollen extract with 10% experiencing positive APT reactions to the same extract.[92] Given the clear reduction in the likelihood of both IgE- and T cell—mediated adverse reactions, a preliminary dose-finding phase IIa study was initiated to evaluate the safety and efficacy of BM32.[93] Using a dosing regimen of three subcutaneous injections administered 3—4 weeks apart, 71 grass-allergic patients were randomized to one of the three BM32 doses (10, 20, and 40 μg) or placebo. The preliminary endpoint was the change in total nasal symptom scores (TNSS) following a 6-hour grass pollen challenge in the Vienna Challenge Chamber before and after treatment. At 4 weeks following the last injection, only the 20 and 40 μg groups showed a significant reduction in TNSS (24% and 20%, respectively, from baseline) compared with placebo.[93] Treatment with BM32 led to a robust IgG antibody response to each of the four major timothy grass pollen allergens. When combined with patients' PBMCS, these antibodies strongly inhibited grass pollen—induced T cell proliferation when compared with antibodies from placebo-treated patients. The occurrence of reported injection site reactions, most of which were late phase, was also comparable between placebo (94.4%) and active treatment (94.4%—100% for all three doses) groups. The most common systemic treatment—associated AE was grade I AR affecting seven BM32-treated patients compared with none in the placebo group. Alongside allergen-specific IgG antibodies, treatment with BM32 also led to an increase in PreS-specific IgG antibodies.[93] BM32-induced PreS-specific IgG titers were significantly greater than titers reported in chronic HBV-infected patients, and strongly inhibited HBV infection of liver cells in vitro.[94]

In a subsequent randomized double-blind, placebo-controlled phase IIb study, the clinical efficacy of 2 years of treatment with BM32 was evaluated over two grass pollen seasons.[95] Grass-allergic patients were randomized to two doses of BM32 administered using a preseasonal dosing regimen of three subcutaneous injections (20 or 40 µg), a booster injection after the first pollen season, and another three subcutaneous injections at the 20 µg dose prior to the second pollen season. Compared to placebo, trending improvements in mean daily symptom medication scores during the pollen season were observed in the 20 µg group at year 1 and 2. Both doses of BM32-induced comparable titers of grass-specific IgG antibodies significantly reduced the elevated grass-specific IgE response seen during the grass pollen season compared to the placebo group. Similar to the phase IIa study, AEs were primarily late-phase local reactions which exhibited a higher frequency 1 year after treatment (88.7% and 86.7% in 20 and 40 µg groups, respectively) compared to year 2 (55.8% in BM32 pooled group). Systemic late-phase AEs were also more frequent in the active treatment groups compared with placebo (28.3% and 21.7% vs. 9.4%) in year 1 and were primarily graded as 1 or 2 in severity. After 2 years of treatment, the frequency of systemic AEs was comparable between active treatment and placebo groups, thus demonstrating the safety and tolerability of a 2-year treatment regimen with low- or high-dose BM32.[95]

Finally, a recent study compared the immunogenicity of BM32 to that of four registered natural allergen extract−based grass pollen allergy vaccines (Pollinex grasses + rye Quattro Plus, Alutard SQ grass mix, Allergovit grass, and Phostal grass + rye).[96] Following immunization of rabbits using dosing regimens recommended by the manufacturers, three subcutaneous injections of BM32 induced robust IgG antibody responses against Phl p 1, 5, and 6, which were comparable with the registered vaccines that required eight or more injections. Moreover, titers of Phl p 2−specific IgG antibodies were higher following vaccination with BM32 and demonstrated significantly greater inhibition of patients' IgE binding to rPhl p 2 compared with the registered vaccines (>80% inhibition vs. < 40% across all four vaccines).[96] Thus, treatment with BM32 may provide superior protection of allergic symptoms induced by group 2 timothy grass pollen allergens.

Summary and conclusion

Significant progress has been made in the field of AIT ever since its first use by Noon and Freeman for the treatment of grass pollen allergy in 1911.[1] The form of allergen used during AIT often impacts both the clinical efficacy and length of treatment required to induce adequate long-term tolerance. For traditional AIT, natural allergen extracts are chosen as they are directly purified from raw material and contain the relevant allergenic components responsible for the allergic symptoms. However, natural extracts are often heterogeneous and contain nonrelevant compounds inherent to the source material used. Thus, natural extract−based AIT can be variable in efficacy and be accompanied by relatively frequent immediate and late-phase allergic reactions due to intact IgE and T cell epitopes, respectively.

Genetically modified forms of native allergens have been developed to address the allergenicity inherent to natural allergen extracts. Preliminary modifications first focused on reducing the amount of reactive conformational IgE-binding epitopes present. These included modifying the conformation of various proteins in the extract itself (e.g., allergoids), isolating major IgE-reactive proteins (e.g., recombinant wild-type allergens), and modifying the specific amino acid sequences encoding major allergens (e.g., recombinant hypoallergenic derivatives). Eventually, synthetic peptides derived from immunodominant T cell epitopes were evaluated as a possible AIT treatment that completely lacked IgE reactivity (e.g., SPIREs and COPs). However, treatment with the aforementioned modified allergens still induced late-phase allergic reactions, likely mediated by the intact T cell epitopes originally preserved to retain immunogenicity of the treatment. B cell epitope—based peptides were later constructed as a safer alternative that exhibited reduced IgE- and T cell—mediated reactivity.

Together, these modifications have a unified purpose of reducing allergenicity and improving clinical efficacy. By lowering the occurrence of IgE- and T cell—mediated adverse reactions, higher doses of allergen can be administered to patients at one time, often leading to shorter dosing regimens with comparable potencies to that of their natural extract counterparts. To date, modified hypoallergenic derivatives have been developed and evaluated for many common environmental allergens, as well as for selected food allergens. AIT based on modified allergens represents a possible treatment for AR and perhaps allergic asthma.

References

1. Noon L. Prophylactic inoculation against hay fever. *Lancet*. 1911;177(4580):1572–1573.
2. Dhami S, Nurmatov U, Arasi S, et al. Allergen immunotherapy for allergic rhinoconjunctivitis: a systematic review and meta-analysis. *Allergy*. 2017;72(11):1597–1631.
3. Dhami S, Kakourou A, Asamoah F, et al. Allergen immunotherapy for allergic asthma: a systematic review and meta-analysis. *Allergy*. 2017;72(12):1825–1848.
4. Curin M, Garib V, Valenta R. Single recombinant and purified major allergens and peptides: how they are made and how they change allergy diagnosis and treatment. *Ann Allergy Asthma Immunol*. 2017;119(3):201–209.
5. Canonica GW, Bousquet J, Casale T, et al. Sub-lingual immunotherapy: world allergy organization position paper 2009. *Allergy*. 2009;64(Suppl 91):1–59.
6. Cox L, Nelson H, Lockey R, et al. Allergen immunotherapy: a practice parameter third update. *J Allergy Clin Immunol*. 2011;127(1 Suppl):S1–S55.
7. Tscheppe A, Breiteneder H. Recombinant allergens in structural biology, diagnosis, and immunotherapy. *Int Arch Allergy Immunol*. 2017;172(4):187–202.

8. Epstein TG, Calabria C, Cox LS, Dreborg S. Current evidence on safety and practical considerations for administration of sublingual allergen immunotherapy (SLIT) in the United States. *J Allergy Clin Immunol Pract.* 2017;5(1):34−40.e2.

9. Passalacqua G, Nowak-Wegrzyn A, Canonica GW. Local side effects of sublingual and oral immunotherapy. *J Allergy Clin Immunol Pract.* 2017;5(1):13−21.

10. Cox LS, Larenas Linnemann D, Nolte H, Weldon D, Finegold I, Nelson HS. Sublingual immunotherapy: a comprehensive review. *J Allergy Clin Immunol.* 2006;117(5): 1021−1035.

11. Epstein TG, Liss GM, Murphy-Berendts K, Bernstein DI. Risk factors for fatal and nonfatal reactions to subcutaneous immunotherapy: national surveillance study on allergen immunotherapy (2008−2013). *Ann Allergy Asthma Immunol.* 2016;116(4), 354−359.e2.

12. Rodríguez Del Río P, Vidal C, Just J, et al. The european survey on adverse systemic reactions in allergen immunotherapy (EASSI): a paediatric assessment. *Pediatr Allergy Immunol.* 2017;28(1):60−70.

13. Calderón MA, Vidal C, Rodríguez Del Río P, et al. European survey on adverse systemic reactions in allergen immunotherapy (EASSI): a real-life clinical assessment. *Allergy.* 2017;72(3):462−472.

14. Trivedi B, Valerio C, Slater JE. Endotoxin content of standardized allergen vaccines. *J Allergy Clin Immunol.* 2003;111(4):777−783.

15. Curin M, Reininger R, Swoboda I, Focke M, Valenta R, Spitzauer S. Skin prick test extracts for dog allergy diagnosis show considerable variations regarding the content of major and minor dog allergens. *Int Arch Allergy Immunol.* 2011;154(3):258−263.

16. Kespohl S, Maryska S, Zahradnik E, Sander I, Brüning T, Raulf-Heimsoth M. Biochemical and immunological analysis of mould skin prick test solution: current status of standardization. *Clin Exp Allergy.* 2013;43(11):1286−1296.

17. Focke M, Marth K, Flicker S, Valenta R. Heterogeneity of commercial timothy grass pollen extracts. *Clin Exp Allergy.* 2008;38(8):1400−1408.

18. Sander I, Fleischer C, Meurer U, Brüning T, Raulf-Heimsoth M. Allergen content of grass pollen preparations for skin prick testing and sublingual immunotherapy. *Allergy.* 2009;64(10):1486−1492.

19. Focke M, Marth K, Valenta R. Molecular composition and biological activity of commercial birch pollen allergen extracts. *Eur J Clin Investig.* 2009;39(5):429−436.

20. Brunetto B, Tinghino R, Braschi MC, Antonicelli L, Pini C, Iacovacci P. Characterization and comparison of commercially available mite extracts for in vivo diagnosis. *Allergy.* 2010;65(2):184−190.

21. Casset A, Mari A, Purohit A, et al. Varying allergen composition and content affects the in vivo allergenic activity of commercial Dermatophagoides pteronyssinus extracts. *Int Arch Allergy Immunol.* 2012;159(3):253−262.

22. van Ree R. Indoor allergens: relevance of major allergen measurements and standardization. *J Allergy Clin Immunol.* 2007;119(2):270−277. quiz 278-279.

23. Moreno Benítez F, Espinazo Romeu M, Letrán Camacho A, Mas S, García-Cózar FJ, Tabar AI. Variation in allergen content in sublingual allergen immunotherapy with house dust mites. *Allergy.* 2015;70(11):1413−1420.

24. Marth K, Focke-Tejkl M, Lupinek C, Valenta R, Niederberger V. Allergen peptides, recombinant allergens and hypoallergens for allergen-specific immunotherapy. *Curr Treat Options Allergy.* 2014;1(1):91−106.

25. Olivier CE. The use of allergoids and adjuvants in allergen immunotherapy. *Arch Asthma Allergy Immunol.* 2017;1(1):040−060.

26. Patel P, Holdich T, Fischer von Weikersthal-Drachenberg KJ, Huber B. Efficacy of a short course of specific immunotherapy in patients with allergic rhinoconjunctivitis to ragweed pollen. *J Allergy Clin Immunol.* 2014;133(1), 121−129.e1-2.

27. Pfaar O, Hohlfeld JM, Al-Kadah B, et al. Dose-response relationship of a new Timothy grass pollen allergoid in comparison with a 6-grass pollen allergoid. *Clin Exp Allergy.* 2017;47(11):1445−1455.

28. Pfaar O, Lang S, Pieper-Fürst U, et al. Ultra-short-course booster is effective in recurrent grass pollen-induced allergic rhinoconjunctivitis. *Allergy.* 2018;73(1):187−195.

29. Hüser C, Dieterich P, Singh J, et al. A 12-week DBPC dose-finding study with sublingual monomeric allergoid tablets in house dust mite-allergic patients. *Allergy.* 2017;72(1): 77−84.

30. Suphioglu C. What are the important allergens in grass pollen that are linked to human allergic disease? *Clin Exp Allergy.* 2000;30(10):1335−1341.

31. Jutel M, Jaeger L, Suck R, Meyer H, Fiebig H, Cromwell O. Allergen-specific immuno-therapy with recombinant grass pollen allergens. *J Allergy Clin Immunol.* 2005;116(3): 608−613.

32. Klimek L, Schendzielorz P, Pinol R, Pfaar O. Specific subcutaneous immunotherapy with recombinant grass pollen allergens: first randomized dose-ranging safety study. *Clin Exp Allergy.* 2012;42(6):936−945.

33. Pauli G, Larsen TH, Rak S, et al. Efficacy of recombinant birch pollen vaccine for the treatment of birch-allergic rhinoconjunctivitis. *J Allergy Clin Immunol.* 2008;122(5): 951−960.

34. Nony E, Bouley J, Le Mignon M, et al. Development and evaluation of a sublingual tablet based on recombinant Bet v 1 in birch pollen-allergic patients. *Allergy.* 2015; 70(7):795−804.

35. Kinaciyan T, Nagl B, Faustmann S, et al. Efficacy and safety of 4 months of sublingual immunotherapy with recombinant Mal d 1 and Bet v 1 in patients with birch pollen-related apple allergy. *J Allergy Clin Immunol.* 2018;141(3):1002−1008.

36. Senti G, Crameri R, Kuster D, et al. Intralymphatic immunotherapy for cat allergy in-duces tolerance after only 3 injections. *J Allergy Clin Immunol.* 2012;129(5): 1290−1296.

37. Niederberger V, Horak F, Vrtala S, et al. Vaccination with genetically engineered aller-gens prevents progression of allergic disease. *Proc Natl Acad Sci USA.* 2004;101(Suppl 2):14677−14682.

38. Reisinger J, Horak F, Pauli G, et al. Allergen-specific nasal IgG antibodies induced by vaccination with genetically modified allergens are associated with reduced nasal allergen sensitivity. *J Allergy Clin Immunol.* 2005;116(2):347−354.

39. Pree I, Reisinger J, Focke M, et al. Analysis of epitope-specific immune responses induced by vaccination with structurally folded and unfolded recombinant Bet v 1 allergen derivatives in man. *J Immunol.* 2007;179(8):5309−5316.

40. Purohit A, Niederberger V, Kronqvist M, et al. Clinical effects of immunotherapy with genetically modified recombinant birch pollen Bet v 1 derivatives. *Clin Exp Allergy.* 2008;38(9):1514−1525.

41. Campana R, Vrtala S, Maderegger B, et al. Hypoallergenic derivatives of the major birch pollen allergen Bet v 1 obtained by rational sequence reassembly. *J Allergy Clin Immu-nol.* 2010;126(5), 1024−1031, 1031.e1-8.

42. Curin M, Weber M, Thalhamer T, et al. Hypoallergenic derivatives of Fel d 1 obtained by rational reassembly for allergy vaccination and tolerance induction. *Clin Exp Allergy.* 2014;44(6):882–894.
43. Chen K-W, Blatt K, Thomas WR, et al. Hypoallergenic Der p 1/Der p 2 combination vaccines for immunotherapy of house dust mite allergy. *J Allergy Clin Immunol.* 2012; 130(2), 435–443.e4.
44. Linhart B, Focke-Tejkl M, Weber M, et al. Molecular evolution of hypoallergenic hybrid proteins for vaccination against grass pollen allergy. *J Immunol.* 2015;194(8): 4008–4018.
45. Swoboda I, Bugajska-Schretter A, Linhart B, et al. A recombinant hypoallergenic parvalbumin mutant for immunotherapy of IgE-mediated fish allergy. *J Immunol.* 2007; 178(10):6290–6296.
46. Zuidmeer-Jongejan L, Huber H, Swoboda I, et al. Development of a hypoallergenic recombinant parvalbumin for first-in-man subcutaneous immunotherapy of fish allergy. *Int Arch Allergy Immunol.* 2015;166(1):41–51.
47. Douladiris N, Linhart B, Swoboda I, et al. In vivo allergenic activity of a hypoallergenic mutant of the major fish allergen Cyp c 1 evaluated by means of skin testing. *J Allergy Clin Immunol.* 2015;136(2), 493–495.e8.
48. Freidl R, Gstoettner A, Baranyi U, et al. Blocking antibodies induced by immunization with a hypoallergenic parvalbumin mutant reduce allergic symptoms in a mouse model of fish allergy. *J Allergy Clin Immunol.* 2017;139(6):1897–1905.e1.
49. Bonura A, Passantino R, Costa MA, et al. Characterization of a Par j 1/Par j 2 mutant hybrid with reduced allergenicity for immunotherapy of parietaria allergy. *Clin Exp Allergy.* 2012;42(3):471–480.
50. Bonura A, Di Blasi D, Barletta B, et al. Modulating allergic response by engineering the major Parietaria allergens. *J Allergy Clin Immunol.* 2018;141(3):1142–1144.
51. Kahlert H, Suck R, Weber B, et al. Characterization of a hypoallergenic recombinant Bet v 1 variant as a candidate for allergen-specific immunotherapy. *IAA.* 2008;145(3):193–206.
52. Meyer W, Narkus A, Salapatek AM, Häfner D. Double-blind, placebo-controlled, dose-ranging study of new recombinant hypoallergenic Bet v 1 in an environmental exposure chamber. *Allergy.* 2013;68(6):724–731.
53. Klimek L, Bachert C, Lukat K-F, Pfaar O, Meyer H, Narkus A. Allergy immunotherapy with a hypoallergenic recombinant birch pollen allergen rBet v 1-FV in a randomized controlled trial. *Clin Transl Allergy.* 2015;5:28.
54. Treudler R, Franke A, Schmiedeknecht A, et al. BASALIT trial: double-blind placebo-controlled allergen immunotherapy with rBet v 1-FV in birch-related soya allergy. *Allergy.* 2017;72(8):1243–1253.
55. Norman PS, Ohman JL, Long AA, et al. Treatment of cat allergy with T-cell reactive peptides. *Am J Respir Crit Care Med.* 1996;154(6 Pt 1):1623–1628.
56. Creticos PS, Hebert J, Philip G, Group ARS. Efficacy of Allervax® ragweed peptides in the treatment of ragweed-induced allergy. *J Allergy Clin Immunol.* 1997;99:S401.
57. Creticos PS. Advances in synthetic peptide immuno-regulatory epitopes. *World Allergy Org J.* 2014;7:71.
58. O'Hehir RE, Prickett SR, Rolland JM. T cell epitope peptide therapy for allergic diseases. *Curr Allergy Asthma Rep.* 2016;16(2):14.
59. Worm M, Lee H-H, Kleine-Tebbe J, et al. Development and preliminary clinical evaluation of a peptide immunotherapy vaccine for cat allergy. *J Allergy Clin Immunol.* 2011; 127(1), 89–97, 97.e1-14.

60. Pawsey S, Hafner RP, Casale TB, et al. Safety, tolerability and efficacy of cat-peptide antigen desensitisation (Cat-PAD) in cat-allergic children — findings from a pilot study. *J Allergy Clin Immunol.* 2017;139(2):AB256.

61. Patel D, Couroux P, Hickey P, et al. Fel d 1-derived peptide antigen desensitization shows a persistent treatment effect 1 year after the start of dosing: a randomized, placebo-controlled study. *J Allergy Clin Immunol.* 2013;131(1), 103-109.e1-7.

62. Couroux P, Patel D, Armstrong K, Larché M, Hafner RP. Fel d 1-derived synthetic peptide immuno-regulatory epitopes show a long-term treatment effect in cat allergic subjects. *Clin Exp Allergy.* 2015;45(5):974–981.

63. *Circassia Announces Top-Line Results from Cat Allergy Phase III Study.* Press Releases [Internet]. Circassia. Available at: http://www.circassia.com/media/press-releases/circassia-announces-top-line-results-from-cat-allergy-phase-iii-study/.

64. Larche M, Hickey P, Hebert J, Hafner R. Safety and tolerability of escalating doses of house dust mite- peptide antigen desensitization (HDM-PAD). *J Allergy Clin Immunol.* 2013;131(2):AB37.

65. Hafner R, Couroux P, Armstrong K, Salapatek A, Patel D, Larche M. Persistent treatment effect achieved at one year after four doses of der p derived synthetic peptide immuno-regulatory epitopes in an exposure chamber model of house dust mite allergy. *J Allergy Clin Immunol.* 2014;133(2):AB289.

66. Hafner R, Salapatek A, Larché M, Ahenkorah B, Patel P, Pawsey S. Initial evidence of sustained efficacy of house dust mite synthetic peptide immuno regulatory epitopes 2 Years after a short course of treatment in house dust mite (HDM) allergic subjects. *J Allergy Clin Immunol.* 2015;135(2):AB142.

67. Hafner RP, Salapatek AM, Larche M, Ahenkorah B, Patel P, Pawsey S. Comparison of the treatment effect of house dust mite synthetic peptide immuno-regulatory epitopes in the environmental exposure chamber and field setting two years after a short course of treatment. *Allergy.* 2015;70(Suppl S101):A55.

68. *Circassia Announces Top-Line Results from House Dust Mite Allergy Field Study.* Press Releases [Internet]. Circassia. Available from: http://www.circassia.com/media/press-releases/circassia-announces-top-line-results-from-house-dust-mite-allergy-field-study/.

69. Hafner RP, Salapatek A, Patel D, Larché M, Laidler P. Validation of peptide immuno-therapy as a new approach in the treatment of allergic rhinoconjunctivitis: the clinical benefits of treatment with Amb a 1 derived T cell epitopes. *J Allergy Clin Immunol.* 2012;129(2):AB368.

70. Ellis AK, Frankish CW, O'Hehir RE, et al. Treatment with grass allergen peptides improves symptoms of grass pollen-induced allergic rhinoconjunctivitis. *J Allergy Clin Immunol.* 2017;140(2):486–496.

71. Ellis A, Frankish CW, Armstrong K, et al. Persistent treatment effect with grass synthetic peptide immuno-regulatory epitopes in grass allergy symptoms in an environmental exposure unit challenge after a second season of natural pollen exposure. *J Allergy Clin Immunol.* 2015;135(2):AB158.

72. Ellis A, Frankish C, Armstrong K, et al. Persistent treatment effect with grass synthetic peptide immuno-regulatory epitopes on grass allergy symptoms in the environmental exposure unit after a third season of natural exposure. *Allergy.* 2015;70(Suppl S101):A81.

73. Prickett SR, Voskamp AL, Phan T, et al. Ara h 1 CD4+ T cell epitope-based peptides: candidates for a peanut allergy therapeutic. *Clin Exp Allergy.* 2013;43(6):684–697.

74. Simms E, Rudulier C, Wattie J, et al. Ara h 1 peptide immunotherapy ameliorates peanut-induced anaphylaxis. *J Allergy Clin Immunol.* 2015;135(2):AB158.

75. Simms E, Wattie J, Waserman S, Jordana M, Larché M. Ara h 1 peptide immunotherapy protects against peanut-induced anaphylaxis in a dose-dependent manner. *J Allergy Clin Immunol*. 2016;137(2):AB410.
76. Valenta R, Campana R, Marth K, van Hage M. Allergen-specific immunotherapy: from therapeutic vaccines to prophylactic approaches. *J Intern Med*. 2012;272(2):144−157.
77. Prickett SR, Rolland JM, O'Hehir RE. Immunoregulatory T cell epitope peptides: the new frontier in allergy therapy. *Clin Exp Allergy*. 2015;45(6):1015−1026.
78. Fellrath J-M, Kettner A, Dufour N, et al. Allergen-specific T-cell tolerance induction with allergen-derived long synthetic peptides: results of a phase I trial. *J Allergy Clin Immunol*. 2003;111(4):854−861.
79. Pellaton C, Perrin Y, Boudousquié C, et al. Novel birch pollen specific immunotherapy formulation based on contiguous overlapping peptides. *Clin Transl Allergy*. 2013;3(1):17.
80. Spertini F, Perrin Y, Audran R, et al. Safety and immunogenicity of immunotherapy with Bet v 1-derived contiguous overlapping peptides. *J Allergy Clin Immunol*. 2014;134(1), 239−240.e13.
81. Spertini F, DellaCorte G, Kettner A, et al. Efficacy of 2 months of allergen-specific immunotherapy with Bet v 1-derived contiguous overlapping peptides in patients with allergic rhinoconjunctivitis: results of a phase IIb study. *J Allergy Clin Immunol*. 2016;138(1):162−168.
82. Haselden BM, Kay AB, Larché M. Immunoglobulin E-independent major histocompatibility complex-restricted T cell peptide epitope-induced late asthmatic reactions. *J Exp Med*. 1999;189(12):1885−1894.
83. Valenta R, Campana R, Niederberger V. Recombinant allergy vaccines based on allergen-derived B cell epitopes. *Immunol Lett*. 2017;189:19−26.
84. Katz DH, Paul WE, Goidl EA, Benacerraf B. Carrier function in anti-hapten immune responses. I. Enhancement of primary and secondary anti-hapten antibody responses by carrier preimmunization. *J Exp Med*. 1970;132(2):261−282.
85. Paul WE, Katz DH, Goidl EA, Benacerraf B. Carrier function in anti-hapten immune responses. II. Specific properties of carrier cells capable of enhancing anti-hapten antibody responses. *J Exp Med*. 1970;132(2):283−299.
86. Focke M, Linhart B, Hartl A, et al. Non-anaphylactic surface-exposed peptides of the major birch pollen allergen, Bet v 1, for preventive vaccination. *Clin Exp Allergy*. 2004;34(10):1525−1533.
87. Chen K-W, Focke-Tejkl M, Blatt K, et al. Carrier-bound nonallergenic Der p 2 peptides induce IgG antibodies blocking allergen-induced basophil activation in allergic patients. *Allergy*. 2012;67(5):609−621.
88. Niespodziana K, Focke-Tejkl M, Linhart B, et al. A hypoallergenic cat vaccine based on Fel d 1-derived peptides fused to hepatitis B PreS. *J Allergy Clin Immunol*. 2011;127(6), 1562−1570.e6.
89. Marth K, Breyer I, Focke-Tejkl M, et al. A nonallergenic birch pollen allergy vaccine consisting of hepatitis PreS-fused Bet v 1 peptides focuses blocking IgG toward IgE epitopes and shifts immune responses to a tolerogenic and Th1 phenotype. *J Immunol*. 2013;190(7):3068−3078.
90. Banerjee S, Weber M, Blatt K, et al. Conversion of Der p 23, a new major house dust mite allergen, into a hypoallergenic vaccine. *J Immunol*. 2014;192(10):4867−4875.

91. Focke-Tejkl M, Weber M, Niespodziana K, et al. Development and characterization of a recombinant, hypoallergenic, peptide-based vaccine for grass pollen allergy. *J Allergy Clin Immunol*. 2015;135(5), 1207-1207.e1-11.

92. Niederberger V, Marth K, Eckl-Dorna J, et al. Skin test evaluation of a novel peptide carrier-based vaccine, BM32, in grass pollen-allergic patients. *J Allergy Clin Immunol*. 2015;136(4), 1101–1103.e8.

93. Zieglmayer P, Focke-Tejkl M, Schmutz R, et al. Mechanisms, safety and efficacy of a B cell epitope-based vaccine for immunotherapy of grass pollen allergy. *EBioMedicine*. 2016;11:43–57.

94. Cornelius C, Schöneweis K, Georgi F, et al. Immunotherapy with the PreS-based grass pollen allergy vaccine BM32 induces antibody responses protecting against hepatitis B infection. *EBioMedicine*. 2016;11:58–67.

95. Niederberger V, Neubauer A, Gevaert P, et al. Safety and efficacy of immunotherapy with the recombinant B-cell epitope–based grass pollen vaccine BM32. *J Allergy Clin Immunol*. 2018;142(2):497–509.

96. Weber M, Niespodziana K, Linhart B, et al. Comparison of the immunogenicity of BM32, a recombinant hypoallergenic B cell epitope-based grass pollen allergy vaccine with allergen extract-based vaccines. *J Allergy Clin Immunol*. 2017;140(5), 1433–1436.e6.

Allergen immunomodulatories

Effect of immunomodulators on allergen immunotherapy

18

Lanny J. Rosenwasser, MD, Neha Patel, MD

Allergy/Immunology, Dept of Medicine, UMKC School of Medicine, KC, MO, United States

Over the last few decades, there has been a growing interest in the role of immunomodulators in a multitude of diseases and conditions. Specific therapies targeting atopic diseases at a molecular level is vastly expanding. Given the significant overlap among patients with asthma and allergic disease, it is likely that these patients may be on multiple immunomodulators at any given time. Our knowledge of the long-term implications of these therapies and interplay between them on the human body is still lacking. Here we discuss the current literature on the effect of immunomodulators on allergen immunotherapy.

Biological agents

Omalizumab

Omalizumab is a well-known humanized monoclonal anti-IgE antibody. It has efficacy in patients with moderate to severe asthma and allergic rhinitis. Mechanism of action involves downregulation of IgE receptors on basophils by binding to free IgE in the circulation.[1] Many patients with asthma and allergic rhinitis may benefit from immunotherapy to treat both conditions simultaneously. Immunotherapy schedules vary from the standard build-up phase to cluster and rush immunotherapy. As expected, rush immunotherapy carries a much greater risk of acute allergic reactions. Casale et al.[2] found that omalizumab pretreatment enhances the safety of rush immunotherapy and may allow more rapid and higher doses of allergen immunotherapy to be given with more efficacy. A subsequent study demonstrated that omalizumab increases the efficacy of allergen immunotherapy by directly blocking IgE binding to CD23[3] (Table 18.1).

A challenge model was used to evaluate the onset of action of omalizumab.[4] Patients with ragweed allergy were given nasal allergen challenge with ragweed, and then omalizumab or placebo followed by rechallenge with ragweed biweekly. They found that the mean IgE levels decreased by 96% ($P < .001$) from baseline within 3 days in the omalizumab group. There was also decreased FcεR1 receptor expression on basophils in the omalizumab group with a median decrease of 73% ($P < .001$) compared with the placebo group. All these changes occurred within

Immunotherapies for Allergic Disease. https://doi.org/10.1016/B978-0-323-54427-6.00018-3

Table 18.1 List of biological agents.

Biological agents	Mechanism of action
Omalizumab	Monoclonal antibody against IgE
Benralizumab	Anti-IL5
Dupilumab	Anti-IL4/IL-13
Pascolizumab	Anti-IL4
Pitrakinra	Anti-IL4
	Anti-TSLP
	Anti-IL33
Others	TNF inhibitor, anti-IL1, anti-IL6, anti-IL7, anti-IL2, anti-IL15, anti-IL23, anti-IL25

2 weeks. It is well documented that omalizumab inhibits the allergen-induced seasonal increases in circulating and tissue eosinophils by decreasing FcεR1 expression on antigen-presenting cells.[5]

The effect on omalizumab on immunotherapy is independent of the type of allergen as shown by its efficacy even in children with grass pollen allergy.[4] In patients with seasonal allergic rhinitis, omalizumab inhibits the allergen-induced seasonal increases in circulating and tissue eosinophils.[5] Omalizumab decreases FcεR1 expression on circulating dendritic cells, which might lead to a reduction in allergen presentation, TH2 cell activation and proliferation. The antiinflammatory effects of omalizumab at different sites of the allergic inflammation show its potential benefit in potentiating efficacy of allergen immunotherapy. These studies show that omalizumab has a role on increasing efficacy of immunotherapy as well as reducing side effects and allowing higher doses of allergen immunotherapy to be administered safely. Many patients with allergic rhinitis have coexisting asthma and, in some patients, poorly controlled asthma has been a limitation in being able to offer allergen immunotherapy safely to these patients. Omalizumab has also been shown to be beneficial in patients with allergic asthma, and it reduces the systemic allergic reactions in these patients allowing for higher doses of allergen immunotherapy to be reached.[6]

The benefits of omalizumab on immunotherapy are not only limited to environmental allergen immunotherapy. Pretreatment with omalizumab has also been shown to reduce side effect of venom immunotherapy especially in patients with underlying mastocytosis.[7] It also has shown efficacy in preventing anaphylaxis in these patients.[8]

Anti-IL-5 therapies

Allergic disease has been characterized as mainly Th2-cell mediated, and in recent years efforts have been made to alter these responses by blocking key cytokines such as IL-4 and IL-5.[8] These newer therapies have been shown to have significant reduction on eosinophil levels. Their effect in allergen immunotherapy is currently unclear. No direct head-to-head studies have been done comparing mepolizumab and reslizumab. The one distinguishing feature of mepolizumab over reslizumab is that mepolizumab has a confirmed oral corticosteroid-sparing effect with a halving of oral corticosteroid dose seen in the SIRIUS study.[9] Benralizumab has a similar steroid sparing effect.[10]

Mepolizumab

Mepolizumab is a neutralizing anti-IL-5 antibody. It was the first anti-IL-5 discovered. Studies have shown effectiveness in inhibiting eosinophilic inflammation induced by allergen as well as the increase in circulating eosinophilia in response to allergen challenge.[11] The MENSA trial enrolled 576 patients with eosinophilic inflammation and recurrent asthma exacerbations despite high doses of inhaled corticosteroids.[12] Patients were randomized to receive IV mepolizumab, subcutaneous mepolizumab, or placebo. The exacerbation rate was reduced by 47% in the IV group and 53% in the subcutaneous group. The mean increase from baseline FEV1 at the end of the study was 100 mL greater than placebo for IV mepolizumab and 98 mL greater for subcutaneous mepolizumab.

The SIRIUS study looked at 135 patients with severe eosinophilic asthma and showed that mepolizumab was associated with a reduction in glucocorticoid dose 2.39x greater than in the placebo group.[9] A large multicenter double-blind placebo-controlled trial enrolling 621 subjects with a history of severe recurrent asthma exacerbations and evidence of eosinophilic inflammation (DREAM Study) showed significantly reduced blood and sputum eosinophil counts in patients treated with IV mepolizumab compared with placebo.[13]

Benralizumab

Benralizumab is a humanized monoclonal antibody to IL-5Rα with enhanced antibody-dependent cell—mediated cytotoxicity.[14] It was formerly known as MEDI-56 and developed by Medimmune AstraZeneca, Gaithersburg, Maryland (USA).[15] It induces antigen-dependent cell cytotoxicity on both eosinophils and basophils.

The first multicenter open-label human study involved 44 subjects with mild asthma receiving a single IV dose of 0.03 mg/kg of benralizumab.[16] These patients were followed for 84 days and were noted to have a robust eosinopenia for at least 84 days in all subjects. There was a similar pattern noted in circulating basophils as well. Another study[17] showed that subcutaneous benralizumab reduced asthma exacerbations and improved lung function and asthma control. A phase IIa study has been reported in adult asthmatics to evaluate the safety and tolerability profiles of multiple doses of benralizumab administered subcutaneously within a few days of administration, and peripheral blood eosinophils were found to be substantially depleted.[14] IL-5 is implicated in disease states that are mediated by eosinophils and therefore may be a novel approach for the treatment of asthma and other allergic disorders; however, further studies are needed to evaluate this.

Reslizumab

Reslizumab (Cinqair) is an IgG4κ monoclonal antibody targeting circulating Il-5 with high affinity.[15] The initial pilot study of 32 patients showed the reslizumab was effective in reducing blood and sputum eosinophil counts.[18] Phase III trials showed significant improvement in FEV1 and asthma symptoms scores.[19] A phase II trial of patients with asthma and nasal polyposis showed significant improvement in asthma symptoms along with asthma control (p- = .012).[20] Cinqair is a second anti-IL-5 biological recently approved as add-on maintenance therapy in asthma. However, its IV administration may be a limiting factor in therapeutics.

Anti-IL-4 therapies

IL-4 was discovered in 1982 and is recognized as a key cytokine necessary to induce the differentiation of TH2 lymphocytes from naïve T cells.[21] Asthma has been recognized as a manifestation of Th2 inflammation and so became a target of investigation for anti-IL-4 therapy.

Dupilumab

Dupilumab has recently been shown to be beneficial in patients with atopic dermatitis and suggests that biologics targeting TH2 cytokines may also be effective across a range of allergic diseases.[22] It has efficacy in reducing skin inflammation.[23] It acts by blocking the signaling of IL-4 and IL-13. It is a fully humanized monoclonal antibody to IL-4Rα. It was initially approved as a treatment for atopic dermatitis and subsequently received approval for moderate to severe asthma. In a phase 2A study of 104 moderate to severe asthmatics, who were randomized to receive dupilumab or placebo, there was an 87% reduction in the proportion of dupilumab-treated subjects who experienced an asthma exacerbation during the 12-week intervention phase, which was the primary end point.[24] This study also showed that single asthma endotype responds well to anti-IL4Rα therapy. Although no studies have been done to date looking at the effect of dupilumab on allergen immunotherapy, its very narrow therapeutic target may limit its effect on the immune system as a whole.

Altrakincept

Altrakincept is a recombinant human IL-4 receptor antagonist. Preliminary studies in steroid-dependent asthmatics appeared promising; however, efficacy could not be demonstrated in phase III trials.[25,26]

Pascolizumab

Pascolizumab is a humanized monoclonal antibody targeting IL-4 that can inhibit upstream and downstream events associated with asthma, inducing TH2 cell activation and IgE production. Pascolizumab inhibited the response of human and monkey T cells to monkey IL-4 and effectively neutralized IL-4 bioactivity when tested against IL-4 responsive human cell lines.[27] However, it was shown to be ineffective in treating asthma.

Anti-IL-13 therapies

It was thought that the reason why anti-IL4 antagonists did not show efficacy was likely due to biological redundancy provided by IL-13. IL-4 and IL-13 are highly homologous to one another and share many signaling pathways. IL-4 is thought to signal primarily within the context of immunologic synapse, while IL-13 is responsible for more distant effects of allergic inflammation and may make IL-13 a more accessible therapeutic target.[21]

Lebrikizumab

Lebrikizumab is a humanized IgG4 monoclonal antibody that binds IL-13 and blocks its action. A large double-blind placebo-controlled trial of 219 subjects with uncontrolled asthma while on inhaled corticosteroids showed that lebrikizumab improved FEV1 across all treated patients compared with controls, although asthma symptom scores were not improved.[28] A phase 2 study of 212 subjects investigated the role of IL-13 and the effect of different doses of lebrikizumab in mild asthmatic patients not receiving inhaled corticosteroids. There were no meaningful changes in FEV1 between lebrikizumab and placebo-control groups.[29]

Tralokinumab

Tralokinumab is an anti-IL-13 humanized monoclonal antibody investigated in a phase II clinical trial of 194 subjects with moderate to severe asthma despite daily inhaled corticosteroid treatment. The primary end point of reduction in symptoms scores was not met.[30]

IMA-638 (Anrukinzumab) and IMA-028

IMA-638 and IMA-028 are humanized IgG1 monoclonal anti-IL13 antibodies. When tested in an allergen challenge model of asthma, IMA-638 was able to attenuate both the early- and late-phase allergic response at 14 days while IMA-028 showed only a nonsignificant improvement in the late-phase response. This study concluded that specifically blocking binding of IL-13 to IL-4Rα1 (IMA-638 action) rather than the IL-13Rα1 (IMA-028 action) may be more effective in preventing allergic responses after allergen challenge.[31]

Pitrakinra

The overlapping nature of IL-4 and IL-13 signaling pathways presents opportunities to inhibit the action of IL-4 and IL-13 simultaneously. Pitrakinra is a recombinant IL-4 and competitive antagonist of IL-4/IL-13 pathways. It was developed by Aerovance and binds to the IL-4Rα subunit.[32] It has reduced inflammation in animal models, and further studies are needed to characterize its role in allergic disease. A phase 2b study looked at the role of pitrakinra in patients with uncontrolled moderate to severe asthma.[33] Patients were randomized to either pitrakinra or placebo for 12 weeks, and the incidence of asthma exacerbations was measured. There was no statistically significant difference found overall; however, there was statistically significant efficacy in asthma patients with eosinophilia.

In an allergen challenge study, nebulized pitrakinra resulted in a decrease in the late-phase allergic response measured by FEV1.[34] In a larger study of 534 symptomatic moderate to severe adult asthmatics using corticosteroids, participants were randomized to inhaled pitrakinra or placebo. No therapeutic benefit was noted in the entire population treated with pitrakinra compared with placebo.[35] Further studies are needed, but this antiinflammatory action of pitrakinra suggests it may have some efficacy in allergen immunotherapy and potentially enhancing its efficacy. The observation that efficacy of pitrakinra is exquisitely sensitive to genetic polymorphisms within IL-4Ralpha suggests that detailed genetic studies may help identify patients that will benefit from this therapy.[21]

Anti-TSLP

TSLP (thymic stromal lymphopoietin) is an epithelial cell—derived cytokine that may be important in inhibiting allergic inflammation. AMG 157 is a human anti-TSLP monoclonal IgG2λ that binds to human TSLP and prevents receptor interaction. A double-blind placebo-controlled study assigned 31 patients with mild allergic asthma to receive 3 monthly doses of AMG 157 or placebo IV and conducted allergen challenges on days 42 and 84 to evaluate the effect of AMG 157 in reducing the maximum % decrease in FEV1.[36] Treatment with AMG 157 reduced allergen-induced bronchoconstriction and indexes of airway inflammation before and after allergen challenge. TSLP induces dendritic cell—mediated TH2- type allergic inflammation.[37] Given that allergic rhinitis is also pathologically characterized by TH2-type allergic inflammation, it may have a role in allergen immunotherapy. Further studies are needed to determine the clinical value of TSLP therapeutics.

Anti-IL31

IL-31 is a tissue signaling cytokine, the receptor of which is mainly found on nonimmune cells. An overabundance of IL-31 has been shown in patients with atopic disorders and therefore represents a promising drug target.[38] A small study did show that IL-31 was able to induce proinflammatory genes such as CCL-2 and granulocyte-colony stimulating factor.

Anti-IL-33

IL-33 has been shown to induce production of T helper 2 cytokines. A study[39] looked at anti-IL-33 antibody in airway inflammation in mice sensitized and challenged to ovalbumin. They found that treatment with anti-IL-33 reduced serum IgE secretions; the numbers of eosinophils and lymphocytes; and concentrations of IL-4, IL-5 and IL-13 in BAL fluid compared with controls. Its role in reducing allergen-induced lung eosinophilic inflammation may show promise in enhancing allergen immunotherapy.

Anti-IL-2 (Daclizumab)

Daclizumab monoclonal antibody against IL-2Rα acts to decrease T cell proliferation and Th2 cytokine production. It is FDA approved for the use in prophylaxis of renal allograft rejection.[40] A double-blind placebo-controlled trial in patients with moderate to severe asthma showed that administration of IV daclizumab every 2 weeks improved FEV1 and decreased peripheral blood eosinophils.[41] Further studies are needed to define its therapeutic role.

Immunomodulators

Multiple immunomodulators have been utilized in immune dysregulation with or without atopic disease. Although only anecdotal, there is no danger to continue allergen immunotherapy despite being on other immunosuppressive therapies. In addition, the circumstances of allergen immunotherapy in these patients have not been reported in any important series (Table 18.2).

A randomized, double-blind, placebo-controlled study looked at the role of methotrexate in steroid-dependent asthma.[42] After 24 weeks of treatment, they found that prednisolone dose was reduced significantly by a greater proportion in the methotrexate group compared with placebo (50% vs. 14%). The reduction was not sustained after the study treatment was stopped suggesting antiinflammatory effects may have a role in allergen-induced processes.

Table 18.2 List of immunomodulators.

Immunomodulators	Mechanism of action
Methotrexate	Antimetabolite
Azathioprine	Antimetabolite
Mycophenolate mofetil	Antimetabolite
6-MP	Antimetabolite
Plaquenil	Antiinflammatory
Gold	Antiinflammatory
Azulfidine	Antimetabolite
Telithromycin	Macrolide antibiotic
Penicillamine	Antiinflammatory
Rapamycin	Immune cyclic inhibitor
Cyclosporin	Immune cyclic inhibitor
Tacrolimus	Immune cyclic inhibitor
Tofacitinib	Kinase inhibitor

References

1. Holgate ST, Djukanovic R, Casale T, et al. Anti-immunoglobulin E treatment with Omalizumab in allergic diseases: an update on anti-inflammatory activity and clinical efficacy. *Clin Exp Allergy.* 2005;35(4):408–416.
2. Casale TB, Busse WW, Kline JN, et al. Omalizumab pretreatment decreases acute reactions after rush immunotherapy for ragweed-induced seasonal allergic rhinitis. *J Allergy Clin Immunol.* 2006;117(1):134–140.
3. Klunker S, Saggar LR, Seyfert-Margolis V, et al. Combination treatment with Omalizumab and rush immunotherapy for ragweed-induced allergic rhinitis: inhibition of IgE-facilitated allergen binding. *J Allergy Clin Immunol.* 2007;120(3):688–695.
4. Lin H, Boesel KM, Griffith DT, et al. Omalizumab rapidly decreases nasal allergic response and FcεRI on basophils. *J Allergy Clin Immunol.* 2004;113:297–302.
5. Holgate S, Casale T, Wenzel S, et al. The anti-inflammatory effects of omalizumab confirm the central role of IgE in allergic inflammation. *J Allergy Clin Immunol.* 2005;115(3):459–465.
6. Massanari M, Nelson H, Casale T, et al. Effect of pretreatment with omalizumab on the tolerability of specific immunotherapy in allergic asthma. *J Allergy Clin Immunol.* 2010;125(2):383–389.
7. Koutou-Fili K. High Omalizumab dose controls recurrent reactions to venom immunotherapy in indolent systemic mastocytosis. *Eur J Allergy Clin Immunol.* 2008;63(3):376–378.
8. Galera C, Soohum N, Zankar N, et al. Severe anaphylaxis to bee venom immunotherapy: efficacy of pretreatment and concurrent treatment with Omalizumab. *J Investig Allergol Clin Immunol.* 2009;19(3):225–229.
9. Bel EH, Wenzel SE, Thompson PJ, et al. Oral glucocorticoid-sparing effect of mepolizumab in eosinophilic asthma. *N Engl J Med.* 2014;371(13):1189–1197.
10. Nair P, Wenzel S, Rabe KF, et al. Oral glucocorticoid-sparing effect of Benralizumab in severe asthma. *N Engl J Med.* 2017;376:2448–2458.
11. Kotsimbos AT, Hamid Q. IL-5 and IL-5 receptor in asthma. *Mem Inst Oswaldo Cruz.* 1997;92:75–91.
12. Ortega HG, Liu MC, Pavord ID, et al. Mepolizumab treatment in patients with severe eosinophilic asthma. *N Engl J Med.* 2014;371(13):1198–1207.
13. Pavord ID, Korn S, Howarth P, et al. Mepolizumab for severe eosinophilic asthma (DREAM): a multicentre, double-blind, placebo-controlled trial. *Lancet.* 2012;380(9842):651–659.
14. Ghazi A, Trikha A, Calhoun WJ. Benralizumab–a humanized mAb to IL-5Rα with enhanced antibody-dependent cell-mediated cytotoxicity–a novel approach for the treatment of asthma. *Expert Opin Biol Ther.* 2012;12(1):113–118.
15. Menzella F, Lusuardi M, Galeone C, et al. The clinical profile of benralizumab in the management of severe eosinophilic asthma. *Ther Adv Respir Dis.* 2016;10(6):534–548.
16. Busse WW, Katial R, Gossage D, et al. Safety profile, pharmacokinetics, and biologic activity of MEDI-563, an anti–IL-5 receptor α antibody, in a phase I study of subjects with mild asthma. *JACI.* 2010;125(6):1237–1244.
17. Park H, Kim M, Imai N, et al. A phase 2a study of benralizumab for patients with eosinophilic asthma in South Korea and Japan. *Int Arch Allergy Immunol.* 2016;169:135–145.

18. Kips JC, O'connor BJ, Langley SJ, et al. Effect of SCH55700, a humanized anti-human interleukin-5 antibody, in severe persistent asthma: a pilot study. *Am J Respir Crit Care Med*. 2003;167(12):1655–1659.

19. Bjermer L, Lemiere C, Maspero J, et al. A randomized phase 3 study of the efficacy and safety of reslizumab in subjects with asthma with elevated eosinophils. *Eur Respir J*. 2014;44(Suppl 58):P299.

20. Gevaert P, Lang-Loidolt D, Lackner A, et al. Nasal IL-5 levels determine the response to anti–IL-5 treatment in patients with nasal polyps. *JACI*. 2006;118(5):1133–1141.

21. Kau AL, Korenblat PE. Anti-interleukin 4 and 13 for asthma treatment in the era of endotypes. *Curr Opin Allergy Clin Immunol*. 2014;14(6):570.

22. Beck LA, Thaçi D, Hamilton JD, et al. Dupilumab treatment in adults with moderate-to-severe atopic dermatitis. *NEJM*. 2014;371(2):130–139.

23. Hamilton J, Ungar B, Guttman-Yassky E. Drug evaluation review: dupilumab in atopic dermatitis. *Immunotherapy*. 2015;7(10).

24. Wenzel S, Ford L, Pearlman D, et al. Dupilumab in persistent asthma with elevated eosinophil levels. *NEJM*. 2013;368(26):2455–2466.

25. Borish LC, Nelson HS, Corren J, et al. Efficacy of soluble IL-4 receptor for the treatment of adults with asthma. *JACI*. 2001;107(6):963–970.

26. Akdis CA. Therapies for allergic inflammation: refining strategies to induce tolerance. *Nature*. 2012;18(5):736.

27. Hart TK, Blackburn MN, Brigham-Burke M, et al. Preclinical efficacy and safety of pascolizumab (SB 240683): a humanized anti-interleukin-4 antibody with therapeutic potential in asthma. *Clin Exp Immunol*. 2002;130(1):93–100.

28. Zeskind B. Lebrikizumab treatment in adults with asthma. *NEJM*. 2011;365(25):2432.

29. Noonan M, Korenblat P, Mosesova S, et al. Dose-ranging study of lebrikizumab in asthmatic patients not receiving inhaled steroids. *JACI*. 2013;132(3):567–574.

30. Piper E, Brightling C, Niven R, et al. A phase II placebo-controlled study of tralokinumab in moderate-to-severe asthma. *Eur Respir J*. 2013;41(2):330–338.

31. Gauvreau GM, Boulet LP, Cockcroft DW, et al. Effects of interleukin-13 blockade on allergen-induced airway responses in mild atopic asthma. *Am J Respir Crit Care Med*. 2011;183(8):1007–1014.

32. Antoniu SA. Pitrakinra, a dual IL-4/IL-13 antagonist for the potential treatment of asthma and eczema. *Curr Opin Investig Drugs*. 2010;11(11):1286–1294.

33. Otulana BA, Wenzel SE, Ind PW, et al. A phase 2b study of inhaled pitrakinra, an IL-4/IL-13 antagonist, successfully identified responder subpopulations of patients with uncontrolled asthma. In: *D101. Asthma Genetics*. American Thoracic Society; May 2011:A6179.

34. Wenzel S, Wilbraham D, Fuller R, et al. Effect of an interleukin-4 variant on late phase asthmatic response to allergen challenge in asthmatic patients: results of two phase 2a studies. *The Lancet*. 2007;370(9596):1422–1431.

35. Slager RE, Otulana BA, Hawkins GA, et al. IL-4 receptor polymorphisms predict reduction in asthma exacerbations during response to an anti–IL-4 receptor α antagonist. *JACI*. 2012;130(2):516–522.

36. Gauvreau GM, O'byrne PM, Boulet LP, et al. Effects of an anti-TSLP antibody on allergen-induced asthmatic responses. *NEJM*. 2014;370(22):2102–2110.

37. Miyata M, Hatsushika K, Ando T, et al. Mast cell regulation of epithelial TSLP expression plays an important role in the development of allergic rhinitis. *Eur J Immunol*. 2008;38(6):1487–1492.

38. Stott B, Lavender P, Lehmann S, et al. Human IL-31 is induced by IL-4 and promotes TH2-driven inflammation. *JACI*. 2013;132(2):446−454.

39. Liu X, Li M, Wu Y, et al. Anti-IL-33 antibody treatment inhibits airway inflammation in a murine model of allergic asthma. *Biochem Biophys Res Commun*. 2009;386(1): 181−185.

40. Long AA. Monoclonal antibodies and other biologic agents in the treatment of asthma. *MAbs*. 2009;1(3):237−246. Taylor & Francis.

41. Busse WW, Israel E, Nelson HS, et al. Daclizumab Asthma Study Group. Daclizumab improves asthma control in patients with moderate to severe persistent asthma: a randomized, controlled trial. *Am J Respir Crit Care Med*. 2008;178(10):1002−1008.

42. Shiner RJ, Nunn AJ, Chung KF, et al. Randomised, double-blind, placebo-controlled trial of methotrexate in steroid-dependent asthma. *Lancet*. 1990;336(8708):137−140.

Anti-IgE therapy

19

Brooke I. Polk, MD [1], Jeffrey R. Stokes, MD [2]

[1]*Assistant Professor, Pediatrics, Washington University, St Louis, MO, United States;* [2]*Professor, Pediatrics, Washington University in St. Louis School of Medicine, St. Louis, MO, United States*

Introduction

Pathophysiology of IgE in atopy

In 1967, Ishizaka and Johansson discovered immunoglobulin E (IgE).[1] IgE has since been established as a crucial mediator in T helper 2 (T_h2)-mediated atopic conditions including asthma, food allergy, allergic rhinitis, and atopic dermatitis (AD).[2,3] Plasma cells of individuals with atopic disease secrete IgE-binding antibodies directed against antigens generally considered harmless, and circulating IgE binds to high-affinity IgE-specific receptors (FcεRI) on basophils and mast cells at the Cε3 region.[4] Subsequent stimulation by the appropriate antigen to the bound IgE leads to cross-linking and receptor activation, resulting in mast cell degranulation and the release of inflammatory mediators including histamine, prostaglandins, and leukotrienes. IgE also promotes mast cell survival, enhances allergen presentation by dendritic cells (DCs), upregulates IgE receptors, and enhances the production of Th2 cytokines during the effector phase of the allergic response.[5,6]

Anti-IgE development

The concept of anti-IgE therapy as a treatment for atopic diseases was first postulated by Chang in 1987.[7] The ideal anti-IgE monoclonal antibody (mAb) should possess appropriate binding specificity to bind circulating IgE, yet not bind basophil or mast cell FcεRI-bound IgE so as to avoid receptor cross-linking and subsequent histamine release.[8,9]

Anti-IgE mAb development originated in two separate pharmaceutical groups. In one program, CGP51901, a chimeric IgG1 monoclonal antibody, and TNX-901, a humanized mAb from the same mouse antibody, demonstrated potential in phase I and II trials for allergic rhinitis and asthma.[10,11] Another group led development of rhuMab-E25, a humanized murine antibody produced in host Chinese hamster ovary (CHO) cells.[12] RhuMab-E25 was chosen for further development when the two programs merged in 1996, and it later became omalizumab.

Immunotherapies for Allergic Disease. https://doi.org/10.1016/B978-0-323-54427-6.00019-5

Omalizumab molecule and mechanism of action

Omalizumab is a humanized, recombinant, DNA-derived IgG1k mAb created via incorporation of the mouse-derived mAb MAE11 complementarity determining region (CDR) into human IgG1k, resulting in a 95% human product.[12] Omalizumab binds to IgE at the Cε3 domain (Fig. 19.1). This is the same site at which IgE binds to FcεRI, thus omalizumab is physically unable to bind to FcεRI-bound IgE and therefore cannot trigger effector cell degranulation. The typical omalizumab-IgE complex is a trimer of two omalizumab molecules per IgE antibody. This omalizumab-IgE immune complex is soluble and is efficiently cleared by the hepatic reticuloendothelial system, though at a lower rate than free IgE.[13] Although free serum IgE is rapidly depleted by almost 99% within 2 hours of omalizumab administration,[2] a rise in total serum IgE is often seen after the initial dose due to slow omalizumab-IgE complex clearance.

As free IgE decreases,[2,14] FcεRI expression on multiple cell types including mast cells, basophils, DCs, and monocytes is significantly reduced.[15–17] Omalizumab reduces expression of FcεRI on basophils within 7 days and basophil responsiveness is reduced by 90% within 3 months.[15] This implies that omalizumab affects not only the early phase of the allergic response, but allergic sensitization as well.

In the case of chronic urticaria (CIU/CSU), a nonatopic condition, the exact mechanism of action of omalizumab is unclear. One hypothesized mechanism involves reduced mast cell survival due to IgE depletion.[18] Other possible mechanisms include a reduction in mast cell sensitivity, improved basophil receptor function, and blockade of IgE directed against a yet-unrecognized antigen, possibly an autoantigen.[19]

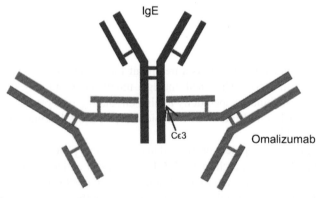

FIGURE 19.1

Omalizumab binding site. Omalizumab binds to the Cε3 region of IgE, most commonly in a trimer of two omalizumab molecules to one IgE molecule.

Anti-IgE therapy in specific diseases
Asthma

IgE plays a pivotal role in the pathogenesis of allergic asthma, and several studies have demonstrated the efficacy and safety of omalizumab therapy for individuals with moderate to severe persistent asthma. An initial phase II study evaluated the effect of two doses (5.8 vs. 2.5 mcg/kg per 1 ng of IgE) of rhuMab-25 (omalizumab) versus placebo in 317 individuals aged 11−50 years with moderate to severe perennial allergic asthma with a baseline oral or inhaled corticosteroid (ICS) requirement.[20] Mean asthma symptom scores were lower in both treatment groups; in addition, both treatment groups were able to decrease or even discontinue inhaled and/or corticosteroid use. Three subsequent phase III trials evaluated 1405 total subjects with a baseline ICS requirement.[21−23] Two studies included symptomatic adolescents and adults, and the third evaluated well-controlled pediatric patients aged 6−12 years. In each study, individuals in the treatment group received omalizumab dosed at 0.016 mg/kg/IgE (IU/mL) subcutaneously with doses ranging from 150 to 375 mg every 2 to 4 weeks. The ICS dose remained stable for 16 weeks followed by an 8-week tapering period to the lowest effective dose, which was maintained for the final 4 weeks of the study. In each study, omalizumab therapy led to lower ICS dose, fewer asthma symptoms, decreased rescue inhaler utilization, and improved quality of life. Omalizumab was well-tolerated, with no serious adverse events noted. These results contributed to omalizumab's approval in 2003 by the United States Federal Drug Agency (FDA) for individuals aged 12 years and above with uncontrolled moderate to severe perennial allergic asthma.[24]

Numerous studies followed to determine characteristics of individuals most likely to benefit from omalizumab. A metaanalysis of all three phase III trials evaluated a subgroup of 254 patients with "high-risk" asthma, defined as an emergency room visit or hospitalization in the preceding year or ever requiring intubation.[25] The authors concluded that omalizumab improved symptom scores, lung function, and quality of life. In addition, omalizumab reduced asthma exacerbations by 56% in this population. It was concluded that treating five patients with omalizumab was needed to keep one patient free of an exacerbation during the 28-week study period. Pooled analysis of the two adolescent/adult phase III trials concluded that emergency asthma treatment in the preceding year was the strongest predictor of response; high baseline ICS dose and a low FEV1 were also prognostic.[26] In a T_h2 biomarker subgroup analysis of 848 adults and adolescents with severe, uncontrolled asthma enrolled in the 48-week EXTRA study, patients with elevated periostin (>50 ng/mL), exhaled nitric oxide (F_{ENO}, >19.5 ppb), and/or blood eosinophils (>260/mcL) experienced a greater reduction in protocol-derived exacerbations than those with low biomarkers.[27] The relationship between elevated blood eosinophils (>300/mcL) and successive improvement on omalizumab was reproduced in a 24-week postmarketing analysis of adolescents and adults and in a subsequent subgroup analysis of phase III trials.[28,29]

A 24-week open-label extension of a previous phase III pediatric trial [27] of 334 subjects demonstrated a continued ICS-sparing effect and 55% of children did not experience an exacerbation.[30] A reduction in F_{ENO} was also seen, despite the significant reduction in ICS dosing.[31] A pivotal 52-week randomized, double-blinded placebo controlled trial (RDBPCT) studied 627 children aged 6 to <12 years with moderate to severe persistent perennial allergic asthma with frequent or severe exacerbations and inadequately controlled symptoms despite at least medium dose ICSs.[32] Omalizumab significantly reduced exacerbations by 43% in this population. Similar results were obtained in 419 adolescent and pediatric patients with persistent asthma by the Inner-City Asthma Consortium (ICAC). It was noted that fall seasonal peaks of asthma exacerbations were nearly eliminated.[33] This led to the ICAC Preventative Omalizumab or Step-Up Therapy for Fall Exacerbations (PROSE) study, which showed that omalizumab, compared with placebo, significantly decreased fall exacerbation rates in inner-city children with asthma.[34] Omalizumab was also superior to an increase in inhaled steroid therapy for a subgroup of children who had experienced an exacerbation in the run-in period; this subgroup was characterized by elevated peripheral eosinophil counts (280/uL) and F_{ENO} (29 ppb) versus those who did have an exacerbation in the run-in period, indicating higher baseline levels of T_H2 inflammation. Overall, the results from studies in children aged 6 to <12 years were consistent with adolescent and adult studies, and omalizumab was consequently FDA-approved for moderate to severe persistent perennial allergic asthma in children aged 6 to <12 years in 2016.

Multiple prospective, open-label, "real-world" studies have shown continued efficacy and safety with prolonged use of omalizumab in both children and adults,[35–38] with evidence for reduced asthma symptoms, emergency room visits, and improved pulmonary function testing and quality of life (Table 19.1). Studies examining patients on baseline oral corticosteroids (OCSs) treated with omalizumab noted a steroid-sparing potential,[39,40] and a 2017 metaanalysis demonstrated omalizumab's effectiveness in reducing both inhaled and OCS utilization when used as an add-on therapy.[38] Interestingly, omalizumab was shown to be effective for individuals with weight or total IgE above the recommended dosing criteria in one

Table 19.1 Benefits of omalizumab in the treatment of perennial allergic asthma.

Decreased asthma symptoms
Decreased inhaled and oral corticosteroid use
Decreased need for rescue inhaler use
Improved quality of life
Improved lung function (FEV1)
Reduced asthma exacerbations

Australian study (IgE >1500).[41] In regard to other outliers, case series show that omalizumab may be effective for those with allergic asthma with total IgE less than 30 kU/L,[42] or even in individuals with severe, nonallergic asthma.[43,44]

There are no solidified recommendations regarding the duration of omalizumab therapy for individuals with asthma, though recent data show some persistence of therapy after withdrawal. The XPORT (Evaluating the Xolair Persistency of Response After Long-Term Therapy) study, a large RDBPCT, studied the results of 12 months of omalizumab continuation versus withdrawal (placebo injections) in 176 individuals with moderate to severe allergic asthma who had received the drug for at least 5 years.[45] The primary outcome was an exacerbation requiring systemic steroids or an emergency room visit. Significantly, less individuals in the continuation group experienced a protocol-defined exacerbation 67% (OR 0.44, 0.23–0.82). Of subjects in the discontinuation group, 47.7% also had no exacerbation. Another open, prospective, "real-life" trial from the Spanish Omalizumab Registry evaluated the persistence and degree of response to omalizumab after withdrawal in subjects who had received omalizumab for 6 years.[46] Of the 49 individuals stopping therapy, 12 experienced an asthma exacerbation requiring corticosteroids within 12 months, and an additional 7 patients relapsed by 48 months. The authors concluded that the effect of 6 years of omalizumab therapy persists after discontinuation in 60% of individuals for at least 4 years.

Chronic urticaria

Chronic idiopathic urticaria/chronic spontaneous urticaria (CIU/CSU) is the only additional condition for which omalizumab is approved by the FDA. The initial case report in 2007 showed that three patients receiving omalizumab for asthma had a coincidental reduction in symptomatic CIU/CSU,[47] leading to a proof of concept study that demonstrated benefit of omalizumab.[48] The ensuing phase II trial in 90 patients with symptomatic CIU despite oral antihistamines demonstrated that the addition of omalizumab reduced itch and urticarial lesions.[49] Subsequently, three pivotal phase III RDBPCTs evaluated a combined 975 individuals aged 12–75 years with physician-diagnosed chronic idiopathic urticaria with elevated urticaria activity score (UAS7) despite use of antihistamines.[50–52] The ASTERIA I (n = 318)[50] and II (n = 322)[51] trials included patients on standard-licensed doses of anti-H1 histamines. Patients were randomized and treated with placebo, 75, 150, or 300 mg omalizumab. The 150 and 300 mg doses led to reduced itch severity score (ISS), with the 300 mg dose being most effective. Inclusion in the GLACIAL trial (n = 335)[52] necessitated failure of "standard combination therapy," consisting of up to four times the approved anti-H1 dose, plus anti-H2, leukotriene receptor antagonists, or a combination thereof, intended to reflect a "real-world" scenario. Patients were randomized and treated with placebo versus 300 mg omalizumab every 4 weeks for 24 weeks. Omalizumab significantly improved ISS and urticaria activity score, with a significant amount of treatment subjects itch-free. As a result, the FDA-approved omalizumab at a dose of either 300 mg or 150 mg every 4 weeks, for individuals aged 12 years and above with refractory chronic urticaria not well-controlled by antihistamine therapy.

A subsequent analysis evaluated response patterns in all three phase III omalizumab trials, demonstrating that improvement was achievable in approximately 60% of patients by week 12, with median time to reach partial and full response of 6 and 12 weeks, respectively.[53] A small group of patients responded after a single dose, though this was not the norm. Experts suggest discontinuing omalizumab if there is no response following a 3-month (12 weeks) trial of 300 mg every 4 weeks.[54] Although initial data reported that baseline serum IgE was not predictive of omalizumab response, later analyses suggest that perhaps those with the lowest IgE may be least likely to respond to therapy.[55]

The Xolair Treatment Efficacy of Longer Duration in Chronic Idiopathic Urticaria (XTEND-CIU) study is an ongoing phase IV multicenter RDBPCT evaluating 206 patients aged 12–75 years with CIU/CSU with frequent symptoms evident by elevated UAS7, with the goal of determining the efficacy of prolonged omalizumab administration and effects of therapy following treatment cessation.[56] All patients received omalizumab 300 mg every 4 weeks for 24 weeks; after this period, subjects were stratified into "responders" (UAS7 $\leq$ 6) and "nonresponders" (UAS7 > 6). After 24 weeks of omalizumab, 65% of subjects were categorized as responders. Weaning the dose and/or interval has been successful, with a suggestion to wean slowly and to withhold therapy and reevaluate once a patient has reached a dose of 150 mg every 8 weeks.[57] In a recent observational study, CSU patients with initial baseline total IgE >100 were more likely to relapse quickly after stopping omalizumab, with no association between initial IgE and response to therapy.[58] In those who initially respond yet experience relapse in urticaria symptoms following discontinuation of therapy, restarting therapy is safe and effective.[59]

Allergic rhinitis

Omalizumab decreases rhinitis symptoms and improves quality of life in individuals with both seasonal and perennial allergic rhinitis. At a dose of 300 mg every 3 to 4 weeks, omalizumab reduced nasal symptom scores and days missed from work/school and improved quality of life compared with placebo in patients aged 12–75 years with ragweed allergy when dosed pre- and coseasonally.[60] Subjects were later recruited to receive omalizumab for a subsequent ragweed season, and the therapy was well-tolerated.[61] Similar success was demonstrated in 251 birch-allergic subjects randomized to 300 mg omalizumab versus placebo coseasonally.[62] Subjects with moderate to severe perennial allergic rhinitis randomized to omalizumab compared with placebo also experienced significantly lower nasal symptom scores and rescue antihistamine use.[63] In 405 adolescents and adults with moderate to severe persistent asthma and concomitant persistent allergic rhinitis, omalizumab improved quality of life and symptom scores for both diseases.[64] A metaanalysis of

11 studies with 2870 patients confirmed the efficacy of omalizumab in allergic rhinitis via improved symptom relief, quality of life, and decreased rescue medication use.[65]

Due to the potential added benefit of anti-IgE therapy to the mechanism of reduced T_H2 allergic responses achieved with immunotherapy, omalizumab has been used in conjunction with allergen immunotherapy (AIT). The decrease in IgE and the downregulation of FcεRI receptors on immune effector cells afforded by omalizumab may boost the immune tolerance to allergens provided by AIT. The addition of omalizumab improved the efficacy of aeroallergen immunotherapy and allowed individuals with severe or uncontrolled asthma to receive AIT.[66–68] In 221 children with allergic rhinoconjunctivitis, the combination of coseasonal omalizumab with either birch or grass AIT was clinically superior to either treatment alone.[67] A 9-week pretreatment course of omalizumab also augmented the efficacy of rush AIT to ragweed in 123 ragweed-allergic adults.[69] In addition, a fivefold decrease in anaphylaxis due to AIT was observed in the ragweed rush IT study. In 248 patients with allergic asthma, omalizumab halved systemic reactions to perennial allergen cluster immunotherapy.[70] The downregulation of the FcεRI receptor may be the protective factor versus systemic reactions to AIT.

Food allergy

Food allergies affect about 6% of children and 2% of adults, with 1.5 million people in the United States allergic to peanut.[71] Initial evaluation of the effects of anti-IgE therapy on food allergy were performed with the anti-IgE mAb TNX-901. In a phase II trial, high-dose treatment improved peanut tolerance in individuals with IgE-mediated peanut hypersensitivity from 178 mg (0.5 peanuts) to 2805 mg (9 peanuts).[71] It was noted that 25% of patients had no improvement. In a small phase II study of peanut-allergic individuals, 24 weeks of omalizumab increased tolerability to 1000 mg peanut flour in four of nine (44.4%) treated subjects. The change was not statistically significant, and the study terminated early due to two severe anaphylactic reactions on initial challenge.[72]

Recent focus has shifted to the addition of omalizumab to food oral immunotherapy (OIT). Although food OIT has shown some success in desensitization to peanut, egg, and milk,[73] frequent systemic reactions complicate effective administration, and as many as 30% of patients fail to become desensitized with therapy.[74] Food OIT is generally performed by administering incremental doses of the food in three phases: initial dose escalation, multiple months of buildup, and months to years of maintenance therapy.[75] Those who do become desensitized to the maintenance dose often fail to reach the target threshold dose on subsequent oral challenge.[76] Conceivably, the immunomodulatory role of omalizumab could be of benefit in augmenting the desired desensitization effects of food OIT.

The first study to evaluate omalizumab plus OIT was performed in 11 milk-allergic subjects, 9 of whom quickly reached the target 2000 mg maintenance dose and passed double-blind placebo-controlled food challenge (DBPCFC) equivalent to 220 mL cow's milk.[77] A subsequent DBPCT assessed the efficacy and safety of omalizumab plus milk OIT in 57 milk-allergic patients. Omalizumab, when dosed 18 weeks prior to starting open-label milk OIT, did not significantly increase the ability to tolerate a 10 g milk challenge at the end of therapy, though adverse reactions were decreased and the time to reach maintenance dosing was lessened.[78]

Omalizumab has been utilized as an adjuvant to OIT in high-risk peanut-allergic patients. In an open-label pilot study, 13 children aged 8−16 years with severe peanut allergy were treated with 12 weeks of omalizumab before undergoing initial dose escalation, followed by 8 weeks of up-dosing to 4000 mg peanut flour (13−16 peanuts), at which time omalizumab was stopped and the 4000 mg dose was continued.[79] All 12 (one drop-out during build-up) patients passed an 8000 mg peanut flour DBPCFC (26−32 peanuts) after 12 weeks off omalizumab. Notably, no severe reactions to OIT occurred while on omalizumab. An RDBPCT published in 2017 confirmed that 12 weeks of pretreatment with omalizumab, with continued administration during initial dose escalation and up-dosing of peanut OIT to 2000 mg, facilitated rapid OIT up-dosing in as little as 8 weeks,[80] compared with the 41−44 week up-dosing reported in studies utilizing OIT alone.[81] Overall, omalizumab seems to provide key benefits in addition to OIT including faster up-dosing, higher initial tolerated dose, and protection from systemic reactions, though no study has yet evaluated the effect of omalizumab on sustained unresponsiveness from OIT.

Other diseases

Data on the efficacy of omalizumab in other diseases (Table 19.2) is limited to case studies and small clinical trials. In AD, studies have yielded conflicting results. In a small, open case series of seven children with severe AD with mean IgE 16,007 kU/L, 12 months of omalizumab (dosed per manufacturer's guidelines for asthma) significantly improved dermatitis symptoms.[82] Though a similar positive effect has been noted in case studies,[83] findings have not been reproduced by placebo-controlled trials, despite the expected decrease in serum IgE and FcεRI expression. Interestingly, patients with severe, refractory AD treated with omalizumab in a small RDBPCT (n = 4) also developed lower levels of thymic stromal lymphoprotein (TSLP), thymus and activation-regulated chemokine (TARC), and OX40-ligand (OX40L) versus placebo (n = 4), though clinical improvement was comparable between the two groups.[84] A recent systematic review and metaanalysis of 13 studies with 103 patients concluded that less than half (43%) of patients with refractory AD respond to omalizumab, suggesting that anti-IgE therapy may be appropriate for a subset of patients with AD, such as those without a filaggrin mutation.[85,86] Omalizumab has also demonstrated success in the management of the AD-like dermatologic manifestations of a patient with likely autosomal-dominant hyper IgE syndrome.[87]

As allergic bronchopulmonary aspergillosis (ABPA) is an IgE-driven disease process, a series of case reports have evaluated the efficacy of omalizumab in

Table 19.2 Indications for omalizumab.

Strong evidence
Allergic asthma, perennial, moderate to severe
Chronic idiopathic urticaria
Good evidence
Allergic rhinitis
Food allergy (as an adjunct to oral immunotherapy)
Nonallergic asthma
Fair evidence
Atopic dermatitis
Bullous pemphigoid
Eosinophilic granulomatosis with polyangiitis
Poor/limited evidence
Allergic bronchopulmonary aspergillosis
Eosinophilic gastrointestinal disorders
Food allergy (as solo therapy)

ABPA treatment. One review summarized eight case reports of ABPA in children with cystic fibrosis and asthma, concluding that omalizumab improved FEV1, respiratory symptoms, and systemic corticosteroid requirement.[88] This was the only trial that met criteria for a 2013 Cochrane review,[89] thus a lack of evidence was concluded.

Case reports and small studies have also demonstrated the efficacy of omalizumab in systemic mastocytosis,[90,91] eosinophilic granulomatosis with polyangiitis (EGPA, formerly termed Churg-Strauss),[92] exercise-induced anaphylaxis,[93] bullous pemphigoid,[94,95] and chronic eosinophilic pneumonia.[96] Omalizumab has demonstrated only limited benefit in eosinophilic gastrointestinal diseases.

Practical matters
Dosing

The only commercially available anti-IgE therapy is omalizumab (Xolair®, Genentech/Novartis), a lyophilized, sterile powder in a single-use 150 mg vial (75 mg vials also available in Europe and other countries) given via subcutaneous injection. Recommended dosing for allergic asthma is a minimum of 0.016 mg/kg per IU of IgE every 4 weeks, at either 2- or 4-week intervals, per a dosing chart included in the packaging insert.[97] Although some doses in the insert may be significantly higher than the recommended minimum dose, the manufacturer recommends utilizing the chart for optimal dosing.[98] In CIU, omalizumab is dosed at either 300 mg or 150 mg every 4 weeks, regardless of total IgE level or patient weight.

Cost

As with other biologics, omalizumab comes with a substantial monetary cost. With an average wholesale price of $541 per vial, the monthly cost ranges from $541 to $2706.[99] A study out of Brazil concluded that omalizumab is cost-effective versus standard therapy for severe asthmatics,[100] while a recent Canadian matched-cohort study found an increase in healthcare costs of $1796 per person ($P < .001$) in omalizumab users, without a significant change in asthma-related hospitalizations or emergency room visits.[101] In a specific subset of severe asthmatics with frequent emergency visits and/or hospitalizations, omalizumab is likely cost-effective.[102]

Safety outcomes

A multitude of studies have shown that omalizumab is well-tolerated with few adverse drug events (ADEs). Commonly reported reactions include local injection site pain or erythema, viral URI symptoms, headaches, and pharyngitis, generally similar to that of placebo in randomized trials.[103,104] Unlike other biotherapeutic agents, there are no reports of development of demonstrable anti-omalizumab antibodies in individuals receiving prolonged therapy.[103] Other rare yet noted ADEs in post-marketing evaluations include thrombocytopenia and transient self-reported hair loss.[105]

Omalizumab administration is associated with a small (0.1%–0.2%) risk of anaphylaxis, and the package insert includes a black box warning.[106,107] The majority of anaphylaxis episodes occur within a 2-hours window of one of the first three doses.[107] Consequently, in addition to an epinephrine autoinjector prescription, the American Academy of Allergy, Asthma, and Immunology/American College of Allergy, Asthma, and Immunology Joint Task Force (JTF) recommends that omalizumab be administered in a healthcare setting with an observed waiting period of 2 hours following the first three injections followed by a 30-minutes observation period with subsequent injections.[106] The exact pathophysiology of omalizumab-induced anaphylaxis is unclear, yet it does not appear to be an IgE-mediated process; a proposed mechanism is a reaction to the excipient polysorbate.[108,109] Individuals with prior history of anaphylaxis unrelated to omalizumab appear to be at higher risk of omalizumab-induced anaphylaxis.[108] The FDA-approved package insert of Xolair infers that all patients be prescribed an epinephrine autoinjector. However, Cox, the chair of the AAAAI/ACAAI Joint Task Force that develops the safety guidelines, does not believe the very low risk of anaphylaxis warrants the prescribing of epinephrine to all patients (personal communication Linda Cox 6/6/18).

Although initial pooled analysis of phase I to III clinical trials showed a marginally higher rate of malignancy in those treated with omalizumab (0.5 vs. 0.2%),[2,24] subsequent analyses have revealed no association between omalizumab and malignancy risk.[110,111] The EXCELS trial (Epidemiologic Study of Xolair (omalizumab): Evaluating Clinical Effectiveness and Long-term Safety in Patients with Moderate to Severe Asthma) was a phase IV postmarketing long-term safety study that enrolled individuals aged 12 years and above with moderate to severe persistent asthma and perennial allergen sensitization, regardless of omalizumab use, with median follow-up of 5 years. The omalizumab cohort had a higher proportion of patients with severe asthma compared with the nonomalizumab cohort (50.0% vs. 23.0%). There was no significant difference in adjusted malignancy rate between the two groups (hazard ratio 10.9, 0.87—1.38), even when nonmelanoma skin cancer was excluded.[112] Due to initial exclusion of patients with history of cancer or premalignant condition and high study discontinuation rate, a definitive conclusion regarding risk of malignancy with omalizumab could not be determined and the FDA added potential risk of cancer to the omalizumab safety label in 2014.[113] Additionally, the EXCELS data showed a small yet significant increased risk of cardiovascular and cerebrovascular events in omalizumab-treated patients compared with placebo (13.4 vs. 8.1 per 1000 patient years).[114] Differences in asthma severity between cohorts likely contributed to this imbalance, but some increase in risk cannot be excluded. Note number of patients who experienced this events was very small and the events ranged from thrombolic to embolic (personal communication Linda Cox, MD 6/6/18 per FDA advisory meeting for pediatric indication for Xolair).

Conclusions

IgE is a pivotal mediator in T_H2-driven allergic disease, serving as an ideal target for biologic therapies. Omalizumab is an effective, relatively safe, and well-tolerated anti-IgE therapy for moderate to severe allergic asthma and treatment-resistant chronic urticaria, with emerging data for other allergic diseases.

References

1. Ishizaka T, Ishizaka K, Johansson SG, Bennich H. Histamine release from human leukocytes by anti-gamma E antibodies. *J Immunol*. 1969;102:884—892.
2. Stokes J, Casale T. Anti-immunoglobulin E therapy. In: *Middleton's Allergy Principles and Practice 8ed*. 8th ed. Philadelphia, PA: Elsevier Saunders; 2014:1481—1488.
3. de Vries JE, Carballido JM, Aversa G. Receptors and cytokines involved in allergic TH2 cell responses. *J Allergy Clin Immunol*. 1999;103:S492—S496.
4. Presta L, Shields R, O'Connell L, et al. The binding site on human immunoglobulin E for its high affinity receptor. *J Biol Chem*. 1994;269:26368—26373.
5. Schroeder JT, Bieneman AP, Chichester KL, et al. Decreases in human dendritic cell-dependent T(H)2-like responses after acute in vivo IgE neutralization. *J Allergy Clin Immunol*. 2010;125:896—901 e6.

6. Broide DH. Molecular and cellular mechanisms of allergic disease. *J Allergy Clin Immunol.* 2001;108:S65–S71.

7. Chang T. Treating hypersensitivities with anti-IGE monoclonal antibodies which bind to IGE-expressing B cells but not basophils. In: *USPTO.* United States of America; 1996.

8. Chang TW, Davis FM, Sun NC, Sun CR, MacGlashan DW, Hamilton RG. Monoclonal antibodies specific for human IgE-producing B cells: a potential therapeutic for IgE-mediated allergic diseases. *Biotechnology.* 1990;8:122–126.

9. Hook WA, Zinsser FU, Berenstein EH, Siraganian RP. Monoclonal antibodies defining epitopes on human IgE. *Mol Immunol.* 1991;28:631–639.

10. Racine-Poon A, Botta L, Chang TW, et al. Efficacy, pharmacodynamics, and pharmacokinetics of CGP 51901, an anti-immunoglobulin E chimeric monoclonal antibody, in patients with seasonal allergic rhinitis. *Clin Pharmacol Ther.* 1997;62:675–690.

11. Corne J, Djukanovic R, Thomas L, et al. The effect of intravenous administration of a chimeric anti-IgE antibody on serum IgE levels in atopic subjects: efficacy, safety, and pharmacokinetics. *J Clin Investig.* 1997;99:879–887.

12. Presta LG, Lahr SJ, Shields RL, et al. Humanization of an antibody directed against IgE. *J Immunol.* 1993;151:2623–2632.

13. Licari A, Marseglia G, Castagnoli R, Marseglia A, Ciprandi G. The discovery and development of omalizumab for the treatment of asthma. *Expert Opin Drug Discov.* 2015;10:1033–1042.

14. MacGlashan DW, Bochner BS, Adelman DC, et al. Down-regulation of Fc(epsilon)RI expression on human basophils during in vivo treatment of atopic patients with anti-IgE antibody. *J Immunol.* 1997;158:1438–1445.

15. Lin H, Boesel KM, Griffith DT, et al. Omalizumab rapidly decreases nasal allergic response and Fce psilonRI on basophils. *J Allergy Clin Immunol.* 2004;113:297–302.

16. Prussin C, Griffith DT, Boesel KM, Lin H, Foster B, Casale TB. Omalizumab treatment downregulates dendritic cell FcepsilonRI expression. *J Allergy Clin Immunol.* 2003; 112:1147–1154.

17. Beck LA, Marcotte GV, MacGlashan D, Togias A, Saini S. Omalizumab-induced reductions in mast cell Fce psilon RI expression and function. *J Allergy Clin Immunol.* 2004; 114:527–530.

18. Chang TW, Chen C, Lin CJ, Metz M, Church MK, Maurer M. The potential pharmacologic mechanisms of omalizumab in patients with chronic spontaneous urticaria. *J Allergy Clin Immunol.* 2015;135:337–342.

19. Kaplan AP, Giménez-Arnau AM, Saini SS. Mechanisms of action that contribute to efficacy of omalizumab in chronic spontaneous urticaria. *Allergy.* 2017;72:519–533.

20. Milgrom H, Fick RB, Su JQ, et al. Treatment of allergic asthma with monoclonal anti-IgE antibody. rhuMAb-E25 Study Group. *N Engl J Med.* 1999;341:1966–1973.

21. Milgrom H, Berger W, Nayak A, et al. Treatment of childhood asthma with anti-immunoglobulin E antibody (omalizumab). *Pediatrics.* 2001;108:E36.

22. Soler M, Matz J, Townley R, et al. The anti-IgE antibody omalizumab reduces exacerbations and steroid requirement in allergic asthmatics. *Eur Respir J.* 2001;18: 254–261.

23. Busse W, Corren J, Lanier BQ, et al. Omalizumab, anti-IgE recombinant humanized monoclonal antibody, for the treatment of severe allergic asthma. *J Allergy Clin Immunol.* 2001;108:184–190.

24. Xolair (omalizumab) US prescribing information. In: *(FDA) UFaDA.* 2015.

25. Holgate S, Bousquet J, Wenzel S, Fox H, Liu J, Castellsague J. Efficacy of omalizumab, an anti-immunoglobulin E antibody, in patients with allergic asthma at high risk of serious asthma-related morbidity and mortality. *Curr Med Res Opin.* 2001;17:233—240.

26. Bousquet J, Wenzel S, Holgate S, Lumry W, Freeman P, Fox H. Predicting response to omalizumab, an anti-IgE antibody, in patients with allergic asthma. *Chest.* 2004;125:1378—1386.

27. Hanania NA, Wenzel S, Rosen K, et al. Exploring the effects of omalizumab in allergic asthma: an analysis of biomarkers in the EXTRA study. *Am J Respir Crit Care Med.* 2013;187:804—811.

28. Busse W, Spector S, Rosen K, Wang Y, Alpan O. High eosinophil count: a potential biomarker for assessing successful omalizumab treatment effects. *J Allergy Clin Immunol.* 2013;132:485—486 e11.

29. Casale TB, Chipps BE, Rosén K, et al. Response to omalizumab using patient enrichment criteria from trials of novel biologics in asthma. *Allergy.* 2017:1—8. epub ahead of print.

30. Berger W, Gupta N, McAlary M, Fowler-Taylor A. Evaluation of long-term safety of the anti-IgE antibody, omalizumab, in children with allergic asthma. *Ann Allergy Asthma Immunol.* 2003;91:182—188.

31. Silkoff PE, Romero FA, Gupta N, Townley RG, Milgrom H. Exhaled nitric oxide in children with asthma receiving Xolair (omalizumab), a monoclonal anti-immunoglobulin E antibody. *Pediatrics.* 2004;113:e308—e312.

32. Lanier B, Bridges T, Kulus M, Taylor AF, Berhane I, Vidaurre CF. Omalizumab for the treatment of exacerbations in children with inadequately controlled allergic (IgE-mediated) asthma. *J Allergy Clin Immunol.* 2009;124:1210—1216.

33. Busse WW, Morgan WJ, Gergen PJ, et al. Randomized trial of omalizumab (anti-IgE) for asthma in inner-city children. *N Engl J Med.* 2011;364:1005—1015.

34. Teach SJ, Gill MA, Togias A, et al. Preseasonal treatment with either omalizumab or an inhaled corticosteroid boost to prevent fall asthma exacerbations. *J Allergy Clin Immunol.* 2015;136:1476—1485.

35. Bhutani M, Yang WH, Hébert J, de Takacsy F, Stril JL. The real world effect of omalizumab add on therapy for patients with moderate to severe allergic asthma: the ASTERIX observational study. *PLoS One.* 2017;12:e0183869.

36. Brusselle G, Michils A, Louis R, et al. Real-life" effectiveness of omalizumab in patients with severe persistent allergic asthma: the PERSIST study. *Respir Med.* 2009;103:1633—1642.

37. Menzella F, Galeone C, Formisano D, et al. Real-life efficacy of omalizumab after 9 Years of follow-up. *Allergy Asthma Immunol Res.* 2017;9:368—372.

38. Alhossan A, Lee CS, MacDonald K, Abraham I. "Real-life" effectiveness studies of omalizumab in adult patients with severe allergic asthma: meta-analysis. *J Allergy Clin Immunol Pract.* 2017;5:1362—1370.

39. Schumann C, Kropf C, Wibmer T, et al. Omalizumab in patients with severe asthma: the XCLUSIVE study. *Clin Res J.* 2012;6:215—227.

40. Molimard M, Buhl R, Niven R, et al. Omalizumab reduces oral corticosteroid use in patients with severe allergic asthma: real-life data. *Respir Med.* 2010;104:1381—1385.

41. Hew M, Gillman A, Sutherland M, et al. Real-life effectiveness of omalizumab in severe allergic asthma above the recommended dosing range criteria. *Clin Exp Allergy.* 2016;46:1407—1415.

42. Ankerst J, Nopp A, Johansson SG, Adedoyin J, Oman H. Xolair is effective in allergics with a low serum IgE level. *Int Arch Allergy Immunol.* 2010;152:71–74.
43. Bourgoin-Heck M, Amat F, Trouvé C, et al. Omalizumab could be effective in children with severe eosinophilic non-allergic asthma. *Pediatr Allergy Immunol.* 2018;29(1): 90–93.
44. Çelebi Sözener Z, Aydın Ö, Mısırlıgil Z, et al. Omalizumab in non-allergic Asthma: a report of 13 cases. *J Asthma.* 2017:1–8.
45. Ledford D, Busse W, Trzaskoma B, et al. A randomized multicenter study evaluating Xolair persistence of response after long-term therapy. *J Allergy Clin Immunol.* 2017; 140, 162-9.e2.
46. Vennera MDC, Sabadell C, Picado C, Registry SO. Duration of the efficacy of omalizumab after treatment discontinuation in 'real life' severe asthma. *Thorax.* 2018; 73(8):782–784.
47. Spector SL, Tan RA. Effect of omalizumab on patients with chronic urticaria. *Ann Allergy Asthma Immunol.* 2007;99:190–193.
48. Kaplan AP, Joseph K, Maykut RJ, Geba GP, Zeldin RK. Treatment of chronic autoimmune urticaria with omalizumab. *J Allergy Clin Immunol.* 2008;122:569–573.
49. Saini S, Rosen KE, Hsieh HJ, et al. A randomized, placebo-controlled, dose-ranging study of single-dose omalizumab in patients with H1-antihistamine-refractory chronic idiopathic urticaria. *J Allergy Clin Immunol.* 2011;128, 567-73.e1.
50. Saini SS, Bindslev-Jensen C, Maurer M, et al. Efficacy and safety of omalizumab in patients with chronic idiopathic/spontaneous urticaria who remain symptomatic on H1 antihistamines: a randomized, placebo-controlled study. *J Investig Dermatol.* 2015;135: 67–75.
51. Maurer M, Rosén K, Hsieh HJ, et al. Omalizumab for the treatment of chronic idiopathic or spontaneous urticaria. *N Engl J Med.* 2013;368:924–935.
52. Kaplan A, Ledford D, Ashby M, et al. Omalizumab in patients with symptomatic chronic idiopathic/spontaneous urticaria despite standard combination therapy. *J Allergy Clin Immunol.* 2013;132:101–109.
53. Kaplan A, Ferrer M, Bernstein JA, et al. Timing and duration of omalizumab response in patients with chronic idiopathic/spontaneous urticaria. *J Allergy Clin Immunol.* 2016; 137:474–481.
54. *Chronic Urticaria: Treatment of Refractory Symptoms.* UpToDate, Inc.; 2017. Available from: https://www.uptodate.com/contents/chronic-urticaria-treatment-of-refractory-symptoms.
55. Straesser MD, Oliver E, Palacios T, et al. Serum IgE as an immunological marker to predict response to omalizumab treatment in symptomatic chronic urticaria. *J Allergy Clin Immunol Pract.* 2018;6(4):1386–1388.
56. Casale TB, Win PH, Bernstein JA, et al. Omalizumab response in patients with chronic idiopathic urticaria: insights from the XTEND-CIU study. *J Am Acad Dermatol.* 2018; 78(4):793–795.
57. Uysal P, Eller E, Mortz CG, Bindslev-Jensen C. An algorithm for treating chronic urticaria with omalizumab: dose interval should be individualized. *J Allergy Clin Immunol.* 2014;133, 914-915.e2.
58. Ertas R, Ozyurt K, Ozlu E, et al. Increased IgE levels are linked to faster relapse in patients with omalizumab-discontinued chronic spontaneous urticaria. *J Allergy Clin Immunol.* 2017;140:1749–1751.

59. Metz M, Ohanyan T, Church MK, Maurer M. Retreatment with omalizumab results in rapid remission in chronic spontaneous and inducible urticaria. *JAMA Dermatol*. 2014; 150:288–290.

60. Casale TB, Condemi J, LaForce C, et al. Effect of omalizumab on symptoms of seasonal allergic rhinitis: a randomized controlled trial. *JAMA*. 2001;286:2956–2967.

61. Nayak A, Casale T, Miller SD, et al. Tolerability of retreatment with omalizumab, a recombinant humanized monoclonal anti-IgE antibody, during a second ragweed pollen season in patients with seasonal allergic rhinitis. *Allergy Asthma Proc*. 2003;24: 323–329.

62. Adelroth E, Rak S, Haahtela T, et al. Recombinant humanized mAb-E25, an anti-IgE mAb, in birch pollen-induced seasonal allergic rhinitis. *J Allergy Clin Immunol*. 2000;106:253–259.

63. Chervinsky P, Casale T, Townley R, et al. Omalizumab, an anti-IgE antibody, in the treatment of adults and adolescents with perennial allergic rhinitis. *Ann Allergy Asthma Immunol*. 2003;91:160–167.

64. Vignola AM, Humbert M, Bousquet J, et al. Efficacy and tolerability of anti-immunoglobulin E therapy with omalizumab in patients with concomitant allergic asthma and persistent allergic rhinitis: solar. *Allergy*. 2004;59:709–717.

65. Tsabouri S, Tseretopoulou X, Priftis K, Ntzani EE. Omalizumab for the treatment of inadequately controlled allergic rhinitis: a systematic review and meta-analysis of randomized clinical trials. *J Allergy Clin Immunol Pract*. 2014;2, 332-40.e1.

66. Kuehr J, Brauburger J, Zielen S, et al. Efficacy of combination treatment with anti-IgE plus specific immunotherapy in polysensitized children and adolescents with seasonal allergic rhinitis. *J Allergy Clin Immunol*. 2002;109:274–280.

67. Rolinck-Werninghaus C, Hamelmann E, Keil T, et al. The co-seasonal application of anti-IgE after preseasonal specific immunotherapy decreases ocular and nasal symptom scores and rescue medication use in grass pollen allergic children. *Allergy*. 2004;59: 973–979.

68. Casale TB. Experience with monoclonal antibodies in allergic mediated disease: seasonal allergic rhinitis. *J Allergy Clin Immunol*. 2001;108:S84–S88.

69. Casale TB, Busse WW, Kline JN, et al. Omalizumab pretreatment decreases acute reactions after rush immunotherapy for ragweed-induced seasonal allergic rhinitis. *J Allergy Clin Immunol*. 2006;117:134–140.

70. Massanari M, Nelson H, Casale T, et al. Effect of pretreatment with omalizumab on the tolerability of specific immunotherapy in allergic asthma. *J Allergy Clin Immunol*. 2010; 125:383–389.

71. Leung DY, Sampson HA, Yunginger JW, et al. Effect of anti-IgE therapy in patients with peanut allergy. *N Engl J Med*. 2003;348:986–993.

72. Sampson HA, Leung DY, Burks AW, et al. A phase II, randomized, double-blind, parallel-group, placebo-controlled oral food challenge trial of Xolair (omalizumab) in peanut allergy. *J Allergy Clin Immunol*. 2011;127, 1309-13010.e1.

73. Lin C, Lee IT, Sampath V, et al. Combining anti-IgE with oral immunotherapy. *Pediatr Allergy Immunol*. 2017;28:619–627.

74. Anagnostou K, Clark A, King Y, Islam S, Deighton J, Ewan P. Efficacy and safety of high-dose peanut oral immunotherapy with factors predicting outcome. *Clin Exp Allergy*. 2011;41:1273–1281.

75. Yu W, Freeland DMH, Nadeau KC. Food allergy: immune mechanisms, diagnosis and immunotherapy. *Nat Rev Immunol*. 2016;16:751–765.

76. Labrosse R, Graham F, Des Roches A, Bégin P. The use of omalizumab in food oral immunotherapy. *Arch Immunol Ther Exp*. 2017;65:189–199.

77. Nadeau KC, Schneider LC, Hoyte L, Borras I, Umetsu DT. Rapid oral desensitization in combination with omalizumab therapy in patients with cow's milk allergy. *J Allergy Clin Immunol*. 2011;127:1622–1624.

78. Wood RA, Kim JS, Lindblad R, et al. A randomized, double-blind, placebo-controlled study of omalizumab combined with oral immunotherapy for the treatment of cow's milk allergy. *J Allergy Clin Immunol*. 2016;137, 1103-10.e11.

79. Schneider LC, Rachid R, LeBovidge J, Blood E, Mittal M, Umetsu DT. A pilot study of omalizumab to facilitate rapid oral desensitization in high-risk peanut-allergic patients. *J Allergy Clin Immunol*. 2013;132:1368–1374.

80. MacGinnitie AJ, Rachid R, Gragg H, et al. Omalizumab facilitates rapid oral desensitization for peanut allergy. *J Allergy Clin Immunol*. 2017;139, 873-81.e8.

81. Bird JA, Feldman M, Arneson A, et al. Modified peanut oral immunotherapy protocol safely and effectively induces desensitization. *J Allergy Clin Immunol Pract*. 2015;3, 433-435.e1-3.

82. Lacombe Barrios J, Bégin P, Paradis L, Hatami A, Paradis J, Des Roches A. Anti-IgE therapy and severe atopic dermatitis: a pediatric perspective. *J Am Acad Dermatol*. 2013;69:832–834.

83. Vigo PG, Girgis KR, Pfuetze BL, Critchlow ME, Fisher J, Hussain I. Efficacy of anti-IgE therapy in patients with atopic dermatitis. *J Am Acad Dermatol*. 2006;55:168–170.

84. Iyengar SR, Hoyte EG, Loza A, et al. Immunologic effects of omalizumab in children with severe refractory atopic dermatitis: a randomized, placebo-controlled clinical trial. *Int Arch Allergy Immunol*. 2013;162:89–93.

85. Wang HH, Li YC, Huang YC. Efficacy of omalizumab in patients with atopic dermatitis: a systematic review and meta-analysis. *J Allergy Clin Immunol*. 2016;138, 1719-17122.e1.

86. Hotze M, Baurecht H, Rodríguez E, et al. Increased efficacy of omalizumab in atopic dermatitis patients with wild-type filaggrin status and higher serum levels of phosphatidylcholines. *Allergy*. 2014;69:132–135.

87. Chularojanamontri L, Wimoolchart S, Tuchinda P, Kulthanan K, Kiewjoy N. Role of omalizumab in a patient with hyper-IgE syndrome and review dermatologic manifestations. *Asian Pac J Allergy Immunol*. 2009;27:233–236.

88. Tanou K, Zintzaras E, Kaditis AG. Omalizumab therapy for allergic bronchopulmonary aspergillosis in children with cystic fibrosis: a synthesis of published evidence. *Pediatr Pulmonol*. 2014;49:503–507.

89. Jat KR, Walia DK, Khairwa A. Anti-IgE therapy for allergic bronchopulmonary aspergillosis in people with cystic fibrosis. *Cochrane Database Syst Rev*. 2013: CD010288.

90. Lieberoth S, Thomsen SF. Cutaneous and gastrointestinal symptoms in two patients with systemic mastocytosis successfully treated with omalizumab. *Case Rep Med*. 2015;2015:903541.

91. Broesby-Olsen S, Vestergaard H, Mortz CG, et al. Omalizumab prevents anaphylaxis and improves symptoms in systemic mastocytosis: efficacy and safety observations. *Allergy*. 2017;73:230–238.

92. Aguirre-Valencia D, Posso-Osorio I, Bravo JC, Bonilla-Abadía F, Tobón GJ, Cañas CA. Sequential rituximab and omalizumab for the treatment of eosinophilic granulomatosis with polyangiitis (Churg-Strauss syndrome). *Clin Rheumatol*. 2017;36:2159–2162.

93. Christensen MJ, Bindslev-Jensen C. Successful treatment with omalizumab in challenge confirmed exercise-induced anaphylaxis. *J Allergy Clin Immunol Pract*. 2017; 5:204—206.

94. Balakirski G, Alkhateeb A, Merk HF, Leverkus M, Megahed M. Successful treatment of bullous pemphigoid with omalizumab as corticosteroid-sparing agent: report of two cases and review of literature. *J Eur Acad Dermatol Venereol*. 2016;30:1778—1782.

95. Fairley JA, Baum CL, Brandt DS, Messingham KA. Pathogenicity of IgE in autoimmunity: successful treatment of bullous pemphigoid with omalizumab. *J Allergy Clin Immunol*. 2009;123:704—705.

96. Kaya H, Gümüş S, Uçar E, et al. Omalizumab as a steroid-sparing agent in chronic eosinophilic pneumonia. *Chest*. 2012;142:513—516.

97. FDA, ed. *XOLAIR ® (omalizumab) for Injection, for Subcutaneous Use*. 2016.

98. Jaffe JS, Massanari M. In response to dosing omalizumab in allergic asthma. *J Allergy Clin Immunol*. 2007;119:255—256.

99. Davydov L. Omalizumab (Xolair) for treatment of asthma. *Am Fam Physician*. 2005;71: 341—342.

100. Suzuki C, Lopes da Silva N, Kumar P, Pathak P, Ong SH. Cost-effectiveness of omalizumab add-on to standard-of-care therapy in patients with uncontrolled severe allergic asthma in a Brazilian healthcare setting. *J Med Econ*. 2017;20:832—839.

101. Tadrous M, Khuu W, Lebovic G, et al. Real-world health care utilization and effectiveness of omalizumab for the treatment of severe asthma. *Ann Allergy Asthma Immunol*. 2017;120:59—65.

102. Dal Negro RW, Tognella S, Pradelli L. A 36-month study on the cost/utility of add-on omalizumab in persistent difficult-to-treat atopic asthma in Italy. *J Asthma*. 2012;49: 843—848.

103. Corren J, Casale TB, Lanier B, Buhl R, Holgate S, Jimenez P. Safety and tolerability of omalizumab. *Clin Exp Allergy*. 2009;39:788—797.

104. Milgrom H, Fowler-Taylor A, Vidaurre CF, Jayawardene S. Safety and tolerability of omalizumab in children with allergic (IgE-mediated) asthma. *Curr Med Res Opin*. 2011;27:163—169.

105. Konstantinou GN, Chioti AG, Daniilidis M. Self-reported hair loss in patients with chronic spontaneous urticaria treated with omalizumab: an under-reported, transient side effect? *Eur Ann Allergy Clin Immunol*. 2016;48:205—207.

106. Cox L, Platts-Mills TA, Finegold I, et al. American Academy of allergy, asthma & Immunology/American College of allergy, asthma and Immunology Joint Task Force report on omalizumab-associated anaphylaxis. *J Allergy Clin Immunol*. 2007;120: 1373—1377.

107. Lieberman PL, Umetsu DT, Carrigan GJ, Rahmaoui A. Anaphylactic reactions associated with omalizumab administration: analysis of a case-control study. *J Allergy Clin Immunol*. 2016;138, 913-915.e2.

108. Lieberman PL, Jones I, Rajwanshi R, Rosén K, Umetsu DT. Anaphylaxis associated with omalizumab administration: risk factors and patient characteristics. *J Allergy Clin Immunol*. 2017;140:1734—1736.

109. Lieberman P. The unusual suspects: a surprise regarding reactions to omalizumab. *Allergy Asthma Proc*. 2007;28:259—261.

110. Busse W, Buhl R, Fernandez Vidaurre C, et al. Omalizumab and the risk of malignancy: results from a pooled analysis. *J Allergy Clin Immunol*. 2012;129, 983-989 e6.

111. Chipps BE, Lanier B, Milgrom H, et al. Omalizumab in children with uncontrolled allergic asthma: review of clinical trial and real-world experience. *J Allergy Clin Immunol*. 2017;139:1431–1444.

112. Long A, Rahmaoui A, Rothman KJ, et al. Incidence of malignancy in patients with moderate-to-severe asthma treated with or without omalizumab. *J Allergy Clin Immunol*. 2014;134, 560-7.e4.

113. Li J, Goulding M, Seymour S, Starke P. EXCELS study results do not rule out potential cancer risk with omalizumab. *J Allergy Clin Immunol*. 2015;135:289.

114. Iribarren C, Rahmaoui A, Long AA, et al. Cardiovascular and cerebrovascular events among patients receiving omalizumab: results from EXCELS, a prospective cohort study in moderate to severe asthma. *J Allergy Clin Immunol*. 2017;139, 1489-95.e5.

Index

'Note: Page numbers followed by "f" indicate figures and "t" indicates tables.'

Printed and bound by CPI Group (UK) Ltd, Croydon, CR0 4YY

03/10/2024

01040300-0011